P9-APK-025

WITHDRAWN

OXFORD MEDICAL PUBLICATIONS

Handbook of Sleep-Related
Breathing Disorders

Handbook of Sleep-Related Breathing Disorders

J. R. Stradling

Consultant Physician and Wellcome Senior Research Fellow,
Osler Chest Unit, Churchill Hospital, Oxford

OXFORD · NEW YORK · TOKYO
OXFORD UNIVERSITY PRESS
1993

Oxford University Press, Walton Street, Oxford OX2 6DP
Oxford   New York   Toronto
Delhi   Bombay   Calcutta   Madras   Karachi
Kuala Lumpur   Singapore   Hong Kong   Tokyo
Nairobi   Dar es Salaam   Cape Town
Melbourne   Auckland   Madrid
and associated companies in
Berlin   Ibadan

Oxford is a trade mark of Oxford University Press

Published in the United States
by Oxford University Press Inc., New York

© J. R. Stradling, 1993

All rights reserved. No part of this publication may be
reproduced, stored in a retrieval system, or transmitted, in any
form or by any means, without the prior permission in writing of Oxford
University Press. Within the UK, exceptions are allowed in respect of any
fair dealing for the purpose of research or private study, or criticism or
review, as permitted under the Copyright, Designs and Patents Act, 1988, or
in the case of reprographic reproduction in accordance with the terms of
licences issued by the Copyright Licensing Agency. Enquiries concerning
reproduction outside those terms and in other countries should be sent to
the Rights Department, Oxford University Press, at the address above.

A catalogue record for this book is available from the British Library

Library of Congress Cataloging in Publication Data
Stradling, John R.
Handbook of sleep-related breathing disorders/J. R. Stradling.
Includes bibliographical references and index.
1. Sleep apnea syndromes—Handbooks, manuals, etc.   I. Title.
[DNLM: 1. Sleep Apnea Syndromes—handbooks.   2. Sleep—physiology-
handbooks.—wf 39 S895h 1993]
RC737.5.S77   1993   616.2—dc20   93-20557
ISBN 0–19–261834–2

Typeset by Advance Typesetting Ltd, Oxford
Printed in Great Britain on acid-free paper
by St Edmundsbury Press Ltd, Bury St Edmunds, Suffolk

Acknowledgements

The Oxford work described in this book has been carried out by many people over the last few years. The Osler Chest Unit has been extremely lucky to have a succession of talented and dedicated research staff. This book would be considerably poorer without their input. Particular thanks are due to three research nurses, Joy Crosby, Gill Thomas, and Debby Pitson and three research fellows, Anthony Warley, Nabeel Ali, and Robert Davies. No unit functions well without an excellent secretary and I am particularly grateful to Denise Roberts who has managed to nurse the manuscript to the publishers in addition to keeping the Unit's disorder at a very low level.

Some of the Oxford work described in this book was generously supported by grants from the Wellcome Trust and the British Lung Foundation.

Devilbiss UK very kindly sponsored the cost of producing the colour plates.

My wife and children have had to endure the neglect inevitable during the preparation of this book and I hope they will forgive me.

Oxford   J.R.S.
1993

Contents

1 Introduction

1.1 Why another book on sleep-related breathing disorders?

The field of sleep medicine has advanced and increased in size enormously over the last 20 years. This has been due largely to the recognition of sleep and breathing disorders, as well as an appreciation of the severe effects that excessive sleepiness and poor vigilance can have on work performance. Most people are aware how even one night of sleep disruption (or deprivation) can affect their daytime performance, particularly, for example, long-distance driving. Many of the patients presenting to sleep clinics have months or years of persistently disrupted sleep such that they almost never have normal vigilance. Unfortunately when daytime sleepiness affects driving it is often not reported by patients, for fear that they will be told to stop driving and lose their licence.

The advances in these fields, particularly in understanding sleep apnoea, have been rapid but controversial. The specialty has been dominated by the writings of specialist centres in North America. This has led to firm guidelines and recommendations, particularly about investigative techniques, that are perhaps more related to how medicine is financed[256] than to what many now realize is really required to diagnose these conditions. These protocols persuaded many in other countries that investigative facilities for sleep-related breathing disorders were too expensive and beyond their reach, particularly in a health system such as the British National Health Service where limited funding has been present for many years. The enormous cost of the recommended full investigative techniques has led to an inability, even in North America, to provide such a service for all those who need it. Thus, one of the interesting developments occurring now is the validation and clinical use of many different simpler systems that allow more patients to be investigated at lower cost.

The investigation of sleep-related breathing is no different from any other medical condition in that history, examination, and a progressive approach to diagnosis and treatment dependent on symptom severity is appropriate, rather than a standard package of management.

This short book seeks to fill a gap in the literature on sleep-related breathing disorders. There are many state of the art texts on the subject with extremely good academic reviews of physiology and pathophysiology.[197,379,525,603]

There are also many didactic accounts of what is 'mandatory' in this area.[184,443,528,728] There seem to be very few texts to guide a reader, seeking to set up a sleep and breathing service, on the fundamental principles of diagnosis and treatment. It is hoped that this book will be a useful starting point for those interested in providing a service for patients.

The pronoun 'he' is used throughout for a patient with sleep apnoea for convenience and because obstructive sleep apnoea is probably about 15 to 20 times more common in men than women.

1.2 Historical background

Charcot, referring to sex-linked muscular dystrophy, wrote 'how come that a disease so common, so widespread, and so recognisable at a glance—a disease which has doubtless always existed, how come that it is only recognised now? Why did we need M Duchenne to open our eyes?' In retrospect the same can be said of sleep apnoea. Here is a condition, severe versions of which are found in probably over 0.3 per cent of adult men,[661] producing significant disability that was only properly recognized in recent times in 1966 by Gastaut *et al.*[215] in France. Long before this there had been sporadic descriptions of what was clearly sleep apnoea. For example, this account by Broadbent[78] in 1877 from St Mary's Hospital, London, is very descriptive and can hardly be bettered today:

Many years ago I observed something very like Cheyne—Stokes respiration during sleep in a gentleman now more than eighty years of age. When a person, especially advanced in years, is lying on his back in heavy sleep and snoring loudly, it very commonly happens that every now and then the inspiration fails to overcome the resistance in the pharynx of which stertor or snoring is the audible sign, and there will be perfect silence through two or three or four respiratory periods, in which there are ineffectual chest movements; finally, air enters with a loud snort, after which there are several compensatory deep inspirations before the breathing settles down to its usual rhythm. In the case to which I allude there was something more than this. The snoring ceased at regular intervals, and the pause was so long as to excite attention, and indeed alarm; and I found, on investigation, that there was not simply obstruction by the falling back of the tongue, but actual cessation of all respiratory movements; these then began gradually but did not at first attain sufficient force to overcome the pharyngeal resistance.

In 1956 Burwell and colleagues[92] described a patient with hypoxia and hypercapnia who in retrospect probably had sleep apnoea and they resurrected the term 'Pickwickian Syndrome' because of the associated obesity. The similarity of the sleepy fat patient to Dickens's character Joe was first noted by Christopher Heath in the discussion following a paper by Caton[1] in 1889 and then enshrined in Osler's[505] medical textbook. However, the key role played by sleep-induced upper airway collapse and episodic nocturnal hypoxaemia in their patient was not appreciated by Burwell and colleagues. The ability to monitor overnight oxygen levels was possible even then and an article by Lovett Doust and Schneider[420] in 1952 described how oxygen levels fell in a snorer when monitored with an early Millikan[472] oximeter. Also, some years earlier, monitoring of the electro-encephalograph (EEG) during sleep from surface electrodes was developing and being used to stage sleep.[418] In 1953 Aserinsky and Kleitman[28] described the electrophysiological characteristics of rapid eye movement (REM) sleep (dreaming sleep). These developments allowed sleep to be described and measured, which in turn led to the publication of a didactic manual of sleep scoring which tried to standardize the way different laboratories were working.[554] There is no doubt that an interest in breathing disorders during sleep first developed in laboratories already skilled in measuring and scoring the EEG during sleep. Laboratory facilities already existed in many centres both for research purposes and for the investigation of patients with insomnia and depression. These circumstances probably account for the heavy bias towards measuring the EEG, electromyogram (EMG), and electro-oculogram (EOG) (all used to stage sleep) that has persisted in this newer area of sleep and breathing disorders.

Elio Lugaresi (an Italian neurologist) and colleagues[122,123,429] first studied the cardiorespiratory physiology of patients with sleep apnoea in a systematic way and indeed hosted the first conference on sleep-related respiratory problems in 1972.[595] Christian Guilleminault (also a neurologist, working at the Stanford University Sleep Laboratory) was one of the first to recognize the full importance and frequency of these conditions. His review of 62 cases in 1976[265] was probably the first widely read account of these disorders and persuaded many people to turn their attentions to them. Finally, it was the arrival of a highly effective non-surgical treatment for obstructive sleep apnoea (nasal continuous positive airway pressure), invented by Colin Sullivan[680] in 1981 in Sydney that made physicians realize that there was no longer any excuse for ignoring these patients with serious problems.

Readers interested in the early accounts of sleep apnoea and why it was ignored for so long will enjoy reading two historical articles by Lavie[397] and Kryger.[378]

1.3 Area to be covered

This short text will cover useful points to know when looking after patients with sleep and breathing disorders. Where differential diagnoses are important, then these are discussed, even if they are not respiratory in origin (for example, narcolepsy). This is because, inevitably, such patients will come to clinics where sleepiness is an important symptom. Both adults and children are dealt with since a sleep clinic is likely to be asked to see patients of all ages. Very young children and sudden infant death syndrome are not covered.

There has been criticism of sleep units that concentrate mainly on sleep and breathing disorders and have less expertise in other sleep disorders. This however, simply reflects the fact that the majority of problems seen at general sleep clinics turn out to be due to sleep apnoea and its variants.[87,461,484,764] This is not to say that other sleep problems are not important and perhaps the dominance of sleep apnoea has pushed the other problems such as insomnia into the background. Ultimately it is the fact that so much can be done for patients with sleep and breathing disorders that has led to the establishment of many specialist centres, which in Britain are usually run by chest physicians and much less often by anaesthetists, neurologists, ENT surgeons, and psychiatrists.

2 Normal sleep and breathing

2.1 Sleep states

At the heart of the pathophysiology of sleep and breathing disorders are the changes in ventilatory control that occur with the transition from wakefulness to quiet sleep and again from quiet sleep to dreaming sleep. Before describing these ventilatory changes, a brief description of sleep is appropriate.

Before electrophysiological monitoring was available, sleep was essentially defined by behavioural criteria and regarded as uniform throughout. The classical hallmarks of sleep are lack of movement, reduced postural muscle tone, closed eyes, lack of response to limited stimuli, and subtle changes in breathing—more regular, expiration more relaxed, and an increase in upper airway noise. All these features can be used to assess if someone is likely to be asleep. However, the accuracy of simple observation is limited, and although the repeated and vigorous movements of rapid eye movement (REM) sleep can usually be seen under the eyelids, adequate quantification by observation of REM and non-REM sleep is not really possible for most research purposes.

The use of the electroencephalograph (EEG), electromyogram (EMG), and electro-oculogram (EOG) has allowed sleep to be classified into various stages based on fairly arbitrary criteria which have stood the test of time.[554]

Wakefulness is characterized by a high frequency, apparently random, low amplitude EEG, often with superimposed muscle activity picked up from the temporalis muscle. The EEG electrical activity is picked up conventionally from three electrodes, one on the mastoid, one on the contralateral scalp (Fig. 2.1)—forming the input to a differential amplifier—referenced to a third electrode, commonly on the other mastoid. The only dominant frequency in the awake EEG is alpha and this usually has a frequency between 8 and 12 Hz. Alpha is only present when the eyes are closed and the subject is beginning to get drowsy. As a subject becomes very relaxed prior to sleep then the EMG activity falls (usually monitored from muscles under the chin). As drowsiness or stage 1 occurs, the alpha EEG activity disappears, the overall frequency falls, so-called theta waves may appear (3–7 Hz), and the eyes usually begin to roll slowly from side to side. Stage 1 in normal subjects only lasts a few minutes. These eye movements

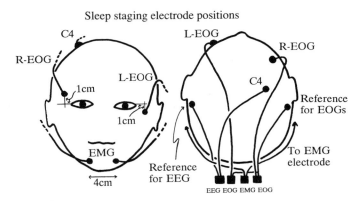

Fig. 2.1 Conventional electrode positions for monitoring sleep and its stages. The eye electrodes (EOG) are displaced horizontally relative to each other to record vertical, as well as horizontal, eye movements.

are picked up electrically from eye electrodes (Fig. 2.1) or small piezo-electric transducers mounted on the eyelids that register actual movement. Both systems register blinks, but these are usually recognizably different. The true moment of sleep onset is not possible to define because there is a period of gradual transition rather than an abrupt switch.

Stage 2 sleep is defined by the appearance of so-called spindles (Fig. 2.2) that are short (>0.5 and usually up to 3 s) bursts of waves at $12-14$ Hz and thus consist of approximately $6-25$ actual complete waves. In addition, K complexes appear that are effectively one big wave lasting approximately 1 s. There may be two types of K complex—those that appear in response to external stimuli (a noise in the bedroom, for example) and those that are probably the beginning of deeper slow wave sleep (SWS).

Stages 3 and 4 sleep (also known as slow wave sleep or delta sleep) are characterized by the appearance of big (>75 μV peak to peak) and slow ($0.5-2$ Hz) waves, during which increasing depth is defined by an increasing percentage of the tracing period being occupied by these big waves (stage 3, $20-50$ per cent and stage 4, >50 per cent).

Because many of these features occur sporadically or it takes a certain length of time to be sure they are present, sleep has been classically staged in epochs, $20-30$ s being used for convenience. Herein lies the major deficiency of this approach—the resolution of the sleep staging is limited to the epoch length. For example, during a 30 s analysis period, if >15 s contain adequate slow waves, then it can be scored stage 3 even if the other 14 s may contain a short arousal (Fig. 2.3). The consequence of this is that a hypnogram (Fig. 2.4) describing the whole night's sleep gives only a

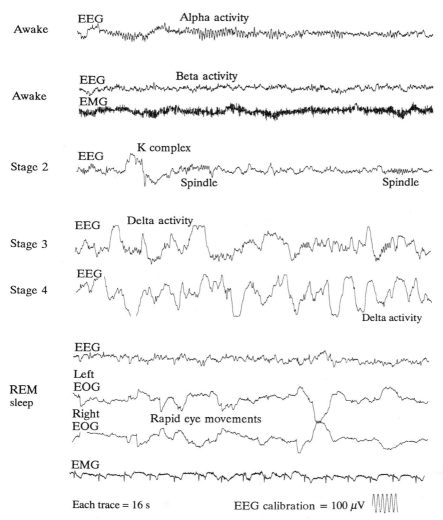

Fig. 2.2 Examples of EEG, EOG, and EMG activity during the different sleep stages.

macroscopic impression of sleep, and may be relatively normal in the presence of hundreds of short (5−10 s) arousals. Although the scoring criteria drawn up by Rechtschaffen and Kales[554] allow for the scoring of 'movement arousals', this was not encouraged and is extremely arduous to do by hand, hence it is often not done. Furthermore, very short arousals,

EEG$_c$

EOG

EEG$_o$

EMG

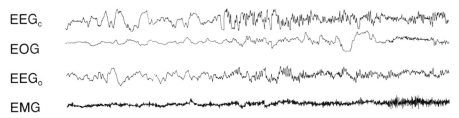

Fig. 2.3 Approximately 20 s of recording (two EEG channels and one composite EOG) showing just over half the epoch occupied by wakefulness. If the wakefulness had been just under half of this epoch, then it would be staged as 3 or 4 (SWS).

perhaps apparent only on the EEG (Fig. 2.5) and lasting under 5 s, are often not logged at all.

The final sleep stage not yet discussed is REM sleep. In going from wakefulness to non-REM sleep (stages 1, 2, 3, and 4) the EMG decreases, but as REM sleep approaches it decreases further and usually completely disappears in established REM sleep. The start of a fall in EMG is often the first indication that REM sleep is approaching, followed a few minutes later by loss of sleep spindles and K complexes and a return of the EEG to a pattern virtually indistinguishable from stage 1 or even wakefulness, that is, much higher frequencies (but no real alpha) and lower amplitude. The characteristic rapid bursts of eye movement usually come later, sometimes a few minutes after the EMG first began to fall. Thus, there is a gradual transition period from non-REM to REM sleep, but the conventional criteria often only 'allow' REM sleep to be scored well into this early transition period. When eye movements and EMG spikes of activity are present this is called phasic REM sleep and may be accompanied by visible twitching of the limbs. The REM sleep periods later on in the night usually have a much higher density of these phasic periods with a great deal of eye activity. Early on in the night the eye movements may be so sparse as to prevent the recognition that it really is REM sleep. These periods of REM sleep are called 'tonic', an unfortunate name since the postural muscles are still inhibited and certainly have no more tone than the phasic REM sleep periods; perhaps 'non-phasic' would have been a better term.

The overall 'sleep architecture' as it is called (Fig. 2.4), follows a certain pattern in normal people. Initially there is fairly rapid descent into SWS through stages 1 and 2. After about 90 min REM sleep commences, sometimes only for a few minutes, before there is a return to SWS. This 90 min cycle continues for the rest of the night but with the REM sleep periods getting longer (maybe up to 1 h or more) and the non-REM periods getting shorter and lighter such that stages 3 and 4 (SWS) may not be entered at all in the latter part of the night, only stages 1 and 2.

Examples of hypnograms

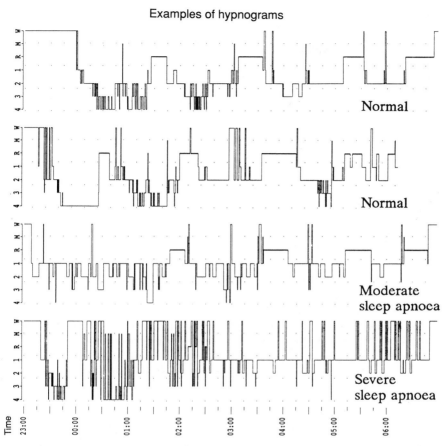

Fig. 2.4 Examples of classic hypnograms (based on 20 s epochs). Two normal subjects are followed by two patients with sleep apnoea of increasing severity. W, awake; M, movement (awake); R, REM sleep; 1 to 4, stages 1, 2, 3, and 4 of non-REM sleep.

Once a hypnogram has been constructed from these 20 or 30 s epochs, then certain other derivatives can be calculated. Table 2.1 lists some of these derivatives that the reader may see used in other literature.

This system of sleep analysis was designed to standardize manual scoring, a very laborious process taking as long as 3 or 4 h. With the advent of cheap and fast desk-top computers, a new approach is both available and desirable. The rules of the manual system of scoring are very hard to imitate by computer and this does not make the best use of the computer's ability to do repetitive and sophisticated number crunching. New approaches that can

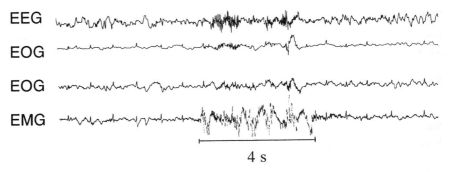

EEG

EOG

EOG

EMG

4 s

Fig. 2.5 An example of a brief 4 s arousal during REM sleep.

characterize sleep on a second by second basis will become more useful in the future and are described later.

2.2 Functions of sleep

There is still no good understanding of why we sleep. Many theories exist and they have been extensively reviewed by Jim Horne[305] in his book *Why we sleep*. The only obvious reason we sleep is to prevent sleepiness. The long-term consequences of inadequate sleep are varied but severely reduced performance, bizarre behaviour, and (in animal experiments) eventual death are all recognized.

Current evidence suggests that adequate SWS is needed in order to feel refreshed. This sleep stage is the one reclaimed most after sleep deprivation.[341] Its importance in mammals is exemplified by the curious strategies adopted by some species to obtain sleep under adverse conditions. For example, dolphins, being mammals, have to breathe at the surface to stay alive. If they stop swimming then they may drown or be swept away from their feeding areas. The Indus dolphin, living in fast running river mouths, has to remain alert and swim continuously in order to avoid debris and stay close to its food.[530] To achieve this it allows itself only short 'micro-sleeps', when the swimming action reduces considerably, before waking up and swimming again. Other dolphin species sleep with each cerebral hemisphere alternately and, because both sides of the body are innervated by both hemispheres, they can thus swim all the time.[480]

If sleep is so important then what is it doing? The difference in total energy consumption between being awake and resting compared to being asleep is very small and unlikely to be the benefit. However, even during quiet wakefulness the brain is working with an energy consumption only

Table 2.1 Derivatives from classical sleep staging

Time in bed (TIB)	Settling time until EEG recording stopped the following morning
Sleep period time (SPT)	TIB less the time to fall asleep initially and less the time awake prior to stopping the EEG recording
Sleep latency	Time to first fall asleep
Wake after sleep onset (WASO)	Time spent awake during the sleep period time (SPT)
Total sleep time (TST)	SPT less WASO
Sleep efficiency index	TST divided by TIB
Number of stage changes	Number of times the sleep state changed— index of disturbed sleep
Number of awakenings	Number of times after sleep onset that periods of wakefulness were scored
Number of REM periods	Usually three to five per night
REM latency	Time to first REM period
Latency (in minutes) to each sleep stage	That is, time to stages 1, 2, 3, and 4
Per cent (or minutes) of each sleep stage time	That is, of stages 1, 2, 3, and 4, REM, and movement

slightly reduced compared to active wakefulness. SWS may be a 'shut-down' period when routine maintenance is carried out. Enforced arousal from SWS requires the highest stimulus intensity and is attended by the most confusion and disorientation while recall of any thoughts or dreams is the least of any sleep state. Horne thus views SWS as 'core' sleep essential for the normal continuance of cerebral function.[305]

However, not all non-REM sleep is SWS and the overall length of sleep can be altered to suit current circumstances. For example, subjects can voluntarily sleep more or less hours per night, within certain limits, without apparent affects. This has led to the concept of 'optional' sleep that can be added on to the vital core sleep if appropriate and would consist mainly of stages 1 and 2. Whether this optional sleep is any more than a 'gap-filler' is not clear. Recent evidence from Horne's laboratory suggests that persistent deprivation of 'optional' sleep leads only to sleepiness and reduced vigilance that can be overcome if the subject is adequately motivated (we are all aware of being able to uprate our performance if really necessary, even after several nights of disturbed sleep). However, deprivation of 'core' sleep may produce true cerebral impairment with reduced cognitive performance

that is not reversible however hard the subject tries.[305,306] These twin
effects of sleep deprivation have been compared to the twin effects of food
deprivation. Initially, long before the body really needs more food, there is
a behavioural drive to eat—the sensation of hunger. However, as food
deprivation continues the hunger often fades to be replaced by physical
weakness and physiological decline. This would parallel the behavioural
drive of sleepiness to seek somewhere to lie down and go to sleep, but if
sleep deprivation continues then true cerebral dysfunction develops.

The function of REM sleep is even more mysterious. Because of its
association with the most vivid dreaming periods many theories abound
about whether it has some important subconscious purpose or is merely a
precursor of television. Some mammals (including the dolphin) appear to
have little or no REM sleep, perhaps because they cannot afford to be
paralysed and stop swimming, as discussed earlier.[480] Most tricyclic antidepressants can abolish REM sleep.[173] In normal subjects given these
tricyclic antidepressants there are no apparent effects from this near
abolition of REM sleep. After total sleep deprivation for several days REM
sleep is only partially reclaimed during the recovery period, unlike
SWS.[341] This all suggests that REM sleep may not be that important. Early
studies purporting to show serious mental problems after selective REM
sleep deprivation probably significantly affected SWS as well, so that they
are not in fact evidence for a vital function for REM sleep.

A simple suggestion, again by Horne, is that REM sleep is merely a brain
alerting mechanism, but without actual physical arousal.[305] As mentioned
earlier, arousal during SWS is attended by disorientation, perhaps because
the cognitive areas of the brain have been 'shut down' for repairs. In a
hostile environment this would be disadvantageous. During REM sleep,
arousal by external stimuli is much easier and equivalent to about stage 1
or 2.[553] Perhaps the brain needs to be aroused every so often during SWS
to prevent serious 'unarousability' in the event of an external threat.
However, recurrent full awakenings during the night would be pointless.
Thus, REM sleep could be viewed as a non-specific cortical arousal
mechanism, emanating from the pons and hippocampus, but with the body
'cut off' by the postural muscle inhibition referred to earlier. This
hypothesis has the merit of possibly explaining two other features of REM
sleep. The nature of dreams is often bizarre and random with incorporation
of previous experiences and current preoccupations. External noises can be
incorporated into dreams without arousal apparently being necessary. The
non-specific cortical arousal mechanism may simply be activating the brain
randomly and therefore what appears in the dream imagery will depend on
what is activated (perhaps more recent or important events are more likely
to be so), the arrival of any external stimuli, and finally the brain's attempt
to make sense of it all. The reduction of muscle tone in REM sleep may be

necessary to 'cut off' the body from the brain. The atonia of REM sleep is a very specific phenomenon and depends on the activity of a particular area in the pons, the locus coeruleus.[337] This area hyperpolarizes the lower motorneurones of postural muscles via inhibitory reticulospinal pathways. This is why the baseline, tonic EMG activity of postural muscles disappears during REM sleep. This atonia may be necessary to prevent the highly active cortex from producing body movements which would be inappropriate during 'sleep' in the middle of the night. This atonia is variable between species and most people are familiar with the barking and scrabbling that dogs often perform during REM sleep compared to the total immobility of cats. It has also been shown that if this REM sleep atonia area in the pons is destroyed, then a range of complex behaviours can occur during REM sleep.[292,478]

These simple explanations of SWS and REM sleep have the merit of simplicity, face validity, and some experimental evidence, but we are a long way from having any conclusive proof about why we sleep.

2.3 Sleep and ventilation

2.3.1 Spontaneous ventilation

2.3.1.1 Non-REM sleep

The effect that sleep has on ventilation is not completely understood, but some of the changes are predictable from what we know about sleep physiology, while others are not.

During wakefulness ventilation is driven by the brainstem respiratory control centres (mainly concerned with chemical control and integration of other respiratory reflexes—vagal etc.) as well as by the cortex. The breathing apparatus has other functions besides ventilating the lungs, for example, vocalizing. These clearly need to override the chemical control up to a point. The evidence that there are these two control pathways comes mainly from disease processes that selectively destroy parts of the brain. In 1958 Plum and Swanson[532] described patients with poliomyelitis who lost chemical control of breathing (no response to CO_2) but who could take breaths quite normally on command. Conversely, there are a few patients who have had cerebrovascular accidents involving the high brainstem that produced the so-called 'locked-in syndrome'. In this condition the patient is conscious but has no control over any part of the body except sometimes the eyes. Despite complete loss of voluntary motor control, ventilation continues in a normal rhythmic way and responds to CO_2.[284]

This wakefulness control disappears, of course, with the onset of sleep and thus breathing becomes much more regular, particularly during SWS.

Table 2.2 Causes of a fall in ventilation and rise in CO_2 during sleep

---

Reduced 'wakefulness' drive into respiratory centre. Fixed amount, equivalent to approximately 4 or 5 l/min

Reduced CO_2 drive. Probably similar to above effect

Reduced general muscle tone. Therefore, a given respiratory centre output to muscle anterior horn cell results in less ventilatory action

Reduced muscle tone to upper airways reduces their calibre and increases upper airway resistance

---

The removal of this extra, additional drive would alone be expected to lower the overall minute ventilation, which is indeed what happens.[658] On average, in normal people, minute ventilation falls by approximately 10−15 per cent and P_{aCO_2} rises by 3−8 mmHg which is not quite the predicted amount, due to a small fall in metabolic rate. There may also be a non-specific wakefulness drive with an input into the chemical control centres or related areas, the removal of which also reduces ventilation.[503] This is discussed further under the section on CO_2 drive (p. 17). There are probably two further factors contributing to the rise in CO_2 and reduced ventilation that occur with sleep onset (Table 2.2). The first is due to the partial withdrawal of muscle tone that occurs for all postural muscles.[112] This is very variable in the respiratory muscles and may be small, since a large fall may already have occurred with the onset of relaxed wakefulness. However, the effect of this reduced muscle tone will be to reduce the activity of the intercostal muscles and other respiratory muscles that also have a postural input, unless there is extra loading (such as increased upper airway resistance) which will lead to their increased activation again. Figure 2.6 represents an anterior horn cell supplying a respiratory muscle. Muscles other than the diaphragm (which has no resting tone and no function as a postural muscle) have, in addition to phasic respiratory input, tonic postural input and the level of activity will vary depending on circumstances. Whether the anterior horn cell fires depends upon whether the sum of the excitatory inputs (versus the inhibitory inputs) is enough to reach the threshold firing potential. Withdrawal of postural tone may mean that an unchanged respiratory signal now no longer causes the anterior horn cell to fire, thus, an EMG electrode at the muscle will show apparent loss of respiratory activity. Recordings of diaphragm activity do not show very much reduction in respiratory activity with sleep onset but the intercostals may do. However, as mentioned above, the usual increase in the resistance of the upper airway with sleep may alter the final level of activity that both the diaphragm and intercostals attain.[419,692] This loss of tone in the inter-

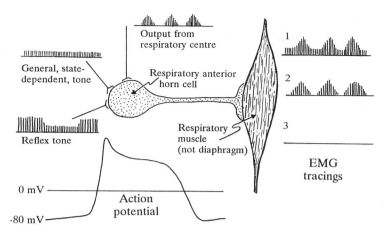

Fig. 2.6 Diagrammatic representation of the various inputs to an anterior horn cell supplying a respiratory muscle (other than the diaphragm). The various inputs summate to determine if the membrane potential reaches its critical level and fires. Thus, the disappearance of respiratory activity measured at EMG level may be due to withdrawal of any of the various anterior cell inputs, not just the phasic, respiratory, one.

costal muscles probably increases chest wall compliance thus allowing the diaphragm to elevate the rib-cage more easily (compared to pushing against the abdominal contents and wall) and hence an increase in rib-cage contribution to ventilation compared to abdominal contribution[658] (Fig. 2.7). Finally, again because of this reduction in the postural input to respiratory muscles, there may be an increase in upper airway resistance that adds a load to inspiration.[419,745] This will be discussed fully in the later section on sleep apnoea (p. 23). Because the pharynx is a muscular tube that relies on tonic and phasic respiratory activity to stay open, any reduction in the background tone will allow pharyngeal narrowing and produce an increase in upper airway resistance. At one stage this increase in upper airway resistance, combined with inadequate load compensation, was advanced as the only reason for a rise in P_{aCO_2} during non-REM sleep.[745,746] However, there are three pieces of evidence to show that although this may be a contributory factor, there is definitely a reduction in central output as well. First, there is a rise in non-REM P_{aCO_2} in tracheotomized dogs where upper airway resistance is clearly irrelevant,[663] second, there is a fall in measured central respiratory output in cats,[503] and third, there is a rise in the P_{aCO_2} level at which inspiratory muscles are turned on in ventilated patients.[323] This last paper studied patients on ventilators and measured the inspiratory muscle response to a rise in P_{aCO_2} induced by adding CO_2 to the circuit. On

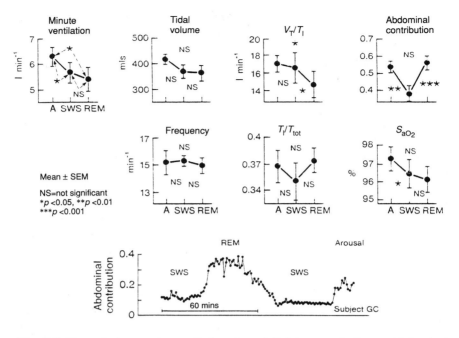

Fig. 2.7 Normal changes in ventilation, its subdivisions, and rib-cage/abdominal contributions in normal young men during sleep. A, awake; SWS, slow wave sleep; REM, rapid eye movement sleep. The change in abdominal contribution (mainly due to diaphragm activity) is also shown for one individual on a minute by minute basis as he goes from SWS to REM, back to SWS and finally on arousal. With permission from Stradling *et al.* (1985).[658]

average the 'CO$_2$ recruitment threshold', as the authors called it, was about 38.3 mmHg awake, 42.2 mmHg in non-REM, and 41.0 mmHg in REM. In this experiment, of course, the upper airway resistance or lung and chest wall mechanics cannot have been implicated in the P_{aCO_2} rise, thus indicating a central mechanism. The rise of 4 mmHg was perhaps a little less than normally seen in non-REM so increased upper airway resistance may play an additional role.

2.3.1.2 *REM sleep*

During REM sleep, breathing becomes less regular often with erratic patterns, somewhat like wakefulness. Indeed it may be that the cortex is able to control the diaphragm again so that ventilation may reflect dream content in some way. It is unlikely, though, that the fluctuations in respiratory excursions reflect dream imagery, but are probably random, in the same way that the rapid eye movements themselves do not seem to be purposefully screening the visual dream image.[304] During the periods when there are no eye movements (the so-called tonic REM sleep referred to earlier) breathing may still be fairly regular but the reduction in postural muscle tone usually means that there is now virtually no respiratory activity in the intercostal muscles.[692] This is reflected in an increase in the abdominal contribution to breathing again, compared to SWS (Fig. 2.7).[658,692] During the phasic periods of REM sleep when the eyes are moving there is often a transient reduction in ventilation (particularly from the rib-cage component) followed by a compensatory recovery.[237,473] Overall minute ventilation may be only slightly reduced compared to SWS but the breath by breath and minute to minute variability is greatly increased, thus allowing fluctuations in P_{aO_2} and P_{aCO_2}. In the study on ventilated patients described in the previous section[323] the CO_2 recruitment threshold was not higher in REM than non-REM sleep, again indicating no significant change in the CO_2 set point.

2.3.2 Carbon dioxide sensitivity

Compared to wakefulness the ventilatory responses to CO_2 during non-REM sleep are reduced, affecting both position and slope (Fig. 2.8). The degree of the fall has differed between studies, [47,91,169,235,323,556,726] but this may reflect the inconsistency of wakefulness measurements, which will be variably influenced by level of arousal and mouthpiece effect. The actual ventilatory responses to CO_2 during SWS have been remarkably similar across studies whereas the awake values have not. It is difficult to know why the CO_2 response has decreased. All the arguments discussed in the section on non-REM sleep (p. 14) as to why ventilation might have dropped and resting P_{aCO_2} risen apply here. There may be a true reduction of central sensitivity, which seems unlikely or there may be an *apparent* decline because of the reduced wakefulness drive to both the central controller or the intercostal muscles. If there were interactions between wakefulness and CO_2 response at the central chemoreceptor, then removal of wakefulness could affect both the slope and position of the CO_2 response curve rather than just the position. Increases in upper airway resistance would apparently influence the CO_2 response too, but alterations of slope and position are also seen in tracheotomized dogs where the upper airway is effectively bypassed.[527]

Whether there are further CO_2 sensitivity changes during REM sleep is not clear. Early work, where phasic REM sleep was used specifically to ensure accurate sleep state characterization,[169,527] suggested marked further reductions in CO_2 sensitivity compared to SWS. However, because of the irregularity of tidal volumes during these periods, CO_2 sensitivities measured by short rebreathing experiments may be difficult to interpret.[726]

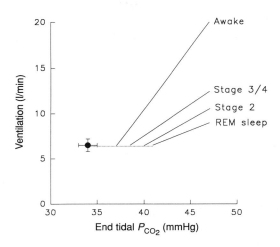

Fig. 2.8 Ventilatory response to rising end tidal CO_2 levels in normal humans, demonstrating the reduction in slope compared to wakefulness. Redrawn with permission from Douglas *et al.* (1982).[169]

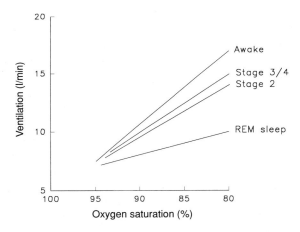

Fig. 2.9 Ventilatory response to falling arterial oxygen levels in normal humans, demonstrating the reduction in slope compared to wakefulness. Redrawn with permission from Douglas *et al.* (1985).[163]

Later work done in tonic REM sleep[684] and across REM sleep as a whole[663,665,726] suggested that there is no further reduction and that if ventilation is reduced during phasic periods then there is compensation during the tonic ones.[41,726]

2.3.3 Hypoxic sensitivity

As with the CO_2 sensitivity, there is a reduction in the response to isocapnic hypoxia during non-REM sleep when measured with a rebreathing technique.[46,168] The percentage fall is approximately the same as the fall in CO_2 sensitivity (Fig. 2.9). All the uncertainties about the mechanism discussed under CO_2 sensitivity also apply here. During REM sleep there appears to be a further reduction again[46,565] but no studies have been done during tonic REM sleep only, or across REM sleep as a whole. Since the apparent falls in hypoxic sensitivity are similar to those observed for hypercapnia during *phasic* REM sleep, it may be that if hypoxic response could be assessed over the whole REM period, it too would be much less affected.

2.3.4 Other ventilatory reflexes

2.3.4.1 Added respiratory load

Measurement of the ventilatory responses to added respiratory load (resistive or elastic) is very variable between subjects and from day to day. It is likely that much of this variation is due to conscious perception of the load, particularly since the P_{aCO_2} often falls during these types of experiments indicating an excessive response. Thus, it is not surprising that during sleep the responses seem much reduced and more consistent[320,325,746,759] and actually absent in dogs.[526] Nevertheless, there is clearly still some response to added resistive loading in humans during non-REM sleep, sufficient to defend ventilation to an extent.[225] This load-compensation ability is critical if blood gases are to be defended when there is an added resistance due to narrowing of the upper airway with sleep onset,[313,419,745] especially when this rise in resistance is particularly large, as it is in heavy snorers.[635] During REM sleep the response to added load is more erratic, but is probably further reduced compared to non-REM sleep.

2.3.4.2 Noxious stimuli to the upper airway

Noxious stimuli (such as fluid or citric acid) normally provoke coughing during wakefulness. During non-REM sleep the response is rapid (arousal followed by coughing) to doses that are not much larger than would provoke

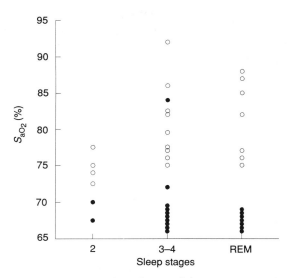

Fig. 2.10 This graph shows how low the arterial oxygen saturation had to fall in individual subjects during different sleep stages before they awoke. The filled circles are experimental runs that had to be aborted, prior to any arousal, for safety reasons. Redrawn with permission from Berthon-Jones and Sullivan (1982).[46]

coughing normally. During REM sleep in dogs the response is much impaired and sometimes apnoea and laryngeal closure may result rather than arousal and coughing.[682,683] In humans the arousal and cough response to citric acid is reduced during non-REM sleep but apparently is not reduced any further during REM sleep.[329]

2.3.4.3 *Arousal responses*

In the face of a respiratory problem, arousal may be the most appropriate response to improve matters. It is of course the recurrent arousal response in the sleep apnoea syndromes that stops the patient asphyxiating, but produces the sleep fragmentation with consequent daytime sleepiness. Hypercapnia, hypoxia, and increased inspiratory load all provoke arousal to a varying degree in different individuals.[46,47,168,169,286,320,325] In some (for example, see Fig. 2.10), there is poor arousal to hypoxaemia even down to 70 per cent S_{aO_2}. In REM sleep the arousal to hypercapnia and hypoxaemia is probably less, but may be better to added resistive loads[320] or occlusion.[325] This apparent difference may be explained by recent observations from Gleeson *et al.*[224,225] that arousal may occur more as a result of the actual ventilatory effort to hypoxia or hypercapnia (measured from pleural pressure swings) rather than to the stimulus or subsequent ventilation itself. Thus, if the ventilatory responses to these stimuli were reduced in REM sleep then arousal to them would appear depressed too, whereas that to occlusion itself might not. This cannot be the whole story because patients with central apnoea wake to hypoxia and hypercapnia when there is no ventilatory effort and the arousal can be delayed by giving extra oxygen.

It is likely that in most patients seen in the sleep laboratory, with sleep disturbed by respiratory problems, that the stimulus to awaken is mixed and that the arousals do not depend on just one physiological signal.

2.3.5 Ventilatory vulnerability during sleep

The very existence of sleep-related breathing disorders shows that the changes with sleep can produce unsatisfactory nocturnal ventilation. The preceding sections have described the relevant physiological changes and summarized below are the aspects that predispose to adverse respiratory consequences during sleep.

1. Reduction in overall drive to breathe with the onset of sleep:
   a. To the diaphragm, producing an overall drop in ventilation. This will not be important unless oxygenation is critical to start with, either in terms of supply to vital organs or near to the arousal threshold for hypoxaemia.
   b. To the upper airway musculature, producing an increase in upper airway resistance.

2. Reduction in general postural muscle tone with onset of sleep:
   a. To the upper airway musculature also producing an increase in upper airway resistance.
   b. To the accessory muscles of ventilation, producing bigger drops in ventilation if the patient is particularly reliant on these muscles.

3. Reduction in ventilatory drives from rising CO_2 and hypoxia—this is closely linked with the resting drive to breathe but:
   a. There will be a less vigorous response to further deteriorations in gas exchange (for example, from sputum retention, postural effects on gas exchange, etc.).

4. The requirement for wakefulness to return, before avoidance manoeuvres can be made, means that the exact arousal threshold becomes important.
   a. Arousal in response to gas exchange deterioration is variable between individuals.

   b. Arousal can be seriously suppressed (for example, by sedatives, sleep deprivation, etc.).

5. The further loss of postural muscle tone in REM sleep produces the same problems as in 2a and b above.

3 Pathophysiology of obstructive sleep apnoea

Obstructive sleep apnoea (OSA) is now the main condition investigated in specialist sleep clinics.[87] Many thousands of patients have been shown to have this condition and have been successfully treated with nasal continuous positive airway pressure (NCPAP). Despite this success story many aspects of OSA are still far from clear and, in particular, 'what constitutes a problem' and 'how should it be diagnosed and monitored?' The current answer to these questions changes from month to month and depends on whom one asks, thus, it is impossible to give firm guidelines. These uncertainties will be discussed extensively because to understand why these areas of disagreement exist improves the understanding of this condition's pathophysiology.

3.1 Upper airway function

The upper airway, extending from the soft palate to the larynx, has to serve two functions, swallowing and breathing, that require very different design features. When only air needs conducting, then the trachea can afford to be a rigid open tube that resists collapse. When only food and liquids are transported, the oesophagus is a muscular, permanently collapsed tube that propels its contents by peristalsis. For the pharynx to conduct both air and propel solids or liquids, requires an open tube most of the time that can be converted to a collapsible peristaltic tube when required. This is achieved by having a collapsible tube that is normally held open by muscular action pulling in appropriate directions on the pharyngeal walls.[86,560] During swallowing these pharyngeal dilators relax and allow the pharyngeal constrictors to propel the food by a wave of activity into the oesophagus. These pharyngeal dilator muscles have a mixture of inputs. There is the tonic component that provides a relatively fixed level of activity (varying with the sleep/wake state) and the phasic component in time with inspiration that braces the pharynx against collapse (Fig. 3.1). During inspiration the intraluminal pressures in the pharynx will fall below atmospheric, because of the pressure drop across the nasal resistance and this partial vacuum

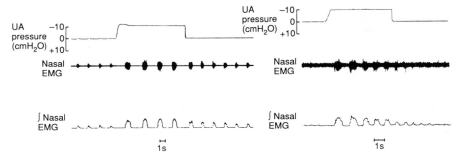

Fig. 3.1 Example (in an anaesthetized rabbit) of the increase in upper airway dilator muscle tone (here a nasal dilator, raw, and integrated EMG) in response to a negative intrapharyngeal pressure (UA pressure). (a) The nasal dilator shows only phasic activity that is enhanced during the fall in pressure. (b) Tonic activity is present initially and respiratory activity only appears during the stimulus period. With permission from Mathew (1984).[448]

will tend to suck in the pharyngeal walls unless adequate opposing forces are available.

There are several muscles that contribute to maintaining the patency of the upper airway (Fig. 3.2). They include genioglossus (keeping the tongue forward and out of the pharyngeal lumen[601]), those attached to the hyoid pulling it forward and upward (geniohyoid, mylohyoid, stylohyoid, and digastric), those connecting the hyoid to the anterior part of the pharynx and larynx (thyrohyoid and omohyoid), and sternohyoid which helps to bring the hyoid forward in concert with geniohyoid. Palatopharyngeus acting alone will pull the soft palate forwards and maintain the patency of the nasopharynx. In conjunction with tensor palati and levator palati then palatopharyngeus may hold open the oropharynx rather like a tent with supporting guy ropes. Tensor palati may also be important as it holds the soft palate up and may prevent it 'plugging' the space behind the tongue.[696] All these muscles essentially work in concert to stabilize the upper airway and resist collapse.[574] Another, more visible, example of muscles being used to open the upper airway is of course the nasal entrance which can be

Fig. 3.2 Diagrammatic representations of most of the muscles involved in pharyngeal patency. Some muscles have direct pharyngeal dilator activity (for example, genioglossus and levator veli palati) whereas others stabilize the pharynx and protect it against collapse (for example, thyrohyoid and styloglossus). The action of many of the other muscles is hard to predict and their exact action on the pharynx will depend on the activity of other muscles working in concert.

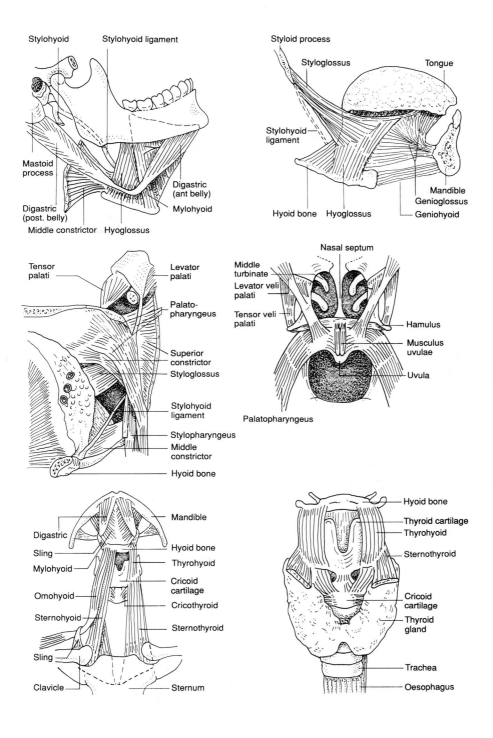

Stylohyoid   Stylohyoid ligament

Mastoid process

Digastric (post. belly)

Middle constrictor   Hyoglossus

Digastric (ant belly)

Mylohyoid

Styloid process

Styloglossus   Tongue

Stylohyoid ligament

Hyoid bone   Hyoglossus

Mandible
Genioglossus
Geniohyoid

Tensor palati   Levator palati

Palato-pharyngeus

Superior constrictor

Styloglossus

Stylohyoid ligament

Stylopharyngeus

Middle constrictor

Hyoid bone

Nasal septum

Middle turbinate

Levator veli palati

Tensor veli palati

Hamulus

Musculus uvulae

Uvula

Palatopharyngeus

Digastric

Sling

Mylohyoid

Omohyoid

Sternohyoid

Sling

Clavicle

Mandible

Hyoid bone

Thyrohyoid

Cricoid cartilage

Cricothyroid

Sternothyroid

Sternum

Hyoid bone

Thyroid cartilage

Thyrohyoid

Sternothyroid

Cricoid cartilage

Thyroid gland

Trachea

Oesophagus

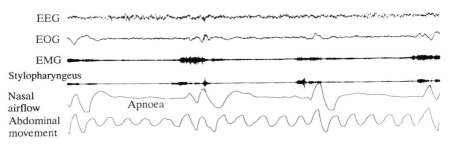

Fig. 3.3 Example of an early tracing showing the activity of pharyngeal dilator and stabilizer muscles disappearing during an apnoea and reappearing shortly before the apnoea ends. With permission from Guilleminault *et al.* (1978).[266]

flared by the alae nasi to reduce inspiratory resistance. These upper airway muscles are activated slightly in advance of the diaphragm, presumably to guard against collapse at the beginning of inspiration.[675]

If these upper airway muscles are not activated by respiratory drive they may allow occlusion of the pharyngeal lumen. This was nicely demonstrated in a patient requiring nocturnal ventilatory support in the form of diaphragm pacing. When breathing on his own there was no obstruction, but once ventilation was taken over by diaphragm pacing then brainstem ventilatory drive and presumably upper airway dilator action fell, allowing obstructive events to develop that prevented successful use of this technique.[318]

In the early stages of the investigation of OSA it was not clear whether the obstruction in the pharynx was due to active contraction of the pharyngeal constrictors or inadequate action of the pharyngeal dilators. However, most EMG data have shown a decrease in overall dilator muscle action during apnoeas and a return of activity when breathing resumes with arousal[254,560] (Fig. 3.3). There has been no good evidence that the pharyngeal constrictors go into spasm as was suggested some years ago.[733] In addition, the obstruction is only on inspiration, with expiration able to occur unimpeded when the expiratory muscles become recruited towards the end of an apnoea.

Once it was realized that failure of adequate pharyngeal dilator action during sleep was the cause of OSA the arguments then centred on whether there was something wrong with the *activation of these muscles*, for example, a brainstem control problem or whether there were *anatomical abnormalities* that provoked obstruction when the normal reduction in upper airway muscle tone with sleep meant their activity was no longer adequate to maintain patency. Diagrams such as Fig. 3.4, illustrating the balance of forces influencing upper airway size, appeared in many reviews with arguments for and against each contributing factor.

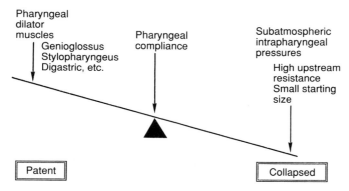

Pharyngeal
dilator
muscles
Genioglossus
Stylopharyngeus
Digastric, etc.

Pharyngeal
compliance

Subatmospheric
intrapharyngeal
pressures

High upstream
resistance
Small starting
size

Patent

Collapsed

Fig. 3.4 Diagrammatic representation of the 'balance of forces' that are thought to be involved in controlling pharyngeal patency.

3.1.1 Neuromuscular failure

In favour of a defect of neuromuscular control was the EMG evidence that the activity of muscles such as genioglossus decreased at apnoea onset and returned with resumption of ventilation. However, this fall in EMG activity occurs in normal people so a similar fall in OSA patients cannot be taken as evidence for an abnormality. An ingenious study[326] in patients with OSA looked at the ability of the pharynx to hold itself open during progressively increased ventilatory efforts against obstructed inspiration. This study found that the upper airway could only hold itself open down to a certain intra-pharyngeal pressure and would then shut off. The negative pressure in the pharynx, needed to provoke collapse, did not become even more negative through an apnoea, despite increasing ventilatory effort. This suggested to the authors that, despite the increasing drive to the diaphragm, there was a simultaneous failure to increase the drive to the upper airway dilator muscles. This was taken as evidence for an abnormality of control of these muscles. However, as will be discussed later, there is the alternative explanation that these muscles were already being driven maximally by the respiratory centre at the point of collapse and there was no further possibility of making them contract any harder (Fig. 3.5).

There are reports in the literature of patients with clear evidence of a primary neuromuscular problem (from brainstem lesions to myopathies) that have had associated OSA.[251] In these cases it seems reasonable to ascribe the OSA to neuromuscular failure, but they are rare and other evidence of neuromuscular dysfunction is usually present, which of course is not true of the majority of patients with OSA.

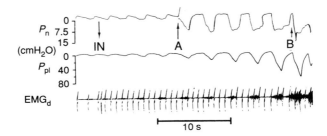

Fig. 3.5 This tracing is from a patient with obstructive sleep apnoea on nasal continuous airway pressure treatment. P_n is nasal pressure, P_{pl} is oesophageal pressure indicating pleural pressure (different scale to P_n) and EMG_d is a diaphragmatic surface EMG. The time bar is 10 s and the sleep stage is SWS. Between A and B the nasal airway is occluded. There is an immediate increase in inspiratory effort, as evidenced by the P_{pl} and EMG_d tracings. However, the increasingly negative intrathoracic pressures are not transmitted all the way up to the intranasal pressure transducer. At about -7.5 cm H_2O the fall in nasal pressure suddenly stops, despite a continuing fall in the intrathoracic pressure, indicating that there has been collapse of the airway between the nose and the trachea (presumably at the pharyngeal level). This was used initially as evidence to suggest abnormal control of pharyngeal dilators, but could also be interpreted as failure of the dilators despite maximum possible activation. With permission from Issa and Sullivan (1984).[326]

The other concept that developed early on was that there could be a discoordination of diaphragm and upper airway control.[83,417,501] For example, following a period of hyperventilation during sleep a central apnoea (that is, no evidence of ventilatory effort at all) will occur. During this period of central apnoea the blood gases will deteriorate and ventilatory drive gradually appears. Peripheral evidence of this returning drive is first seen in the diaphragm and a little later in the upper airway muscles. This delay sometimes allows one or two obstructed breaths to occur until the drive to the upper airway is adequate to overcome the negative pressures in the pharynx induced by diaphragm activity.[11] In normal subjects the induction of periodic breathing during sleep by administering hypoxic mixtures, in conjunction with inspiratory resistive loads to challenge the pharynx, can induce obstruction to the pharynx which will not occur without this periodicity provoked by the hypoxia.[499] However, the obstructive events are brief and few, quite unlike real OSA.

In animal studies[729] it can be shown that ventilatory drive to the genioglossus muscle, during elevations of arterial CO_2, initially increases much less than the diaphragm drive but seems to 'catch up' at higher CO_2 levels (Fig. 3.6). This kind of study was originally interpreted as showing upper airway drive to be more precarious than diaphragmatic drive.

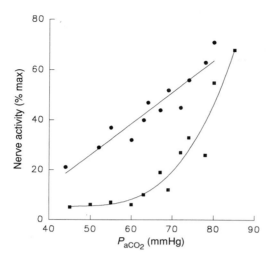

Fig. 3.6 Different behaviour of the phrenic nerve (circles) compared to the hypoglossal nerve (squares) in response to rising arterial CO_2 levels. Nerve activity to the tongue appears not to get under way compared to the diaphragm until higher levels of CO_2 are reached. With permission from Weiner *et al.* (1982).[729]

Unfortunately it is virtually impossible to imply mechanical function of a muscle from its EMG activity because of the complex relationship between actual firing of a muscle fibre and the end-product, such as pharyngeal dilation: the curves in Fig. 3.6 may simply be describing the EMG to function relationships of the diaphragm and genioglossus muscles with the end-products being perfectly matched.

Thus, although instability of ventilatory control can induce some obstructive events it is unlikely to be the underlying cause of OSA. Further evidence for this comes from the observation that most OSA patients following successful treatment with nasal CPAP do not show irregular ventilation during non-REM sleep.[441]

If there is an element of neuromuscular failure contributing to OSA then a possible reason might be failure of upper airway reflexes that could detect pharyngeal collapse and increase power to dilator muscles. In the pharynx there are certainly receptors that consist of a ramification of fibres under and between the squamous cells of the epithelium[186] which link up with myelinated fibres. It is likely that these receptors are capable of responding to stretch and collapse of the pharynx and that non-myelinated fibres respond to nociceptive stimuli. The pharyngeal muscles themselves may also be able to signal proprioceptive information (from muscle spindles) that influence the eventual motor tone to these dilator muscles.

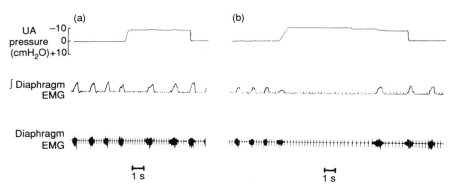

Fig. 3.7 Two traces showing the effect of sudden falls in intrapharyngeal pressures (UA press) on respiratory timing in an anaesthetized rabbit. Note the slowing and apnoea evident on the diaphragm EMG traces. With permission from Mathew and Farber (1983).[450]

A variety of ingenious experiments, both in animals and man, demonstrate that there are surface receptor-induced upper airway protective responses to a subatmospheric, collapsing, pressure in the pharynx. These protective responses include increased upper airway dilator muscle activity[307,308,448,449] and a reduction of inspiratory effort (sometimes even apnoea) which is viewed as protective because this will lessen the intraluminal subatmospheric, collapsing pressure.[450]

Figure 3.7 shows the effect of exposing the upper airway of a rabbit to −10 cm H_2O. Note the increase in tonic and phasic tone of a dilator muscle (in this case the laryngeal dilator, posterior cricoarytenoid) and the effect on inspiratory effort. Figure 3.8 shows the abrupt rise in genioglossus EMG to a −15 cm H_2O drop in pharyngeal pressure. Although this study[308] was done in conscious man the speed of the reflex is too fast to be via conscious perception.

The abolition of inspiratory effort by stimulation of the pharyngeal receptors is interesting because it may have a clinical counterpart. Some patients sound as if they will have OSA from their histories and indeed on their sides they may have snoring and classical obstructive events. However, when supine they appear to have central apnoeas and make no effort to breathe.[328] At the end of the apnoea an opening, sucking noise is usually heard with the first breath suggesting the upper airway was in fact closed. These central apnoeas respond to nasal continuous positive airway pressure and can be converted to classic obstructive events by topically anaesthetizing the upper airway.[328] Why the majority of patients fight their apnoeas while others do not is unknown.

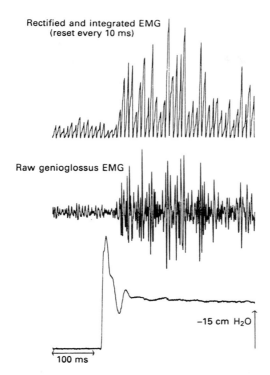

Rectified and integrated EMG
(reset every 10 ms)

Raw genioglossus EMG

−15 cm H$_2$O

100 ms

Fig. 3.8 Response of the genioglossus muscle in a conscious human to a sudden fall in intrapharyngeal pressure. The time delay (approximately 50 ms) is too short to be due to a cortical response and is presumably a spinal cord reflex. With permission from Horner *et al.* (1991).[308]

An alternative signal to the upper airway that it is in trouble may be the vibration of snoring itself. It has been pointed out[679] that the sub-atmospheric pressures needed to experimentally collapse a snorer's pharynx during sleep may be very small, perhaps only −5 cm H$_2$O,[327] yet when he is snoring loudly he is resisting pressures perhaps as low as −80 cm H$_2$O.[426,428] Externally applied vibrations of 30 Hz have been shown to activate upper airway dilator and stabilizer muscles during sleep in both normal subjects and those with OSA,[293] there being no suggestion though that they were actually deficient in the latter. Thus, it is conceivably possible that snoring serves a useful 'purpose' as an early warning system of pharyngeal collapse which turns on protective mechanisms.[679] The presence of these upper airway reflexes, particularly that due to snoring, has been used as a theoretical argument against the use of pharyngeal operations, for example, uvulopalatopharyngoplasty (UPPP), which may interfere with them. Some possible evidence for this comes from two sources. Oropharyngeal anaesthesia in snorers increases the number of obstructive episodes they have[107] and following UPPP obstructive episodes may get worse.[136,536,566]

3.1.2 Anatomical abnormalities

On the other side of the balance of forces (Fig. 3.4) are the anatomical abnormalities that might provoke upper airway collapse. For an anatomical abnormality to provoke collapse it needs to narrow the upper airway all the time (awake as well) so that the *normal* loss of upper airway muscle tone and airway narrowing is now enough to occlude the airway. In addition, narrowing in a compliant segment of the pharynx will result in a greater tendency to narrow further through the Bernoulli effect. Where an airway narrows the speed of the air has to increase, leading to a local fall in pressure which tends to suck the walls further together. This tends to be an unstable process (if complete collapse is possible), because once airflow ceases the reduced pressure rises again allowing airway reopening. This leads to vibration of the upper airway, at a frequency depending mainly on upper airway compliance and is the main mechanism of snoring.

Alternatively the anatomical abnormality needs to load the upper airway in a way that requires increased dilator activity to successfully oppose it, a compensatory action, which is then lost with sleep onset: there are other examples of ventilatory compensation reducing considerably with sleep onset, for example, the diminished response to an external resistive load which was mentioned in the section on added respiratory loads (p. 19). During wakefulness expiratory muscles are used to keep functional residual capacity (FRC) normal during either negative external pressure, positive end expiratory pressure or CO_2-stimulated ventilation: a compensation mechanism also lost during non-REM sleep.[58,719]

Many case reports have shown that obvious anatomical abnormalities can provoke OSA. These range from acquired changes such as large tonsils,[652] acromegaly,[521] oedema,[664] myxoedema,[243] the mucopolysaccharidoses,[520] lymphomas, or other tumours[767] to congenital deformities such as retro- or micrognathia.[322] In adults the tonsils usually atrophy but may remain (Plate 1), causing OSA that is fully treated by their removal.[652] However, the majority of patients with OSA do not have these obvious anatomical abnormalities. Most, though, are overweight. The relevance of being overweight seemed initially to be understated by those in the field, probably because there was an overrepresentation of the rarer causes in early series. Now most series of patients with OSA find being overweight to be extremely common. For example, in 1978 Guilleminault et al.[266] found that about 35 per cent of patients with OSA were >30 per cent overweight but by

1988 this had risen to 66 per cent of such patients.[252] In a recent publication on sleep apnoea and echocardiographic findings the *mean* body mass index was 33.5 kg/m^2 (approximately 106 kg in a man of average height).[261] In all series, looking at the risk factors for sleep apnoea, body weight or an obesity index has been the dominant risk factor. The degree of variance in the sleep apnoea measured that can be 'explained' by obesity has often been in excess of 40 per cent.[143,348] What has been less obvious is how the excess fat is contributing to the pathogenesis of sleep apnoea. It had been suggested that they might both be the result of a primary problem, such as a hypothalamic disorder, but there is no evidence for this. Imaging of the upper airway using computerized tomography (CT) or magnetic resonance (MR) techniques has shown very little excess fat actually in the pharyngeal tissues immediately under the mucosa that could contribute to airway encroachment,[276] and certainly no more than in weight-matched controls.[309] However, despite this apparent lack of fat in the immediately surrounding tissues there is still a good correlation between body weight, OSA severity, and pharyngeal narrowing.[276,310,572] The explanation for this is probably simply that fat masses elsewhere in the neck cause both static compression (and therefore diurnal narrowing) as well as dynamic loading (and therefore overwhelm the residual pharyngeal dilator action at night). Although Horner *et al.*[309] did not find excess fat in the submucosa in patients with OSA compared to weight-matched controls using MR imaging there was excess fat, particularly posterolaterally to the retropalatal airspace in the vicinity of the carotid vessels. A different group have also shown these fat pads and, in addition, that the pharyngeal airway in OSA patients is narrower from side to side compared to the pharynx in normal non-obese subjects which is narrower front to back,[578] perhaps suggesting lateral pressure.

The really striking aspect of patients with OSA is that the majority have big necks, even if not particularly obese. The published imaging studies have all tended to concentrate on peripharyngeal fat deposition rather than where the bulk of the fat is—anteriorly and subcutaneously. The study by Horner *et al.*[309] shows enormous amounts of fat all around the neck in the subcutaneous tissues, as is also seen in Fig. 3.9.

It was for these reasons that we asked the simple question 'is neck circumference, a surrogate measure of neck fat, a better predictor of sleep apnoea than overall obesity?' Four groups have shown this to be so[143,348,436,705] lending support to the idea that obesity causes sleep apnoea through excess fat in the neck. For example, in our study[143] neck circumference (measured at the level of the cricothyroid membrane) accounted for 42 per cent of the variation in OSA severity with no extra predictability coming from the obesity index, when analysed with multiple linear regression techniques. Figure 3.10 shows the relationship between neck

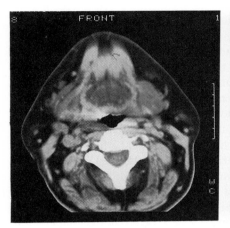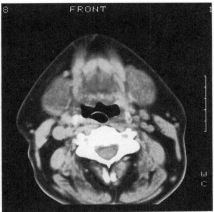

Fig. 3.9 Transverse computerized tomography sections at the retroglossal level (second scan just catching the epiglottis) in a patient with obstructive sleep apnoea. Note the absence of fat (black) immediately around the airway, but extensive subcutaneous deposits for a considerable proportion of the neck circumference.

circumference and OSA severity in a sleep clinic population and there is the suggestion of a threshold effect above which OSA severity increases rapidly. An epidemiological study also showed that neck obesity was a better predictor of snoring than overall obesity.[661]

Indirect evidence for the vulnerability of the upper airway to mass loading comes from an experiment which showed that very small extra weights applied externally over the pharynx easily produced airway collapse in anaesthetized rabbits.[361] A case report of a neck lipoma provoking OSA and its cure by surgical resection, is interesting in this respect too.[364] Although height-corrected neck circumference and general obesity are clearly related, Fig. 3.11 shows that this correlation is not particularly strong ($r = 0.75$). Thus, only about 60 per cent of the variance in neck obesity can be accounted for on the basis of general obesity; this means that some non-overweight individuals can have big necks and vice versa. Figure 3.11 shows only males; females on the whole have smaller necks for a given degree of obesity. This gynaecoid lower body distribution of fat may be the simple explanation for the lower prevalence of sleep apnoea and snoring in women. After the menopause, women's androgenous fat distribution and snoring prevalence increase.

Further evidence for the concept that upper airway muscles are simply being overloaded comes from EMG studies of genioglossus awake and asleep. Suratt *et al.*[686] measured EMG activity in young normal subjects and older subjects (obese and non-obese) as well as patients with OSA,

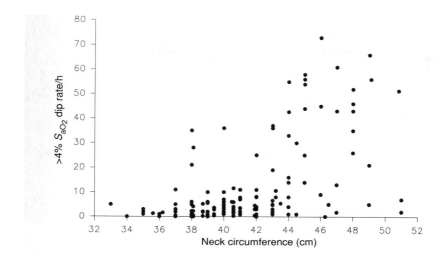

Fig. 3.10 Relationship between neck circumference and the severity of sleep apnoea, measured by the number of >4 per cent S_{aO_2} dips per hour overnight, in 124 sleep clinic patients.

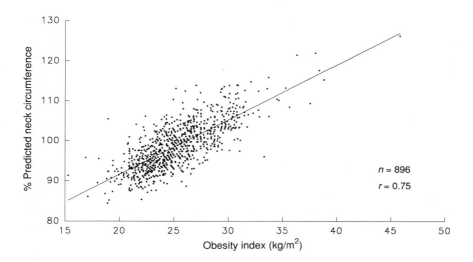

Fig. 3.11 Relationship between obesity and neck circumference (with a minor correction for height) in 896 randomly selected men aged 35–65 years. Note that there are some individuals with big necks who are not particularly obese.

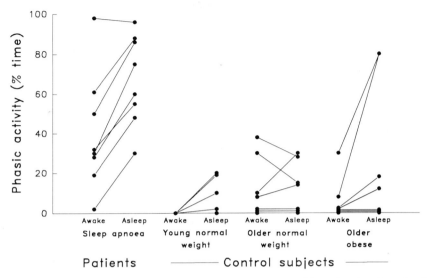

Fig. 3.12 Genioglossus activity (assessed as percentage of breaths showing phasic respiratory EMG activation) in four different groups of subjects, awake and asleep. Note that patients with obstructive sleep apnoea have the highest activity suggesting that this muscle is actually being stimulated more by the respiratory system in these patients, not less. Redrawn with permission from Suratt *et al.* (1988).[686]

awake and asleep. Because comparisons between subjects of EMG activity are not possible they 'quantified' the activity by noting the percentage of breaths showing phasic inspiratory activity (Fig. 3.12). Thus, they were looking mainly at the respiratory input rather than the tonic or 'posture' input. In young normal subjects little activity in genioglossus was present, awake or asleep. In older subjects, particularly the obese, there was more activity which increased further when asleep. In the patients with OSA there was even more activity, particularly asleep. Thus, although the tonic activity probably decreased in genioglossus with sleep, the phasic (respiratory) activity increased. This suggested to the authors that there is a rise in the drive to this muscle as a defence mechanism following the withdrawal with sleep onset of the tonic (postural) inputs.[695] These different inputs to respiratory muscular anterior horn cells were discussed earlier in the section on non-REM sleep (p. 14). Further preliminary evidence for this hypothesis has appeared recently and has also shown that this increased genioglossal activity in patients with OSA disappeared when the OSA was successfully treated with CPAP, presumably making the compensatory activity no longer necessary.[466] Whether genioglossus activity in this context is representative of upper airway dilator activity in general is not clear. EMG studies on tensor palati suggest that this muscle, a palate elevator, does not increase its activity with increasing upper airway resistance in the way that genioglossus does.[696] Indeed there is some correlation between loss of tensor palati action and increases in upper airway obstruction during sleep.

Overall the evidence seems strongly in favour of the majority of OSA in adults being due to mass loading of the upper airway (usually by fat) which can be fended off during wakefulness but, with the withdrawal of postural tone to the dilator muscles during sleep, this compensatory activity becomes inadequate.

However, not *all* adult obstructive sleep apnoea can be explained by neck obesity or the obvious anatomical abnormalities referred to earlier in this section.

Carefully standardized lateral head and neck radiographs (cephalometry) do demonstrate differences between patients with OSA, snorers, and normal subjects, for example, Andersson and Brattstrom.[20] In particular the group at Stanford[258,330] has found several differences (Fig. 3.13): retroposition of the mandible, a more acute angle between the sella to nasion and nasion to supramentale planes (SNB), a downward movement of the hyoid, an elongation of the soft palate, and a narrower anteroposterior distance behind the tongue. Other groups have found the same differences and have also been able to identify many more bony measurements that are less convincingly different in patients with OSA.[674] The retropositioning of the mandible is presumably simply minor retrognathia and can be suspected clinically from the degree of overjet (by how much further forward the top front teeth are compared to the bottom when teeth together) and the presence of teeth crowding. That this should be a risk factor, which is perhaps also suggested by the narrow retroglossal space, is not surprising. From a predictive point of view it is not sensitive or specific enough to diagnose OSA, nor does its discovery lead to a useful outcome unless severe, when facial advancement surgery becomes a possibility. The more acute cranial base flexion is hard to explain and the way in which this may contribute to OSA is also not clear. The elongated soft palate, low hyoid, and enlarged tongue may be nothing to do with the *cause* of OSA at all. Lugaresi *et al.*[427] first suggested that some of the changes in the anatomy of patients with OSA might be secondary to the considerable down-pulling of the pharynx and its associated structures during the frustrated inspiratory attempts or perhaps be adaptive changes. Davies and Stradling[143] showed, after allowing for neck obesity, that soft palate length and hyoid position no longer correlated with OSA severity at all, suggesting that they were therefore secondary phenomena and not causal. If the mandible is surgically shortened for some reason, then the hyoid bone does move down and this has been interpreted as an attempt to pull the root of the tongue out of the now crowded pharynx to improve the lumen.[744] It may be that in patients

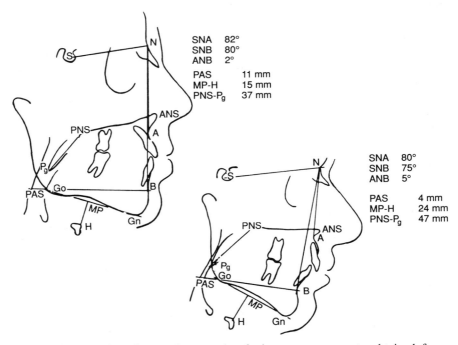

Fig. 3.13 Examples of some bony and soft tissue measurements obtained from cephalometric radiographs. S, sella; N, nasion; A, subspinale; B, supramentale; Gn, gnathion; H, hyoid; MP, mandibular plane; Go, gonion; PAS, posterior airspace; Pg, pogonion (tip of uvula); PNS, posterior nasal spine; ANS, anterior nasal spine. The left subject has normal measurements, but the right subject (with OSA) has a shorter mandible and maxilla (reduced angles SNA and SNB), narrower retroglossal space (PAS), longer soft palate (PNS-Pg) and a more inferiorly placed hyoid bone (MP-H). With permission from Riley *et al.* (1983).[564]

with OSA the hyoid descent is also an adaptive remodelling to reduce crowding in the pharynx and the larger tongue may be hypertrophy of genioglossus and other muscles. Some patients (with snoring or OSA) also describe how their uvulas are big and swollen in the morning, but reduce in size during the day. Because the uvula is sucked down into the retroglossal space and subjected to much vibration, it seems reasonable to postulate that enlargement of the soft palate could also be a secondary phenomenon. There is some evidence that following treatment of OSA with nasal continuous positive airway pressure therapy there is a reduction in soft tissue bulk, both pharyngeal mucosa and the tongue.[592]

Hence, the only clearly pathogenetic craniofacial abnormality seems to be a degree of retrognathia, ranging from very subtle to the full blown Pierre

Robin syndrome, sometimes called the bird-like face syndrome. It is not clear why some people have smaller lower jaws than others, although there is some evidence that mandibular underdevelopment relates to enforced mouth breathing very early on in life. Experimental nasal blockage in primates (forcing oral respiration) from shortly after birth produces gross underdevelopment of the lower jaw with teeth crowding.[471] It is suggested that a predominantly closed mouth with the tongue up against the hard palate is needed to stimulate the correct growth of the lower face.

This leads to an interesting hypothesis that factors present early in life might influence the development of the lower face in a way that predisposes to OSA in later life, particularly if there is additional obesity.[247,257] There is good evidence that nasal obstruction, usually due to adenoidal enlargement, leads to altered facial development in children[315,497,617] which is similar to that thought to contribute to OSA. This is more familiar as the 'adenoidal facies' (increased anterior face height in the lower third of the facial skeleton, posterior buccal cross-bite, high palate, steep mandibular plane, and an overjet or class II occlusion) which resolves following adenoidectomy, if performed early enough.[414,415] In addition, there is evidence that enlarged tonsils retard facial growth which can correct post-tonsillectomy if this is done before the age of 6 years.[316] Later on in this book the possible consequences of falling adenotonsillectomy rates in provoking childhood sleep apnoea are discussed and, in conjunction with these data on adenoidectomy, it makes one wonder if the liberal policy of adenotonsillectomy 30 years ago might not have had its benefits.

In concluding this section on the basic pathophysiological factors leading to OSA in the adult, one has to say that there is more than one contributory cause. Obesity in the neck is clearly a major risk factor, but probably interacts with subtle abnormalities in the shape of the lower facial skeleton. There is no good evidence that pharyngeal dilator muscle activity is deficient relative to normal in any way in the vast majority of patients and these muscles may in fact be working harder than normal.

3.1.3 Other provoking factors

3.1.3.1 Alcohol

As well as the relatively fixed anatomical abnormalities discussed above, there are other factors known to influence pharyngeal collapse more acutely. Alcohol, taken in the evening increases apnoea rates, converts snoring to full apnoea, and delays arousal, which produces longer apnoeas and bigger dips in S_{aO_2}.[324,609,690] The increased snoring from someone who has too much alcohol is unfortunately familiar to many. The main mechanism seems to be through further suppression of upper airway dilator activity.[63,576]

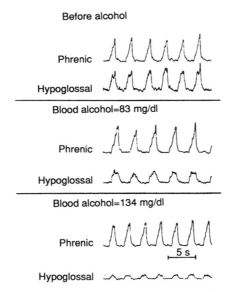

Before alcohol

Phrenic

Hypoglossal

Blood alcohol=83 mg/dl

Phrenic

Hypoglossal

Blood alcohol=134 mg/dl

Phrenic

5 s

Hypoglossal

Fig. 3.14 The effect of raising blood alcohol levels on phrenic (diaphragm) and hypoglossal (genioglossus) nerve activities in an anaesthetized cat. Note the fall in hypoglossal activity, but preservation of phrenic activity. With permission from Bonora *et al.* (1984).[63]

Although phasic respiratory activity in genioglossus is suppressed by alcohol (Fig. 3.14) this does not mean that the respiratory centre is depressed, only that the sum of inputs to the anterior horn cells is decreased (as discussed in the section on non-REM sleep, p. 14). This is likely to be due to alcohol's known muscle relaxing properties, perhaps through a non-specific action on the lipid membranes of the anterior horn cells. Alternatively, the CNS depressant effects may directly influence upper airway respiratory pathways in preference to diaphragmatic pathways[63] but this seems unlikely.

In addition to these acute effects, alcohol may also have longer term effects that in some unknown way contribute to the development of OSA.[694,713] This might be through the recurrent acute provocation of snoring with permanent pharyngeal damage or through some unspecified CNS damage. Long-term alcohol may also be important in contributing to CO_2 retention in OSA.

3.1.3.2 *Sedatives*

Other sedatives have also been shown to worsen sleep apnoea, mainly the benzodiazepines[246,462] but also barbiturates. Again the mechanism is not clear but benzodiazepines do depress hypoxic drive considerably[387] as well as reducing general muscle tone via specific receptor sites in the CNS[561] whose occupation leads to increased activity of the gamma-aminobutyric acid (GABA) inhibitory pathways. In this way they mimic and further lower the reduced tone that occurs with non-REM sleep and even more so with REM sleep.

3.1.3.3 *Sleep deprivation*

Sleep deprivation itself may provoke worsening upper airway obstruction during sleep, again probably by promoting greater reductions in general muscle tone and blunting arousal.[260] Patients' spouses comment that snoring is worse when the patient is very tired although this has not been formally documented. Sleep deprivation has been shown to reduce activation of genioglossus during wakefulness but the mechanism is not clear.[405] Sleep deprivation also reduces the ventilatory response to CO_2,[740] but again the mechanism is not clear. Both these effects could promote obstructive events and prolong apnoeas.

3.1.3.4 *Nasal blockage*

Nasal patency has a role in OSA but just exactly how is not resolved. Most published series of patients with OSA report a high prevalence of nasal pathology.[498] There is often a long history of nasal stuffiness or previous nasal injury. Very occasionally relief of nasal blockage improves OSA.[290] If the nose is semi-blocked then increased inspiratory effort will be required to draw adequate air into the lungs at the expense of lower pharyngeal pressures. This will tend to collapse the pharynx as discussed in the section on anatomical abnormalities (p. 32). However, once collapse is complete, flow stops, the intraluminal subatmospheric pressure returns to zero, and the pharynx opens again (Fig. 3.15): flow restarts, subatmospheric pressures recur, and collapse again occurs. This is a Starling resistor but, if complete collapse can occur when there is no inspiratory flow attempted, then the upstream nasal resistance cannot be important: furthermore, if there is maintained collapse with no reopening and vibration during inspiratory attempts, then again upstream resistance can no longer be important.[639] This presupposes that the pharynx is a Starling resistor, but it is likely that there is hysteresis to the pressure–lumen size relationship, perhaps due to surface tension forces from the wet mucosal surfaces.[326] If the pharynx is not a Starling resistor then high nasal resistances could provoke collapse that then remains because of surface tension forces.

At a clinical level, improving nasal patency often helps snoring but rarely OSA, suggesting that once upper airway collapse problems have reached the severity of OSA then the pharynx stops behaving like a Starling resistor. Thus, the common history of nasal blockage may be important to the

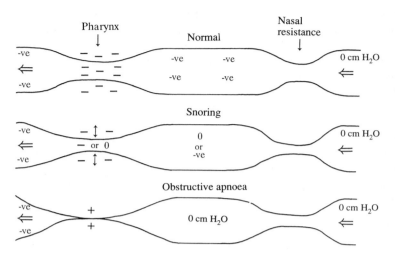

Fig. 3.15 Diagrammatic representation of pharyngeal collapse during snoring and obstructive sleep apnoea. The pressure drop across the nose during inspiration produces a negative collapsing pressure in the pharynx. If this narrows the pharynx enough then snoring occurs. If the pharynx closes off then flow stops, the intraluminal pressures rise back to atmospheric and the pharynx opens again. For complete and sustained collapse to occur requires overwhelming *external* compressive forces and in theory cannot just be due to a high upstream resistance in the nose.

generation of snoring in the years prior to the development of full OSA,[407] perhaps damaging the pharynx and making it more compliant, but once OSA has developed the high nasal resistance is no longer important. As will be discussed later, whether there is complete apnoea or only obstructive hypoventilation with snoring during a sleep study, may influence whether or not nasal surgery is worth trying.

3.2 Definitions

Having discussed the aetiology of OSA we can now consider how much upper airway collapse during sleep constitutes a problem and produces a clinical syndrome worth treating. This is far harder than one might imagine and such definitions are currently not possible. Originally it was observed that patients had repeated episodes of complete cessation of breathing (apnoeas) during sleep that led to recurrent arousal and sleep fragmentation.[215] At this very early stage no attempt was made to define

what was supposedly normal and what was not. Not long after, the group
at Stanford said that an episode of apnoea could only be such if it lasted 10 s
or more and disregarded the secondary events that actually led to symptoms
—arousal and perhaps hypoxaemia. Furthermore, based on a few studies on
young normal subjects, it was decided that a maximum of such events of five
per hour could be regarded as normal. This index of 'apnoeic activity' was
called the apnoea index (AI). The result of this arbitrary approach was to
create quasiscientific limits that made some normal people 'abnormal' and
some abnormal people 'normal'. For example, there is a range of upper
airway problems which do not cause 10 s apnoeas, but can lead to recurrent
arousals. In children particularly, apnoeas can be much less than 10 s and
provoke arousal.[135,542,670] Obstruction in the upper airway can produce
hypoventilation and hypoxaemia without actual apnoea at all, so-called
hypopnoeas.[238] This gave rise to the apnoea—hypopnoea index (AHI).
Finally, obstruction to the upper airway can lead to recurrent arousals
without apnoea, hypoventilation, or hypoxaemia.[264,297,662] This is because
the compensation for this added upper airway resistance is almost perfect,
but the extra inspiratory effort this takes provokes arousal.[224,225,763] This
recently recognized variant of 'sleep apnoea' is discussed later in Chapter 8.
In the opposite direction there are normal respiratory pauses of over 10 s
that do not lead to arousal or hypoxaemia and thus are unimportant. Some
sleep centres have therefore very sensibly changed to logging any
respiratory event that appears to lead to arousal.

The next problem is 'what is an arousal?' The original sleep analysis
technique for characterizing the *macro*-architecture of sleep divided sleep
into 30 s epochs and labelled each epoch according to the dominant
sleep stage present.[554] Because this process was done manually, greater
resolution than 30 s for routine work was impractical. This resulted in
arousals lasting less than 15 s being specifically filtered out. Often the
arousals following apnoeas or hypopnoeas *are* less than 15 s and would
therefore be passed over. Thus, a measure of arousals or sleep discontinuity,
is much more important than macro-sleep architecture. This then leads to the
problem of defining how long a transient event on the EEG or EMG
channels needs to last to be called an arousal. Figure 2.5 (see p. 10) shows
a very short 'arousal'. We do not have enough information to decide if many
such short arousals produce daytime sleepiness. It may not be the arousals
themselves that produce symptoms, but the consequent failure to establish
uninterrupted deeper stages of sleep for any length of time. What aspects of
sleep are required to make it restorative are simply not known, but
uninterrupted SWS is probably very important.[172,305,339] Again arbitrary
criteria have been drawn up to try and define an 'arousal' which has been
set at 3 s or more of EEG/EMG activity suggesting a return towards
wakefulness,[60] but in the absence of adequate data this precision seems

pointless. The best data available found that short arousals, defined as EEG changes for > 1.5 s with any transient increase in EMG, correlated the best with patients' reaction times measured during the day.[114]

The approach to this problem at present should be to ask the following question—'are there sufficient recurrent respiratory events (apnoeas, hypopnoeas, or just loud snoring) leading to detectable arousals that could explain the patient's symptoms and, thus, should lead to a trial of therapy?' At present this is a clinical decision based on soft facts and experience; arbitrary definitions add an undeserved air of precision.

Further uncertainties revolve around the importance of other consequences of OSA. For example, it is not clear whether the *degree* of hypoxaemia with each apnoea is particularly important. Figure 3.16 shows two oximeter tracings from patients with OSA. The patient with the smaller dips is actually more hypersomnolent. It is not known if daytime sleepiness correlates at all with degree of hypoxaemia, but it seems unlikely, once other factors have been allowed for. The depth of the hypoxaemia will of course influence the heart: values lower than 60 per cent S_{aO_2} raise substantially the likelihood of developing arrhythmias.[620]

Recently, attention has been paid to the haemodynamic effects of OSA. These will be discussed later, but negative pleural pressure swings present during the obstructive phase and the rises in blood pressure on arousal, may both have important consequences on health. At present, no good evidence exists to support this hypothesis.

Having been very nihilistic about current definitions of OSA, what approach should be used clinically to guide therapeutic decisions? Because *increased upper airway resistance* during sleep produces problems mainly through *sleep disruption*, these two factors should be monitored directly or indirectly. This will then allow the assessing clinician to decide if there is sufficient sleep disruption due to upper airway obstruction (complete or otherwise) to be commensurate with the patient's daytime symptoms. If there appears to be, then a trial of therapy (usually nasal continuous positive airway pressure therapy—NCPAP) should be instituted which will answer the question. In reality, the majority of sleep studies are either normal with no evidence of upper airway problems or clearly abnormal with recurrent sleep disruption from obstructive apnoeas and hypopnoeas throughout the night. There are however an increasing number of these 'middle ground' patients where rigid definitions are unhelpful.

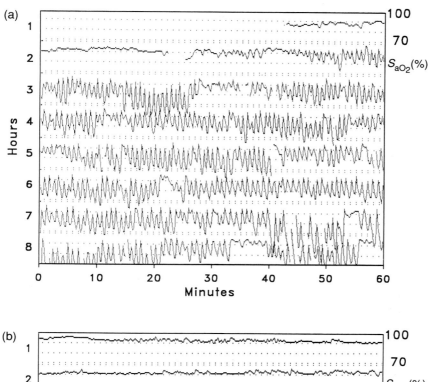

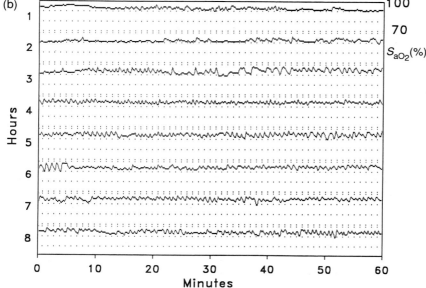

Fig. 3.16 Two overnight oximetry tracings. Each tracing shows eight sequential hours. Each line is on a scale of 70–100 per cent S_{aO_2}. The beginning of the night is top left and the end, bottom right. (a) A man with classical OSA showing very obvious >4 per cent dips in S_{aO_2}. (b) A similar patient with classical OSA but most of the S_{aO_2} dips are less than 4 per cent.

3.3 Short-term consequences of sleep apnoea

3.3.1 An apnoea

An apnoea or period of increased upper airway obstruction, usually commences as sleep develops from awake towards stage 2. In some patients they can obstruct whilst still in stage 1 and be capable of vague limb movements, whereas others need to go a little deeper to compromise the upper airway. This presumably depends on the severity of the factors provoking upper airway collapse. The patient will usually begin to fight the upper airway obstruction with increasing inspiratory efforts, each effort greater than the one before (Fig. 3.5). If the previous apnoea had been followed by a period of overshoot hyperventilation, the P_{aCO_2} will have been driven below the apnoea threshold.[142,158] This means that during the first part of the subsequent apnoea there may be a period of 'central' apnoea where no effort is being made. Once the P_{aCO_2} has climbed enough, then the inspiratory efforts will return against the blocked upper airway. This pattern of central followed by obstructive apnoea used to be called a mixed apnoea, but this category is essentially unhelpful as it is not really diagnostically or therapeutically different from the purely obstructive.

During the inspiratory efforts, intrathoracic pressures drop transiently to subatmospheric values unlikely to be achieved under any other circumstances. These repeated Müeller manoeuvres may be important (see the later section on blood pressure and pleural pressure swings, p. 51). Carbon dioxide levels rise and oxygen levels fall until the subject awakens, thus returning tone to the upper airway and restoring ventilation.

This cycle may be repeated hundreds of times with physiological consequences that are described in the following five sections (Fig. 3.17).

3.3.2 Hypoxaemia and hypercapnia

During an apnoea the time courses of the P_{aO_2} (or S_{aO_2}) and P_{aCO_2} changes are different. The CO_2 evolved from the returning venous blood rapidly raises the P_{aCO_2} in the trapped gas in the lungs to the mixed venous level (within 30 s) and thereafter the P_{aCO_2} rises very slowly (approximately 0.6 kPa/min) because of the large CO_2 stores available throughout the body. The fall in P_{aO_2} is faster and occurs approximately at a fixed rate that depends on the rate of oxygen usage by the body and lung volume at the beginning of the apnoea: a doubling of lung volume would halve the rate of fall which in a normal person, apnoeic at functional residual capacity (FRC), would be approximately 8 kPa per min.[190] During an apnoea the ventilatory drive may rise enough to recruit expiratory muscles. This can produce significant expiratory puffs (because expiration is not obstructed)

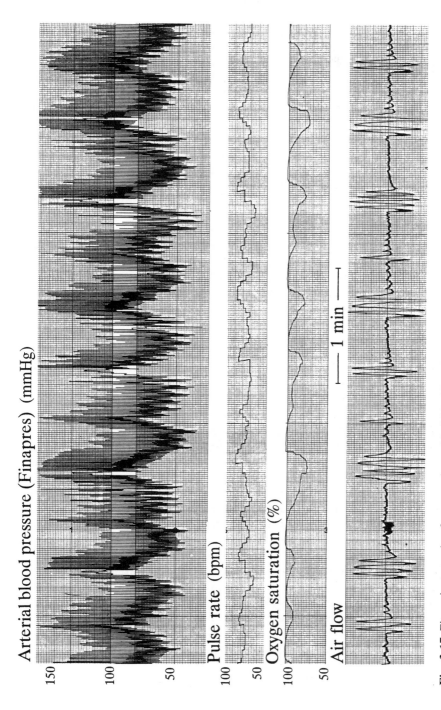

Fig. 3.17 Five minute tracing from a patient with OSA. Note the rises in blood pressure and heart rate with the cessation of each apnoea. During the apnoea each frustrated inspiratory effort is accompanied by a fall in blood pressure (pulsus paradoxus).

that ratchet down the lung volume below FRC (because inspiration remains obstructed), thus reducing the O_2 stores and increasing the rate of fall of P_{aO_2}. Because the fall in P_{aO_2} is approximately linear, the fall in S_{aO_2} looks like the top end of a haemoglobin dissociation curve.

The actual lowest P_{aO_2} or S_{aO_2} value reached thus depends on five main factors: the length of the apnoea, the oxygen consumption rate (higher in the obese), the starting lung volume (lower in the obese), whether expiration is recruited, and, of course, the starting P_{aO_2} or S_{aO_2} at which the apnoea commenced.[72,190] Thus, the actual S_{aO_2} nadir reached in any particular apnoea will vary enormously and not just depend on apnoea length.

The results of this hypoxaemia and hypercapnia are not entirely clear. Because they are transient, with recuperation in between, it is unlikely that any tissues are significantly compromised. For example, even though S_{aO_2} values down to 60 per cent are common, erythropoietic secretion is not augmented,[228] and right ventricular hypertrophy rarely occurs unless daytime hypoxaemia is also present as well.[74] It is possible, though, that the asphyxia leads to increased catecholamine production[120,202,640] and provokes arrhythmias, particularly if the S_{aO_2} falls to less than 60 per cent in patients with pre-existing coronary artery disease.[620]

3.3.3 Sleep disruption

The apparent degree of sleep disruption provoked by sleep apnoea can vary enormously between individuals. From a behavioural point of view the arousal can vary from barely any body movement to violent thrashing around. The EEG change during the arousal can be a very brief rise out of SWS into stage 1 or wakefulness for perhaps only 5 s followed by rapid return to SWS or be a return to full wakefulness for 20 s or so. The effect this has on the overall gross sleep architecture is also very variable (see Fig. 2.4, p. 9). There may be predominantly stage 1 and 2 demonstrating that the patient rarely managed to have more than 10 s or so of SWS at a time or it may show normal amounts of SWS because the arousals were so short and the return to SWS so quick. Thus, almost any pattern of classical sleep architecture is compatible with OSA.

There is no doubt in experimental subjects that increasing the number of arousals and their 'size' reduces daytime performance progressively. For example, arousing individuals every 2 min leads to decreased vigilance the following day. However, if the arousal produced required a verbal response to a question, this impaired vigilance was far more than if only EEG evidence of arousal was produced.[61] At present there is no validated way of measuring sleep disturbance that consistently correlates at all well with daytime performance. Sophisticated computer analysis of EEG holds out the best hope of actually measuring sleep discontinuity rather than simply counting events that cross an arbitrary threshold.

The way in which this sleep disruption affects daytime performance is discussed in the section on daytime sleepiness (p. 65) and how it can be measured in the section on measuring daytime sleepiness (p. 68) in Chapter 4.

The causes of the arousal that actually terminate the apnoeic or hypopnoeic event are not known for certain, but are almost certainly multifactorial. Giving added oxygen to lessen the fall in S_{aO_2} with each apnoea does lengthen them slightly, but this is not impressive and, thus, hypoxaemia cannot be the main arousal mechanism.[224,225,763] However, removing the carotid bodies grossly reduces the arousal response to hypoxaemia in dogs.[69] Since the patient with OSA will wake up at the end of the apnoea, even if fully oxygenated, something must be responsible for the arousal and the CO_2 level seems to be most likely. As mentioned in the previous section, P_{aCO_2} will rise rapidly over the first 20–30 s and much more slowly thereafter.

Recent work has suggested that it is not actually the blood gas tensions that arouse, but more the respiratory effort that is made in response to them. Gleeson et al.[225] showed in normal subjects that arousal to three respiratory loads (hypoxia, hypercapnia, and inspiratory resistance) occurred when the falls in pleural pressure reached were about the same. Although this arousal threshold was consistent within a subject, different subjects had different pleural pressure arousal thresholds (Fig. 3.18). This means that arousal could certainly occur in response to heavy snoring, when pleural pressures can fall to as low as -80 cm H_2O[426] without there necessarily being any accompanying deterioration in gas exchange, a phenomenon discussed further in Chapter 8. Further work from this group,[224] comparing hypercapnia and the ventilatory stimulant adenosine, has confirmed that it is the actual effort that seems to cause arousal rather than any particular level of P_{aO_2} or P_{aCO_2}. In tracheotomized dogs it has been shown that the addition of an added respiratory load during progressive hypoxia provokes earlier arousal at a higher S_{aO_2}, that cannot be explained by the slightly higher levels of P_{aCO_2}.[763] This is probably due to pleural receptors, rather than pharyngeal, since the upper airway was bypassed.

3.3.4 Pulse rate

Except in patients with autonomic neuropathy, the pulse rate tends to fall during an apnoea and rise during the ventilatory and arousal phase (Fig. 3.17). The physiologic factors contributing to this are probably several. Any cause of arousal will increase heart rate because heart rate falls with sleep. This is likely to be a change in sympathetic–parasympathetic

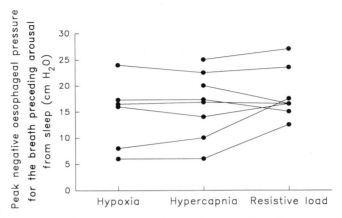

Fig. 3.18 This experiment measured the respiratory effort (from an oesophageal balloon) present on arousing in response to progressive hypoxia, hypercapnia, and an added resistance in normal subjects. Note that, on the whole, each subject woke at a similar respiratory effort, regardless of the stimulus. Redrawn with permission from Gleeson *et al.* (1990).[225]

balance with an increase in sympathetic outflows on arousal and wakefulness. Thus, on return to sleep following an apnoea-generated arousal, one would expect to see the pulse fall again. However, in some patients the fall in pulse rate with the apnoea can be profound, occasionally with cardiac standstill for a few seconds. This is clearly more than just the usual fall in pulse rate with sleep and is probably due to activation of the diving reflex.[24] Hypoxia, in the absence of pulmonary inflation, leads to bradycardia and vasoconstriction especially if accompanied by trigeminal nerve stimulation. This is mediated via the carotid body and the strength of the reflex correlates with hypoxic sensitivity.[446] Thus, a diving mammal, holding its breath underwater and experiencing hypoxia, will convert itself into a heart–brain preparation.[19] The vasoconstriction saves most of the cardiac output for the brain and the bradycardia prevents hypertension. During an obstructive apnoea there is hypoxaemia and little pulmonary inflation, hence this reflex may be activated. In addition, pharyngeal stimulation may enhance this reflex[21] in the same way as stimulation of the face does. In a small number of patients with OSA Zwillich *et al.*[768] showed that the bradycardia correlated with the severity of hypoxaemia and apnoea length, was lessened by alleviating the hypoxaemia with added oxygen, and could be mimicked with breath-holding in normal subjects. Hedner *et al.*[288] have shown increasing sympathetic tone to muscular arterioles during the apnoeas which disappears on arousal and resumption of breathing. The recruitment of this reflex during apnoea is clearly very variable with some patients not reducing their heart rate oscillations following added oxygen at all.[13] This may depend on the previously mentioned dependence of this reflex on hypoxic chemosensitivity.[446] There is also preliminary evidence that patients with OSA may have an enhanced diving reflex, perhaps through recurrent 'use' of it (P. Parchi, personal communication).[21,756]

Thus, the heart rate oscillations seen in OSA represent a swing between vagal slowing during the apnoeas and sleep, to sympathetic acceleration during breathing and wakefulness.

3.3.5 Blood pressure and pleural pressure swings

Figure 3.17 shows the changes in blood pressure that occur with OSA. As with pulse rate, there is a fall in BP with sleep onset and during the beginning of the apnoea, with a rise at arousal and apnoea termination. Superimposed on this are the respiratory swings in BP. Because the heart is in the thorax it is subjected to the swings in pleural pressure of breathing. If pleural pressure falls 20 mmHg then intrathoracic aortic pressure falls 20 mmHg and, because the aorta is simply a column of fluid, peripheral arterial pressure will fall 20 mmHg unless compensation reflexes come into play. Thus, pulsus paradox from a respiratory cause (not cardiac tamponade) is an indirect reflection of respiratory effort. Indeed, there exists a fairly close relation between the size of swings in pleural pressure and the swings in systolic blood pressure (SBP).[404] This effect on blood pressure and cardiac output can be indirectly measured from heart rate-related caudal and cephalic body movements (ballistocardiogram), so that changes in respiratory effort can also be detected using this method.[538]

The mean blood pressure across the course of an apnoea thus depends on the underlying trend and the size of each of the inspiratory dips. Following arousal and the resumption of ventilation, the SBP rises abruptly over a 20−30 s period. The cause of this rise in BP was initially thought to be a response to the hypoxaemia since the degree of rise correlated with the extent of S_{aO_2} fall.[619] However, later work has shown the rise to be independent of hypoxaemia and more dependent on apnoea length.[13,571] The apparent correlation with hypoxaemia was probably due to longer apnoeas causing more oxygen desaturation. Three groups have now shown that rises in SBP occur with arousal alone and are of similar magnitude to those seen in most patients with OSA.[12,146,571,624] Furthermore, the height of the SBP rise depends on the 'size' of the arousal.[146] Arousals in excess of 10 s produce rises in SBP similar to that seen in OSA and even 'arousals' that are hardly recognizable on EEG produce some SBP rise. The dependence of the SBP on degree of arousal may explain the correlation with apnoea length[13] since a long apnoea may imply a greater 'sleep pressure'

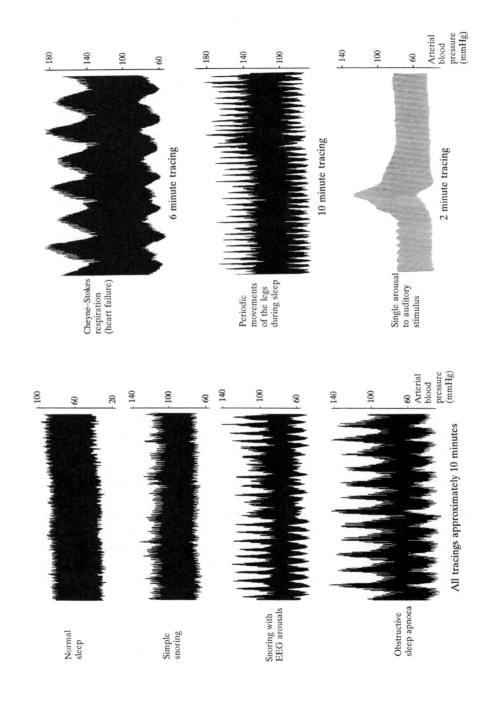

Normal sleep

Simple snoring

Snoring with EEG arousals

Obstructive sleep apnoea

All tracings approximately 10 minutes

Cheyne–Stokes respiration (heart failure)

6 minute tracing

Periodic movements of the legs during sleep

10 minute tracing

Single arousal to auditory stimulus

2 minute tracing

Arterial blood pressure (mmHg)

and would require a larger arousing stimulus to end it.[553] There is also indirect evidence that the usual falls in BP with sleep are more due to the absence of activity rather than sleep and the circadian rhythm *per se*.[119] Figure 3.19 shows some examples of BP rises associated with arousals in both respiratory and non-respiratory situations. There is some evidence that although the cortical response to arousing stimuli may habituate, the autonomic responses (BP rise, pulse rate rise, and skin blood flow changes) may not.[172,335]

The immediate consequences of these SBP rises are not known but the possible long-term results are discussed later (see the section on systemic circulation, p. 57).

The pleural pressure swings that occur with the inspiratory efforts may have profound effects on cardiovascular function. During the falls in pleural pressure the aortic pressure falls and therefore, unless vascular resistance also falls, left ventricular emptying must also be reduced: less head of pressure to a fixed resistance means less flow. Cardiac dilatation during OSA has been demonstrated with cinefluoroscopy and echocardiography,[261,426] but the reliability of such techniques to measure chamber dimensions accurately during the strong repetitive inspiratory efforts is questionable. There is some evidence that some of the cardiac dilatation is actually right-sided, perhaps due to increased venous return provoked by the repeated inspiratory efforts, the so-called 'respiratory pump'. It is far from clear if venous return really does significantly increase in OSA.[390] The original work on venous return suggested that below a certain pleural pressure the veins entering the chest would collapse at the point of entry and limit further 'aspiration' of blood into the chest.[270] This 'pinching off' of the great veins can be demonstrated radiographically[214] and by ultrasound.[483] At what negative intrathoracic pressure the entering veins do collapse depends on the actual starting venous pressure.[483] Thus, a high venous pressure will to some extent protect against collapse and allow the 'aspiration' effect to work down to lower pressures. The echocardiographic work suggests that the right ventricle does enlarge during the course of the apnoea and may even embarrass left ventricular function through interventricular shift.[261] This would tend to reduce cardiac output even further during the apnoea. If there was a build up of blood in the heart during the obstructive apnoea then this would be available at the cessation of apnoea which, together with the tachycardia, would contribute to the post-apnoeic BP rise. However, as mentioned earlier, arousal is likely to be the major cause of post-apnoeic BP

Fig. 3.19 Examples of beat to beat blood pressure trends (top of the trace is systolic and the bottom is diastolic) in normal sleep and various abnormal situations. Refer to the text for explanations.

rises, such as have been demonstrated in a patient with central apnoeas (no inspiratory efforts) and a fixed heart rate due to a pacemaker.[144]

Although these acute changes in myocardial loading and function do occur, there is only a small amount of evidence that any direct long-term consequences result and this is discussed later (see the section on systemic circulation, p. 57).

3.3.6 Hormonal changes

Because sleep is so disrupted it would not be surprising if the secretion of hormones that have a diurnal or circadian pattern was altered by OSA. Several endocrine systems have been looked at with the largest differences occurring in the secretion of growth hormone, testosterone, catecholamines, and possibly atrial natriuretic peptide and insulin.

Growth hormone release has been linked to sleep onset and possibly SWS, for some time.[66,343,616] Particularly in prepubertal children, growth hormone is strongly related to early sleep when SWS is greatest.[193] In children with OSA, growth is stunted and recovers when the OSA is treated.[39,590,670] In adults with OSA there is a depression of insulin-like growth factor I (somatomedin, released from the liver in response to growth hormone) which tends to recover after CPAP therapy[242] (Fig. 3.20). Low growth hormone levels in adults were originally not thought to be a problem. Recently, the importance of growth hormone to the balance between fat and lean mass in the body has been established.[588] It seems that lack of growth hormone produces a shift to more body fat and less muscle and can be corrected by returning growth hormone levels to normal.[588] This has led to the intriguing suggestion that not only does obesity cause OSA, but that OSA might provoke obesity.[383] This would be compatible with clinical experience that patients with OSA often put on much more weight *after* the onset of OSA symptoms; however, there are other explanations for this phenomenon that are discussed in the section on simple approaches to the treatment of OSA in Chapter 7 (p. 118).

Testosterone levels have been known, for many years, to be suppressed by the hypoxaemia of chronic lung disease[612] and this is also true of patients with OSA.[242,600] Whether this is due to the hypoxaemia or sleep disruption is not clear. Following treatment with nasal CPAP or an effective uvulopalatopharyngoplasty (UPPP), there is an improvement in plasma testosterone.[242,600] This is also clinically relevant since impotence is one of the recognized symptoms of OSA which usually improves on nasal CPAP.

There is conflicting evidence about other hormones and the effect of OSA. There is probably no change in luteinizing hormone (LH), follicle stimulating hormone (FSH), prolactin, and thyroxine levels[242] although not all studies agree.[463] Overnight catecholamine secretion is raised by

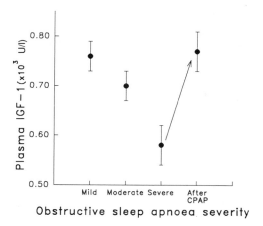

Fig. 3.20 Plasma insulin-like growth factor 1 (old name, somatomedin) levels in normal subjects and patients with obstructive sleep apnoea. Note the rise in the levels of this substance, induced by growth hormone, following nasal continuous positive airway pressure therapy. Data from Grunstein *et al.* (1989).[242]

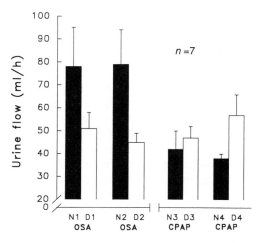

Fig. 3.21 Effect of sleep apnoea (OSA) and its treatment on nighttime (black bars) and daytime (open bars) urine production. When OSA is present during the night (nights 1 and 2, N1 and N2) the urine production is much higher than when the OSA is treated with nasal continuous positive airway pressure (CPAP) on nights 3 and 4 (N3 and N4). Redrawn with permission from Warley and Stradling (1988).[725]

OSA.[120,202,697] Cortisol secretion may be affected: a *decrease* overnight in patients with OSA has been found by some.[242,331,353,469]

Fluid balance-related hormones have been investigated because of the nocturnal polyuria seen in patients with OSA[369,725] (Fig. 3.21), as well as the suggestion that they may be more prone to hypertension. Because of the negative intrathoracic pressure generated by the obstructive episodes it was thought possible that right atrial distension might lead to the release of atrial natriuretic peptide (ANP). There is some evidence for this and most (but not all) groups have found a rise in ANP during OSA or a fall on CPAP therapy.[36,368,370,372,577,727] The effects of CPAP are complicated though, because positive pressure breathing alone can reduce ANP production and lower sodium excretion in normal subjects.[117]

Finally, there is one report of renin production rising after CPAP therapy for OSA.[177] This might account for the reduction of polyuria on CPAP but the mechanism of the altered renin production is not apparent although it might be due to right atrial distension and reduced sympathetic outflow to the kidney.

3.4 Longer term consequences

3.4.1 *Respiratory failure and cor pulmonale*

It is noticeable how many patients with severe OSA and nocturnal hypoxaemia, apparently for many years, have normal daytime P_{aO_2} and P_{aCO_2} values and no evidence of cor pulmonale. However, there are a few patients who do get diurnal respiratory failure, evidence of cor pulmonale with pulmonary hypertension, and polycythaemia. It seems that patients who have OSA alone only rarely get ventilatory failure and the consequences of long-term hypoxia. Another factor, in addition to the OSA, seems to be necessary and this is usually lower airways obstruction.[25] Three series have now shown that associated chronic airways obstruction (CAWO) is the factor that pushes patients with OSA into diurnal ventilatory failure,[74,75,203,373,731] sometimes with a degree of airway obstruction that would not normally be associated with CO_2 retention. This also leads to the converse; that a patient with mild to moderate CAWO, who has unexpected CO_2 retention, should be investigated for possible sleep apnoea. If the two conditions co-exist then clearly both need treating to maximally improve the ventilatory failure.

The mechanism of interaction of OSA and CAWO is not clear, but it has been suggested that the presence of lower airways obstruction prevents full recovery of the blood gases after each apnoeic episode. Normally there is even an overshoot of P_{aO_2} and P_{aCO_2} values because of the vigorous hyperpnoea following apnoea. Thus, increased lower airways resistance could limit this and provoke gradual tolerance of diurnal hypercapnia and hypoxaemia over time. In addition, the severity of the CAWO influences the severity of the nocturnal hypoxaemia,[500] but this is probably through its effect on ventilation perfusion mismatch and daytime P_{aO_2}.

Two other factors that may provoke ventilatory failure in association with OSA are massive obesity and neuromuscular weakness. The mechanism here may be similar to CAWO in that full compensatory hyperventilation between the apnoeas may not be possible.

The practical consequences of this are two-fold. First, if there is some degree of CAWO in a patient suspected of having OSA then it is worth checking the P_{aCO_2} level since if it is raised one would add this to symptoms as a reason for treatment. Second, if a patient with OSA has CO_2 retention, it is worth looking for another cause which will usually be CAWO, but may be due to a neuromuscular problem or particularly gross obesity (perhaps in excess of 150 kg, but there is no evidence for this).

3.4.2 Cardiovascular complications

3.4.2.1 Pulmonary circulation

There is clear evidence that OSA provokes periodic rises in absolute pulmonary artery pressure (PAP) and transmural pulmonary artery pressure (Fig. 3.22). The recurrent subatmospheric pressure swings of OSA make measurements of PAP relative to atmospheric pressure difficult to interpret. There is a progressive rise in transmural PAP during an apnoea, probably due to increasing hypoxaemia and pulmonary vasoconstriction[440] but this may also be due to some increase in venous return (see the section on blood pressure and pleural pressure swings, p. 51). There is no good evidence that this effect on PAP is harmful or that it persists beyond the apnoeas. The situation is probably the same as discussed above for the other features of cor pulmonale and diurnal ventilatory failure; that associated CAWO is necessary to lead to sustained pulmonary hypertension.[373]

3.4.2.2 Systemic circulation

In the section on blood pressure and pleural pressure swings (p. 51) we discussed the acute affects of OSA on systemic blood pressure. However, it is not known if OSA affects the cardiovascular system in any other way. Some evidence exists that there is an increased likelihood of a cardiovascular death in patients with OSA,[234,282,513,515,703] but unfortunately there are no proper matched-control studies looking at mortality in a treated and untreated group of patients with OSA. It is unlikely that this could ever be done since treatment cannot now be withheld because it is so effective for symptoms and is readily available. The data that have been collected are

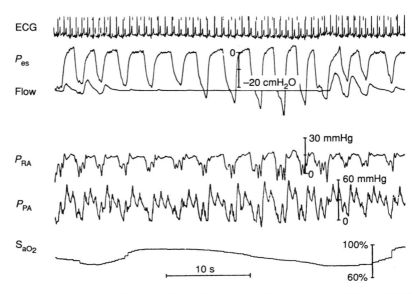

Fig. 3.22 Tracing showing the effect of an obstructive apnoea on right atrial (P_{RA}) and pulmonary artery (P_{PA}) pressure. As the apnoea progresses with increasing respiratory effort (increasing swings in oesophageal pressure P_{es}) these are of course reflected in pulmonary artery pressures measured relative to atmospheric. These swings virtually obscure the small average rise in pulmonary artery pressure towards the end of the apnoea, measured when there is no respiratory effort during expiration. With permission from Podszus *et al.* (1991).[535]

retrospective and depend on poorly or untreated control groups which are not similar to the treated group for a variety of reasons. For example, Partinen *et al.*[515] contacted 198 patients with OSA up to five years post-diagnosis. Tracheostomy had been performed on 71 with complete cure. In the other 127 weight loss had been recommended and/or they had refused tracheostomy. Despite this lack of randomization the tracheostomy group were on the whole more severe than the weight loss group, but had similar levels of pre-morbid cardiovascular disease (including hypertension). Over the five years there were no deaths in the tracheostomy group and 14 in the other group. Eight of these deaths were cardiovascular. This suggested that OSA led to cardiovascular deaths although the problems of unmatched groups has to be remembered. A second publication on the same patients two years later[513] confirmed that at seven years follow up there was still a significant excess cardiovascular mortality in the untreated OSA patients (Fig. 3.23).

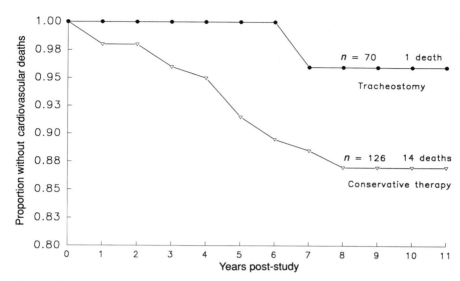

Fig. 3.23 Long-term survival without a cardiovascular death of patients with sleep apnoea. The two groups are defined according to whether tracheostomy was accepted or refused by the patient. Patients not receiving tracheostomy had no specific therapy. Redrawn with permission from Partinen and Guilleminault (1990).[514]

He *et al.*[282] traced 385 male OSA patients (out of 706) up to nine years post-diagnosis and assessed predictors of mortality (Fig. 3.24). Increasing apnoea severity in the untreated patients increased the likelihood of death and treatment with either nasal CPAP or tracheostomy prevented this excess mortality. Patients who had uvulopalatopharyngoplasty (UPPP) as a treatment fared no better than untreated patients (see Fig. 7.9, p. 138) and considerably worse than those receiving nasal CPAP where there were no deaths. Again the problem of non-randomization exists here; patients who refuse treatment are probably different from those who accept. However, the UPPP group are in a sense a placebo-treated group and their failure to derive the same benefits as CPAP-treated patients is fairly convincing.

In a much smaller study of 91 OSA patients, Gonzalez-Rothi *et al.*[234] were not able to show a significantly increased mortality in the 24 untreated OSA patients compared to 35 poorly matched non-OSA controls (who had an unexpectedly high mortality). In a group of OSA patients followed for six and a half years Thorpy and Ledereich[703] found a survival of 85 per cent, lower than would have been expected. Full details of this study are not available.

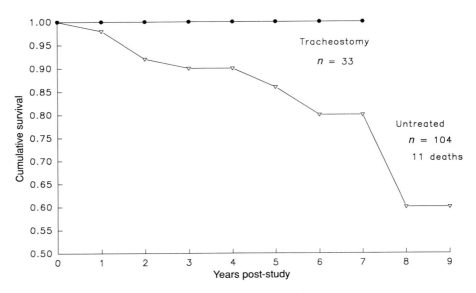

Fig. 3.24 Long-term survival of patients with sleep apnoea depending on whether a tracheostomy was performed or not. Redrawn with permission from He *et al.* (1988).[282]

Taken together it is likely that OSA leads to excess cardiovascular deaths although in the absence of a control group matched for all the other known risk factors (for example, upper body obesity, insulin resistance, cholesterolaemia, and smoking) some doubt must remain.

If there is a link between OSA and cardiovascular death, what might it be? Several suggestions have been made such as sustained hypertension,[249] increased adrenergic activity,[288,289] increased lipids,[205] hypoxaemia and cardiac arrhythmias,[248] and perhaps left ventricular hypertrophy.[535,706]

The evidence for obstructive apnoea leading to diurnal systemic hypertension is poor. Early reports found a high prevalence of hypertension in OSA patients[265] in the region of 30–50 per cent. This was thought to be due to OSA being a stressful condition leading to catecholamine release[120,202,229] and raised sympathetic tone[288,289] with eventual resetting of baroreceptors. In other conditions of increased catecholamine release there can be sustained hypertension.[229,502] It was reasonable to suggest that the hypoxaemia might lead to this catecholamine release[33,640] or that perhaps it was just a result of recurrent arousals.

Most patients with OSA are overweight, in most clinics the mean obesity index (kg/m^2) is more than 30, which is about 30 per cent overweight. Once this confounding variable is taken into account there seems little evidence that OSA provokes hypertension in its own right. It is also important to control for upper body obesity[244,660] since it is this distribution that predisposes to cardiovascular mortality[52,393,730,734] and it is neck obesity that provokes OSA rather than general obesity[143,348] and neck obesity is likely to be a 'marker' of upper body obesity. Hoffstein et al.[300] looking at 372 snorers (some of whom had OSA) found that, compared to obesity and age, the degree of OSA contributed virtually nothing to explaining the level of the systolic BP. Similar results were obtained by Rauscher et al.[552] Escourrou et al.[181] could also find no association between the severity of OSA and the blood pressure in 50 patients with OSA. In 206 adult patients with OSA, Millman et al.[474] could not show that OSA severity affected blood pressure, once age and obesity had been controlled for, except in a small subset of very obese young subjects. In the elderly the presence of higher values of the apnoea—hypopnoea index (AHI) was not associated with increased blood pressure.[360]

More recently Davies et al.[151] compared patients with OSA to control subjects carefully matched for obesity, age, sex, smoking, and alcohol consumption. The daytime blood pressures were assessed with an ambulatory system. There was absolutely no difference in the daytime blood pressures between the two groups (Fig. 3.25).

It has also been stated from uncontrolled studies that the blood pressure falls when CPAP is commenced.[351,453] However, this is probably due to the well recognized regression to the mean of abnormal values on second measurement because when an untreated group has been included there is no evidence for this effect.[550]

Other work cited as evidence for a link between sleep apnoea and hypertension has found an increased prevalence of sleep apnoea in patients originally diagnosed as hypertensive. This early work did not have proper controls or drug-free subjects and did not find particularly severe degrees of OSA.[199,340,400,655,754] Some of the hypertensive drugs can provoke apnoeic episodes, for example, alkalinizing diuretics,[681] beta blockers,[68] and α-methyl dopa.[385] In addition, minor degrees of heart failure can provoke periodic respiration and apnoeas.[274] Two subsequent controlled studies on drug-free individuals have failed to confirm any increased prevalence of sleep apnoea in hypertensive patients.[298,724] Hirshkowitz et al.[298] studied 175 hypertensive men and 110 normotensive men during sleep and found no difference between these groups except that a *treated* subset of the hypertensive men did have slightly higher apnoea indices.

It might be expected to find higher rates of central apnoeic events in hypertensive subjects since these patients, as a group, are found to have increased ventilatory responses to hypoxaemia via the carotid body.[548,714] This increased hypoxic sensitivity and carotid body activity might be expected to provoke periodic ventilation such as occurs at altitude.[558]

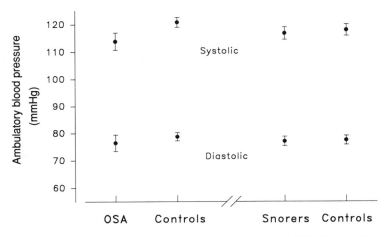

Fig. 3.25 Daytime *ambulatory* blood pressures (means and SEMs) in patients with obstructive sleep apnoea (OSA), snorers, and carefully matched control subjects (for age, sex, weight, alcohol, and cigarette consumption).

There is also some epidemiological evidence linking snoring with hypertension,[425] strokes,[366,509,516,644] myocardial infarction,[699] and angina.[365] Because snoring is assumed to be an epidemiological marker of OSA, these associations have been taken as evidence for an association between OSA and cardiovascular events. Unfortunately snoring is a particularly 'dirty' symptom in that it correlates with many other things such as obesity (in particular upper body obesity[57,244,661]), smoking, alcohol usage, and hypnotics,[57] as well as several other diseases.[496] In the studies mentioned above these confounding variables have not been adequately factored out. Two more recent studies have not found an association between snoring and hypertension.[607,660]

There are limited data on other cardiovascular risk factors such as insulin, cholesterol, and triglycerides. However, the available data suggest that when really carefully matched controls are used then there is no difference in patients with OSA.[150]

If it is correct that OSA leads to increased cardiovascular mortality, but not to sustained diurnal hypertension or other known risk factors, then what is the cause of the deaths? It is unproven, but it seems possible that the nocturnal hypertensive surges discussed in the section on blood pressure and pleural pressure swings (p. 51) are the culprit. Figure 3.17 showed an example of the surges with each apnoea cessation, sometimes increasing systolic BP by up to 100 mmHg, often more than 400 times a night. The average effect of this on nocturnal BP is shown in Figs 3.26 and 3.27.

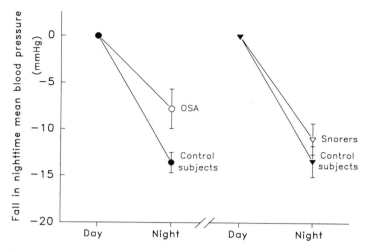

Fig. 3.26 Change in *ambulatory* mean blood pressure between the all day and all night values in patients with obstructive sleep apnoea (OSA), snorers, and carefully matched control subjects (means and SEMs). Note that patients with OSA have smaller falls.

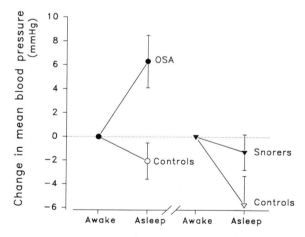

Fig. 3.27 Change in *beat to beat* mean blood pressure between quiet wakefulness (just prior to sleep) and a subsequent sleep period in patients with obstructive sleep apnoea (OSA), snorers, and matched control subjects (means and SEMs). Note that patients with OSA experience a rise in mean blood pressure whereas all the other groups have a fall.

These data come from 19 OSA patients and 19 carefully matched control subjects.[147] The blood pressure was measured with the Finapres device (see the section on blood pressure in Chapter 6, p. 100) that records beat to beat BP non-invasively. On average normal subjects experience a fall in BP with sleep onset of approximately 2 mmHg, whereas the OSA patients have on average a rise of 6 mmHg; one subject had an average rise in his sleeping BP of 20 mmHg. It can be crudely estimated that this extra 8 mmHg rise at night, if equivalent to about a third as large a rise spread over 24 h, might produce an excess cardiovascular mortality which could explain roughly half of the excess mortality observed in the OSA survival studies mentioned at the beginning of this section (see Figs 3.23 and 3.24, pp. 59 and 60). Although this is a very crude calculation, it shows that the nocturnal rises in BP are of the right order to explain the excess mortality even if they were not pulsatile, which is likely to be much more harmful to blood vessels (haemorrhagic strokes, aortic dissection, and atheroma generation) than a steady rise.

An additional factor may be the frustrated inspiratory efforts during OSA that increase left ventricular afterload and would also encourage left ventricular hypertrophy (see the section on blood pressure and pleural pressure swings, p. 51). It has been shown in one study that patients with OSA have abnormally hypertrophied left ventricles, and this is true even in a subgroup who do not have diurnal hypertension,[287] although we have not found this when carefully matched control subjects have also been studied. Other studies have shown that left ventricular hypertrophy correlates better with nocturnal BP than daytime values.[711]

Thus, there are a variety of candidates for the pathological events in OSA that could increase cardiovascular mortality, but correct apportionment is not yet possible.

4 Clinical presentation of obstructive sleep apnoea

Without doubt the dominant symptom of OSA is daytime hypersomnolence. This symptom is often not recognized by patients and their doctors as a specific problem with a differential diagnosis. Too often it is dismissed as the consequence of getting older, not going to bed for long enough, laziness, malingering, etc. The second most important symptom is snoring. If OSA is not known about, neither patient nor doctor will link the two symptoms and ask the relevant questions. Although both symptoms are common, careful questioning does allow the preliminary filtering out of patients with a high probability of having OSA. Table 4.1 shows most of symptoms in OSA ranked according to frequency in our sleep clinic.

4.1 Daytime sleepiness

In the early days of studies on sleep apnoea it was thought that hypoxaemia might play a part in the excessive daytime sleepiness, perhaps more so than the recurrent sleep disruption.[504] However, with better analyses of EEG and appropriate statistical techniques it has been shown that daytime symptoms correlate with sleep disruption and not indices of hypoxaemia.[579]

The daytime sleepiness of OSA is no different to that which we would all experience if denied adequate sleep. We have all experienced the problem of staying awake during boring lectures after a night on the tiles, but come the following evening's entertainment the sleepiness can disappear. This is of course because sleepiness can be overcome if the drive to do so is adequate. A patient developing OSA will initially experience sleepiness only when particularly understimulated at times of normally diminished vigilance, for example, during meetings after lunch. Progressively the sleepiness will impinge on more and more activities such as reading, watching television, as a passenger in a car, sitting on the toilet, in the bath, on the train, etc. Finally there will be difficulty staying awake even during very important activities such as driving and operating machinery. It is important to differentiate between sleepiness and other descriptions of 'fatigue' such as tiredness, lethargy, malaise, and exhaustion. They are often used interchangeably but are not the same. Sleepiness describes the urge to sleep, not just the urge to sit in a chair and do nothing. One can do a hard day's work

Table 4.1 Symptoms of obstructive sleep apnoea

Most common (>60%)	Less common (10–60%)	Rare (<10%)
Loud snoring	Choking or shortness of breath sensations at night	Enuresis
Excessive daytime sleepiness	Reduced libido	Recurrent arousals/insomnia
Restless sleep	Nocturnal sweating	Nocturnal cough
Unrefreshing sleep	Morning headaches	Symptomatic oesophageal reflux
Nocturia		
Apparent personality changes		
Witnessed apnoeas		

and be tired in the evening without necessarily wanting to go to sleep. On the other hand, one can be short of sleep and know that if things are interesting enough the desire will disappear. If the difference between tiredness and sleepiness is explained to a patient then he will usually confidently choose one or the other as best describing his problem. Overwhelming tiredness (without real sleepiness) is rarely a symptom of OSA and is seen more in other debilitating conditions, for example, myalgic encephalitis or ME syndrome.

The sleepiness of OSA is often seen as disinterest and lack of motivation (which in a sense it is) or just laziness. This leads to immense problems at work with promotion prospects diminished or loss of job. At home the spouse becomes disenchanted by the change in her husband's behaviour and his lack of enthusiasm for evening and weekend entertainment. Coupled with a deteriorating temper, failure at work and failure at home, this provides a recipe for marital disharmony.

Another problem is that the sleepiness may have been progressive over many years and may not be seen by the patient as abnormal or be put down simply to age. It is only following treatment that he will realize just how sleepy he was. This denial may unfortunately make the patient unwilling to seek help or accept treatment. Direct questioning such as 'are you ever sleepy during the day?' will not reveal sleepiness under these circumstances, but 'situational' questions such as 'do you fall asleep reading or watching television?' may do. Useful scales of sleepiness based on such questions are described in the following section.

Of particular concern to others who may be driving in the opposite direction, is sleepiness whilst driving. It is difficult sometimes to get patients to admit or discuss this problem for fear of being told to stop driving. One often hears that 'driving is the only time I don't get sleepy', a statement that the wife usually disagrees with. There is now abundant evidence that OSA leads to increased driving accidents.[9,187-189,191,192,217,234,277,647,654,762] These are usually single driver accidents (where the car has gone off the road for no apparent reason) or low speed shunting accidents. Hermann Peter, from the Marburg Sleep Unit, tells the story of a German business man with OSA who never had car accidents in Germany driving his Porsche at high speed. However, whenever he drove in the United States at the legal 50 mph he had great trouble staying awake and had several accidents. Driving a Porsche at over 100 mph kept him awake. On average, patients with OSA seem about five to ten times more likely to have driving accidents.[191,217,234,279] Finding out what proportion of car accidents is due to sleepiness and then what proportion of the sleepiness is due to OSA, will be very difficult but such studies are under way.

There are other, less common, secondary effects of excessive daytime sleepiness. For example, automatic behaviour can occur which is where boring tasks are performed in an automatic fashion with little recall afterwards. During these automatic activities the ability to react quickly and appropriately is much diminished. There is also a failure to register properly what is being said by someone else, thus producing apparent forgetfulness and worries of early dementia.

4.2 Measuring daytime sleepiness

Measuring daytime sleepiness in an objective and meaningful way has proved very difficult. Various questionnaire approaches have been used, trying to identify the key questions to ask. Unfortunately there is no gold standard for sleepiness measurement with which to compare these questionnaires. However, in other areas of medicine symptoms are asked about, their severity judged qualitatively on history, and treatments prescribed commensurate with the assessed severity. For example, angina is not objectively measured, but antianginal preparations are prescribed and altered according to clinical response. The quantitative measurement of daytime sleepiness has been championed by the Stanford group who feel objective measures of sleepiness are required. The clinical advantages of such an expensive test are not clear, other than to weed out malingerers who fabricate their symptoms. The multiple sleep latency test (MSLT) has achieved considerable status as the standard for measuring sleepiness.[100,101,704] This test involves measuring how long it takes for an individual to fall asleep lying down in a darkened room on four or five separate occasions across the day. There are a variety of different ways in which this test is carried out but there is no doubt that they all measure something to do with sleepiness and the average results change as one would expect under a variety of clinical circumstances (Fig. 4.1). This graph also demonstrates the considerable overlap of the MSLT results between normal people and those with pathological and disabling sleepiness, thus limiting its usefulness. It is very labour intensive, sometimes surprisingly short in perfectly normal people, and does not always correlate well with performance tests.[489] It is more suited to research than to clinical use. Its value in the diagnosis of narcolepsy is mentioned in the section on intrinsic causes of sleepiness in Chapter 12 (p. 228). The MSLT tries to measure sleepiness which is only one of the consequences of sleep disruption and deprivation. In terms of daytime performance, the ability to remain vigilant is more important and perhaps more clinically relevant. The problem with measuring vigilance is that the subject will always be able to uprate his performance, at least for a while. Adequate tests of vigilance depend on long boring tasks which highlight lapses of attention.[751] An example is the multiple unprepared reaction time test[752] which measures the reaction time in response to a visual stimulus

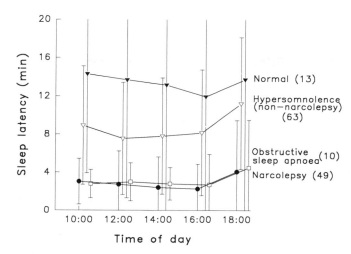

Fig. 4.1 Multiple sleep latency test results on five occasions across a day in a variety of clinical conditions compared to 13 normal subjects. Each point is the mean with *one* SD. Although the means are clearly different, the overlap is considerable. Redrawn with permission from Mitler (1982)[476] and Dement *et al.* (1978).[157]

presented at random between 1 and 10 s after the previous one, over a period of 10–15 min. These sorts of tests probably need to be at least 10 min long and possibly more than 30 min. Figure 4.2 shows the results of this test after one night's sleep deprivation, compared to a control situation. A variety of different vigilance tests have been used on patients with OSA and, although on average they are impaired, there are still patients with bad OSA and major vigilance problems who manage to uprate their performance for the test duration.[659] A variant of the MSLT, called the maintenance of wakefulness test (MWT), asks the subject to try and stay awake rather than try to fall asleep.[534] This is probably more relevant to the clinical problem of poor vigilance and the two tests do not measure quite the same thing.[599]

In the section on functions of sleep in Chapter 2 (p. 10) two different types of sleepiness were discussed—that reversible by effort and the associated cognitive impairment that is only reversed by adequate sleep. Various groups have looked specifically at cognitive function in OSA and have found it impaired[54,55,159,206] although, again, overlap with normal subjects is considerable. There are other research techniques purporting to measure sleepiness, cognitive function, or vigilance which will not be reviewed here, but the reader is referred to Dinges and Broughton.[81] At present there is no clinically suitable objective test of sleepiness that adds anything to simple questioning in the management of OSA.

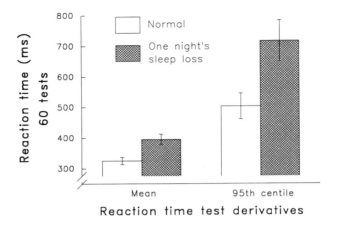

Fig. 4.2 Results of the multiple unprepared reaction time test in 20 nurses at 8.00 a.m., fresh on duty after a night's sleep and after their first night of night duty (which is effectively a night of sleep deprivation). The columns labelled mean are the mean reaction times of the second 60 tests (out of a total of 120 lasting 14 min altogether) and the 95th centile column is the 95th centile of the results for the same period of the test. Each column is the mean and SEM of these derivatives for the 20 nurses. Note the large (and significant) rise in the 95th centile result; over 300 ms longer.

There are several questionnaire-derived scales of sleepiness that help the clinician get a feel for an individual's tendency to sleep, as well as providing a number for comparison purposes. An early version was the Stanford Sleepiness Scale (SSS)[299] which was probably influenced by tiredness as well as sleepiness (Fig. 4.3). Our own department, as well as others, have used simple 'situational' questions[134,145,605] such as 'do you have to pull off the road due to sleepiness while driving?' A recent addition to this approach, the Epworth sleepiness scale,[332] appears to be more intuitively sensible. Our initial impressions are that it 'measures' more closely what the patient is complaining about but is still prone to wilful errors (Fig. 4.4).

4.3 Other daytime consequences

Apparent changes in personality occur with the development of OSA. Whether they are all simply due to the sleepiness or result more directly from the sleep disruption and hypoxemia is not clear. Aggressive and unpredictable behaviour alternating with passive and disinterested periods is common. The patient may want to be left alone and not pestered, so that

Stanford sleepiness scale

1 Feeling active and vital. Alert. Wide awake

2 Functioning at a high level. But not at peak. Able to concentrate

3 Relaxed. Awake. Not at full alertness. Responsive

4 A little foggy, not at peak. Let down

5 Fogginess, beginning to lose interest in remaining awake. Slowed down

6 Sleepiness. Prefer to be lying down. Fighting sleep. Woozy

7 Almost in reverie, sleep onset soon. Lost struggle to remain awake

Fig. 4.3 The Stanford sleepiness scale, designed to assess levels of sleepiness on a seven point scale.

persuading him to seek medical attention may be very difficult. Very rarely a frank psychosis can develop which reverses on effective treatment (Berrettini[42] and unpublished case from our unit). The fact that the wife wants to sleep in another room, because of the snoring and restless sleep, may amplify feelings of paranoia as well. Depression may set in because the patient realizes that his faculties are deteriorating.

Impotence is another common problem that is often put down to advancing age. The cause of the impotence is not completely clear, but disinterest due to the sleepiness, as well as the consequences of low testosterone levels (see the section on hormonal changes in Chapter 3, p. 54), are likely to be the major factors. This problem usually resolves following successful treatment. The improvement of impotence following NCPAP can be used as part of the dialogue to persuade a patient to try this therapy.

As well as sleepiness there may be true cognitive dysfunction. As discussed earlier (see the section on functions of sleep in Chapter 2, p. 10), this may result from prolonged sleep deprivation or perhaps directly from the nocturnal hypoxaemia of OSA. The part played by the hypoxaemia is likely to be small; other conditions causing hypoxaemia are not noted to produce significant deterioration of mental function until very severe. The cognitive dysfunction may be severe enough to raise suspicions of early dementia, thus sending the patient down an investigative pathway unlikely to reveal OSA.

Morning headache has been reported to be common in patients with OSA[265,266] but in our experience this is not so. Only about 10–15 per cent admit to morning headaches and these are rarely complained of spontaneously. Recently a review of symptoms in patients with sleep complaints suggested that headaches were no more common in OSA than in other sleep

Epworth sleepiness scale

Name:...

Date:...

Your age (Yr)................................   Your sex (Male = M/Female = F)..

How likely are you to doze off or fall asleep in the situations described in the box below, in contrast to feeling just tired?

This refers to your usual way of life in recent times.

Even if you haven't done some of these things recently try to work out how they would have affected you.

Use the following scale to choose the most appropriate number for each situation:-

0 = would never doze

1 = Slight chance of dozing

2 = Moderate chance of dozing

3 = High chance of dozing

Situation	Chance of dozing
Sitting and reading	
Watching TV	
Sitting, inactive in a public place (e.g. a theatre or a meeting)	
As a passenger in a car for an hour without a break	
Lying down to rest in the afternoon when circumstances permit	
Sitting and talking to someone	
Sitting quietly after a lunch without alcohol	
In a car, while stopped for a few minutes in the traffic	

(a)   Thank you for your cooperation

Epworth sleepiness scale results

Subjects/diagnoses	Total no. subjects (M/F)	Age in Yr (mean ± SD)	ESS scores (mean ± SD)	ESS scores two SD range	Range
Normal controls	30(14/16)	36.4 ± 9.9	5.9 ± 2.2	1.5 – 10.3	2 – 10
Primary snoring	32(29/3)	45.7 ± 10.7	6.5 ± 3.0	0.5 – 12.5	0 – 11
Obstructive sleep apnoea	55(53/2)	48.4 ± 10.7	11.7 ± 4.6	2.5 – 20.9	4 – 23
Narcolepsy	13(8/5)	46.4 ± 12.0	17.5 ± 3.5	10.5 – 24.5	13 – 23
Idiopathic hypersomnia	14(8/6)	41.4 ± 14.0	17.9 ± 3.1	11.7 – 24.1	12 – 24
Insomnia	18(6/12)	40.3 ± 14.6	2.2 ± 2.0	0.0 – 6.2	0 – 6
Periodic movements of the legs during sleep	18(16/2)	52.2 ± 10.3	9.2 ± 4.0	1.2 – 17.2	2 – 16

(b)

I thought you might be interested in this conversation we overheard while waiting to see you in outpatients—a *very* large gentleman was being asked questions by his wife who was completing your sleepiness questionnaire. They got to the question related to driving and falling asleep while stopped at traffic lights. The man was rather aggressive and said 'say no to that'. 'What do you mean?' the wife said, 'you fell asleep at the wheel at the traffic lights on the way here'. 'Don't be stupid' he said, 'if you put yes I will lose my job, they will stop me from driving'. I just wonder how many people have similar problems and are frightened of mentioning them.

(c)

Fig. 4.4 (a) The Epworth sleepiness scale and (b) the results of its use in different clinical situations. From Johns (1991).[332] (c) An interesting letter from a patient indicating a potential limitation of this approach.

problems.[10] If morning headache is complained of spontaneously, it is likely that significant CO_2 retention is present, probably persisting through the day as well.

Hypnagogic hallucinations (those occurring at sleep onset) are rare in our experience. They usually consist of fleeting and ill-defined images occurring during the struggle to stay awake. Their most serious manifestation has been in a patient who kept 'avoiding people' whilst driving on motorways at night. He saw brief images of people standing on the carriageway in front of him, which instantly disappeared with the jerk awake and the avoidance manoeuvre.

4.4 Nocturnal symptoms

Snoring is virtually universal in OSA. It is a fairly reliable marker of upper airway obstruction and, on average, the louder it is the more the obstruction. There are some important exceptions to this generalization. If there is no witness to the patient's sleep then snoring may simply not be known about, but usually someone at sometime will have told the patient his (or her) snoring was unacceptable! In the later stages of OSA, when respiratory failure has set in, the drive to breathe may be quite impaired. This leads to very little effort being made and the noise made across the narrowed pharynx may be trivial. We have certainly had histories where snoring used to be awful, but has apparently improved recently and a sleep study revealed gross OSA. In fact the sleep study may be misinterpreted as central sleep apnoea because the weak effort fails to move the rib-cage and abdominal monitoring bands. In the section on upper airway function in Chapter 3 (p. 29) it was mentioned that pharyngeal collapse could activate reflexes, possibly through apposition of the mucosal surfaces and could lead to reflex central apnoea. This has been shown to happen clinically in patients with upper airway collapse, usually when they are supine.[73,328] At the end of the apnoea, with the arousal, the airway seems to clear quickly with little, if any, snoring. Thus, despite the aetiology being upper airway obstruction, there is not much snoring when supine, although it may be present when the patient lies on his side. It is our experience that this pattern tends to occur amongst those patients with less severe OSA and not when OSA is present all night.

An idiopathic situation in which absence of snoring does not mean no OSA, is following palatal surgery. Uvulopalatopharyngoplasty (UPPP) removes the uvula and soft palate. The soft palate seems to be necessary to generate characteristic snoring, acting as the 'clapper' in the partially obstructed airstream behind the tongue. Its removal thus may remove much of the noise whilst doing nothing for the obstruction. Sometimes character-istic snoring may be removed by a UPPP, but a different sort of obstructed noise replaces it—more of a higher pitched sucking noise.

A patient with severe OSA usually has snoring all night and every night. In addition, he will snore whenever he is asleep, including daytime naps. Occasionally being asleep in a chair means that the gravity effects on the upper airway are less and it may be the only posture where OSA is not present. This may account for the occasional story one gets that having a quick nap in the car seems more refreshing than a whole night's sleep.

A good witness will be able to describe the apnoeic pauses, followed by explosive snoring, that repeat time after time throughout the night (Fig. 4.5). Failing this the witness may recognize a demonstration of an obstructive apnoea by the physician in the clinic (warn the other staff first!).

Witnessed apnoeas have proved to be very predictive of OSA subsequently confirmed by sleep study.[134] There is no doubt that an audio tape recording of a period of snoring with apnoeas is so characteristic that a confident diagnosis can be made from this alone. A tape recording would be a very sensible first investigation where no special equipment is available, such as in general practice.

The patient's disturbed sleep is often reported by the spouse. This varies enormously from slight head movements with each arousal through to violent awakenings with thrashing about that may injure the spouse. It is not clear what determines the 'degree' of arousal and movement, but it does not seem to relate to severity (that is, degree of hypoxaemia or apnoea length) or length of the illness as estimated from the history. The clinical point is that absence of very restless sleep does not exclude significant OSA. In

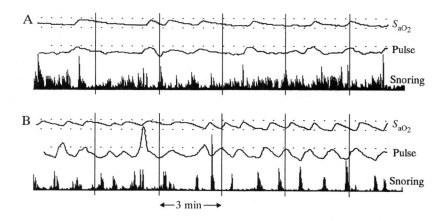

Fig. 4.5 Two tracings of S_{aO_2}, pulse, and snoring level in one subject. The top tracing shows virtually continual snoring with hypopnoea (as evidenced by the falls in S_{aO_2}) and arousals (as evidenced by the rises in pulse rate). Listening and watching the video revealed 'crescendo snoring', that is, a gradually increasing volume of snoring terminating with movement and arousal, followed by a return to sleep with another period of crescendo snoring: these cycles lasted approximately 4–7 min and occurred whilst the patient lay on either side. The second tracing is the same subject supine, now with classical apnoeas as evidenced by the snoring–silence–snoring pattern along with the oscillations in pulse and S_{aO_2}: these cycles lasting approximately 2 min.

our own practice the presence or absence of restless sleep was not at all predictive of a positive sleep study.[145]

The patient himself may not be aware at all that his sleep is restless and disturbed. The total incredulity of patients when they watch a video of themselves asleep makes this point. They often say how sound their sleep is and they cannot understand why they are so sleepy during the day.

Sleep walking has been reported in patients with OSA, but this is rare and when present is usually just a period of partial confusion on awakening.

Waking up feeling *choked* or unable to breathe is reported by some patients. It is remarkable that so few patients are aware of even a few of their hundreds of apnoeas. The upper airway has usually cleared by the time cognitive arousal has occurred and this level of arousal is rarely reached anyway. If an apnoeic episode is perceived by the patient then this unusual event is presumably due to the persistence of blockage for much longer than usual. What we have observed in these patients is episodes of nocturnal coughing that seem to be provoked by aspiration of pharyngeal secretions during the intense explosive snoring following the apnoeas.

Occasionally the perception of these upper airway obstructions can cause panic arousals.[176] This presents sometimes as the only symptom of significance. The patient may be a known snorer and wake suddenly from sleep with acute panic. The episode is usually very brief (a few seconds) before respiration is rapidly re-established and he returns to sleep. This may occur many times during the night with recollection of only a few of these episodes. They are particularly disturbing to the partner as well. This very brief panic arousal should not be confused with the longer (10–30 s) panic arousals associated with laryngeal stridor. These are not necessarily related to snoring and usually seem to be due to acid reflux. Here the patient arouses and is aware of obstruction for many seconds with the obstruction clearing more slowly with inspiratory *stridor* gradually subsiding.

Particular profuse whole body *sweating* is sometimes seen in OSA, such that bedclothes need changing. This presumably results from stimulation of the sweat glands by circulating catecholamines, rather than by sympathetic cholinergic nerve fibres (which are recruited in response to a rise in body temperature).

True nocturnal *polyuria* occurs during OSA.[369,725] Some aspects of this were discussed in the section in Chapter 3 (p. 54) on hormonal changes in OSA because one of the hypotheses for this nocturia is an increase in atrial natriuretic peptide (ANP) production. This is thought to occur because of right atrial distension either from extra venous aspiration into the chest or from the hypoxaemia leading to hypoxic pulmonary vaso-constriction and therefore an increase in afterload to the right ventricle. Different groups have found different changes in ANP but it probably is involved.[36,368,370,372,727] Normally, lying down during the day provokes polyuria but lying down asleep at night does not, an unknown mechanism prevents this happening with obvious benefits. This mechanism is likely to be related to sleep and/or the circadian rhythm, so it would not be surprising if a sleep disruption syndrome led to an increase in nocturnal urine flow. Certainly when continuous sleep is re-established with NCPAP therapy, the nocturnal polyuria diminishes so that once again there is a higher urine production rate during the day than at night (see Fig. 3.21 p. 55).

Enuresis is reported in OSA but in our practice has been rare. Enuresis could be a result of a full bladder with poor arousal or due to the hypoxaemia. It may result from nocturnal fitting, but this is very rare in OSA and perhaps more due to periods of asystole than hypoxaemia.[377]

The large negative intrathoracic pressure swings of OSA should in theory greatly encourage the movement of gastric contents back into the oesophagus, although the arguments about aspiration of blood into the thorax apply here as well (see the section on blood pressure and pleural pressure swings in Chapter 3, p. 53). Symptoms of *reflux* or oesophagitis are rarely reported so it is likely that the cardiac sphincter works well and is aided by collapse of the oesophagus just below the diaphragmatic crura.

Finally it has been reported that the hypoxaemia of OSA can trigger nocturnal *epilepsy*.[377] Because seizures are known to occur more at night in some epileptics anyway, a possible association with OSA may be missed. However, OSA presenting as nocturnal fits must be extremely uncommon. The sleep deprivation of OSA itself may bring out a latent fitting tendency; sleep deprivation is actually used diagnostically to provoke seizure activity.

4.5 Other points in the history

It is useful to ask about the changes in body weight and neck circumference over the years. Usually there has been a large weight gain in recent years but sometimes this has been a gradual process over many. Hypothyroidism and acromegaly ought to be considered since they can cause OSA. Because associated lung disease can combine with OSA to accelerate respiratory failure, smoking and asthma are important. The past medical history may be relevant with previous cardiovascular events suggesting the patient may be more at risk from the hypoxaemia and blood pressure surges of OSA. Angina may be provoked at night by OSA.

It is also worth asking about any orthodontic work done for overcrowding (suggesting micrognathia) and whether the tonsils were removed as a child. A long history of problems with nasal blockage is often obtained.

Finally, a current alcohol and drug history is necessary since sedation aggravates OSA.

Appendix 1 contains an example of the routine clerking sheets used in our Sleep Clinic during the first outpatient appointment (p. 238).

4.6 Examples of case histories

1. A 57 year old chartered accountant came complaining of daytime sleepiness. He had a reputation for nodding off at a moment's notice anytime, anywhere. He transiently nodded off whilst driving which led to his seeking medical attention. He had earlier had to give up a business, in retrospect due to inability to concentrate on the job. His second business was being run by his wife who had essentially taken over the reins of all aspects of his life.

   In addition to the daytime sleepiness, there was loud snoring (every night and all night), restless sleep and nocturia.

   Examination was essentially normal apart from minimal obesity ($kg/m^2 = 27$) but a neck circumference of 48 cm (19 in). The pharynx was characteristically small with crowding from all directions.

   A sleep study revealed over 400 arousals due to complete apnoeas with recurrent hypoxic dips down to 60 per cent S_{aO_2} every minute or so. Nasal CPAP at 9 cm H_2O abolished all respiratory related arousals.

   Over a week, he returned to normal with loss of all sleepiness and a return of his previous enthusiasm for work. He returned to active management which produced considerable problems since his wife had been running the business by herself for so long.

2. A 53 year old supervisor in a factory and City Councillor presented to his GP with snoring and occasional panic arousals to the extent that they were causing considerable marital disharmony. He was referred for ENT evaluation and a uvulopalatopharyngoplasty (UPPP) was performed. Post-operatively his wife expressed satisfaction that the snoring noise was much less and changed in character, but the episodes of stopping breathing were still present along with continuing panic arousals.

   On presentation to the Sleep Clinic he denied any symptoms of daytime sleepiness. He was a little obese ($kg/m^2 = 31$) with a 43 cm (17 in) neck. The retroglossal space appeared small. A sleep study showed silent obstructive sleep apnoea throughout the night with over 400 arousals.

   The absence of sleepiness precluded the acceptance of CPAP and weight loss with posture training was advised. A 4 kg weight loss improved matters a bit and no further action was taken.

   Two years later the snoring had returned and was now a different, more objectionable, high pitched noise. Recurrent dreams of suffocating were complained of (unusual in OSA) and for the first time sleepiness was interfering with his driving. In addition, sleepiness at other times was admitted to. Body weight had risen again by 6 kg.

The sleep study was virtually identical to that two years previously and nasal CPAP was offered. This abolished the apnoeas with full resolution of symptoms and snoring.

3. A 52 year old plumber and builder presented with more than five years of increasing sleepiness. He had fallen asleep talking to clients on the phone and whilst using a blow torch. He had often fallen asleep against his will, particularly whilst driving and as a consequence had not driven for 18 months. All this had had a severe effect on his income. He had been treated with antidepressants and sleeping tablets. He slept 14 h a day with no apparent benefit and was known to toss and turn all night. He was aware that sleeping in a chair was more restful than in a bed (as discussed in the section on nocturnal symptoms, p. 74). Before his wife mentioned apnoeas he was investigated for epilepsy as a possible cause of his sleep attacks during the day. He was finally referred to the Sleep Clinic where the symptoms were clearly those of OSA but, in addition, he had noticed an increase in shoe size from eight to ten over the last few years. He had acromegalic features, a neck circumference of 48 cm (18 in) and a big tongue.

An oral glucose tolerance test showed no growth hormone suppression and the sleep study showed gross sleep apnoea with over 300 hypoxic dips to 70 per cent S_{aO_2}. Nasal CPAP was instituted with relief of symptoms. His acromegaly was treated with trans-sphenoid removal of his pituitary tumour. Despite evidence of clinical and biochemical remission of his acromegaly, his neck size remained at 46 cm (18 in) and repeat sleep studies showed only minor improvement in the degree of sleep apnoea. This is unusual as OSA usually improves markedly following successful treatment of acromegaly. It is assumed that his obesity (kg/m^2 = 34) was the major precipitating factor with acromegaly additive, perhaps through tongue size.

4. A 60 year old retired captain in the Navy had been complaining for many years of excessive daytime sleepiness. This had been labelled narcolepsy and treated intermittently with amphetamines. The sleepiness was disastrous. He had been unable to stay awake during briefings and had eventually been retired early on health grounds despite a wish to progress further up the promotional ladder. He was finally referred when his niece, a medical student, realized what his problem must be. He had been a heroic snorer for as long as anyone could remember.

He was moderately overweight (kg/m^2 = 31) with a neck circumference of 48 cm (18¾ in). Even when only 80 kg his collar size had been 45 cm (17½ in). His pharynx was very crowded but no other abnormalities were found.

Sleep study revealed gross OSA with over 450 complete apnoeas per night and saturations falling to below 50 per cent S_{aO_2}. An initial reluctance to believe this diagnosis, after years of believing it to be narcolepsy, was removed when the patient watched his own sleep video recording.

Nasal CPAP reversed all symptoms allowing him much greater enjoyment of retirement, but unfortunately too late to save his career aspirations.

5. A 56 year old lady presented to the accident and emergency department with a stroke. She was very large (estimated 160 kg, 25 stone) with a history of diabetes and amphetamine treated narcolepsy. She was managed conservatively, making a slow recovery from her stroke. She required 450 units of insulin a day to keep her glucose below 10 mmol/l. During her stay other patients complained of her snoring and it was finally recognized that she had severe sleep apnoea. Overnight oximetry confirmed this with over 400 dips in S_{aO_2} per night down to levels around 60 per cent S_{aO_2}. Her neck circumference was 51 cm (20 in).

Following treatment with nasal CPAP her hypersomnolence disappeared and severe hypoglycaemic episodes appeared. Insulin requirements fell to 100 units a day and areas of acanthosis nigricans regressed.

Her weight has fallen over a year to about 140 kg and the neck circumference reduced to 49 cm (19¼ in). Nasal CPAP therapy is still required.

6. A 54 year old minicab driver on permanent night shift complained of increasing hypersomnolence over 20 years that was originally put down to his night duty. He had initially worked as the controller at the minicab firm but because he constantly fell asleep whilst manning the radio he was transferred to driving a minicab! This had led to crashing four minicabs in one year with many near misses due to sleepiness. His referral to our unit from another Region was initially refused under the extracontractual referral system because the relevant officer had never heard of sleep apnoea. When he finally came with his referral letter this stated that the previous week he had fallen asleep whilst standing up and fallen over.

He had all the symptoms of OSA, sleepiness, snoring, nocturia, restless sleep, apnoeas noticed by his wife, and choking episodes during sleep. He was overweight ($kg/m^2 = 40$, 119 kg) with a neck circumference of 48 cm (19 in). There were slightly enlarged tonsils, a degree of nasal blockage and a very small pharyngeal volume.

Sleep study revealed over 400 complete apnoeas per night with hypoxia down to 60 per cent S_{aO_2}. These were abolished with 12 cm H_2O of nasal CPAP. The effects were, as is usually the case, dramatic with the patient describing a new lease of life. Following nasal CPAP a weight loss of 30 kg has been achieved. Sleep study revealed a persistence of OSA but the CPAP pressure could be reduced to 7 cm H_2O. Hopefully further weight loss will allow him to dispense with CPAP.

7. A 52 year old quality control manager in a large company complained of daytime sleepiness that had led to several warnings of redundancy as well as problems driving. The final warning included a date by which he would have to sort out his problems. This date was five days after his initial outpatient appointment. He had been a snorer for at least 12 years and seriously sleepy for three years (Epworth sleepiness score = 21, Fig. 4.4). His weight had increased to 125 kg (kg/m^2 = 40) and his collar size to 51 cm (20 in). His wife had noticed apnoeas, but despite all this no doctor would take his symptoms seriously and refer him. His wife worked in the biochemistry department of their local hospital and referral to a physician was arranged. On suspicion of OSA he was referred to our sleep unit. Because of his employment problems, an afternoon sleep study was performed after his Friday outpatient appointment. This revealed gross OSA. That evening he was put on nasal CPAP with instant effect. He returned to work on Monday, with complete recovery and the redundancy threat was withdrawn.

5 Examination and investigations

The value of a physical examination is limited when assessing for the *possibility* of OSA. The history of sleepiness is likely to be the main driving force to do a sleep study. The reason for doing a physical examination is to look for causes and consequences of OSA.

5.1 Causes worth looking for

These are shown in Table 5.1. Nasal patency can be assessed simply by sniffing through each nostril in turn. More objectively, the Youlton modified peak expiratory flow meter (Clement Clarke International, Fig. 5.1) can be used. This is a simple technique of limited use but can be used to document, for example, the effect of dilating the anterior nares. Some patients (more relevant to snoring only) have a narrow anterior nares that collapses on sniffing and during sleep. The insertion of the Nosovent device (Plate 2) splints the nasal valve open and allows a higher peak inspiratory nasal flow. If opening the front of the nose does not improve flow then the obstruction lies further back in the territory of the ENT surgeon.

The reason for assessing the teeth and jaw is to assess the degree of retrognathia or micrognathia. This may help explain why, for example, a thin person might have sleep apnoea. But unless considerable, its presence will not lead to differences in management. Absence of wisdom teeth and crowding of other teeth suggest jaw underdevelopment (see the end of the section on anatomical abnormalities in Chapter 3, p. 39). There has been some suggestion that a narrow lower jaw contributes to OSA as well because it prevents the tongue from resting so far forward. To look properly for these jaw abnormalities requires conventional cephalometry, but retrognathia may be obvious on clinical examination, either from a profile view, from the degree of overjet (how much further forward the front incisors are than the bottom), or from the dentition.

Inspection of the palate and pharynx requires some experience and the changes of OSA are difficult to describe. Plate 3 shows a normal and an abnormal pharynx of moderate OSA. The usual changes consist of crowding with a much smaller lumen, mucosal oedema and humping to produce 'redundant folds' of tissue, biggish swollen and elongated soft palate and uvula, and sometimes a reddened and injected appearance. There will be all

Table 5.1 Factors to look for when examining a patient with suspected OSA

Causal		Consequential and possibly consequential	
Obesity	height and weight (BMI = kg/m^2)	Sleepy	nods off in waiting room
Nose	patency and site of any obstruction	Respiratory failure	cyanosis (or S_{aO_2} by oximetry)
Teeth	crowding?		polycythaemia
	wisdom teeth present?		asterixis
	significant overjet?		ankle swelling
Palate	size	Cor pulmonale	raised JVP
	appearance, swollen or oedematous		
Pharynx	size	Hypertension	resting BP
	appearance, swollen, odematous, wrinkled with 'redundant' folds		
	encroaching structures such as tonsils		
Tongue	size		
Neck	circumference at level of cricothyroid membrane		
Voice	inspiratory 'snore' or snort even when awake		
Other diseases	hypothyroid, acromegaly, airways obstruction		
Alcohol	spida naevi		
	alcohol on breath		

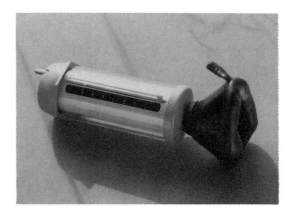

Fig. 5.1 The Youlton nasal inspiratory peak flow meter. This is a simple device (actually a modified Mini-Wright peak flow meter) to estimate nasal patency. The result obtained can be influenced by alae nasi activation (variable from sniff to sniff) and it is important not to let the mask pinch the nose. Photograph courtesy of Clement Clarke International.

degrees of these changes and their absence does not rule out OSA. The presence and size of any tonsillar tissue or other encroaching structures is very important since this may change management considerably. Plate 1 was an example of OSA due to enormous tonsils.

The tongue is harder to assess clinically, although radiographically it is enlarged in patients with OSA.[394,422] Marked ridging of the tongue edge by the teeth suggests enlargement, as sometimes seen in generalized amyloid deposition. The enlargement of the tongue muscle (genioglossus) may well be secondary to OSA rather than a primary causal problem.[427]

Neck circumference has been shown to be a better predictor of likely OSA than any other measurement or question prior to the sleep study.[143,145] This is measured at the level of the cricothyroid membrane. Although a height-corrected reading was minimally more predictive of OSA than the raw figure, the difference was very small and not worth the effort of conversion in routine practice.[143]

The voice and speech of a subject with bad OSA can be characteristic. This is due to almost snoring whilst awake. During the fast inspiration between spoken phrases the upper airway may collapse a little and begin to vibrate, presumably when it is particularly small to start with. This may happen more when the patient is not very alert and the wakefulness stimulus to the upper airway is already being withdrawn. This inspiratory flutter can sometimes be measured on a flow—volume loop, but is not specific enough for OSA to be of clinical value either for making or excluding the diagnosis.[275,301,349,564]

The presence of other contributing problems may first be suspected on clinical examination, such as myxoedema, acromegaly, or heavy alcohol intake. It is worth assessing small airways obstruction, simply with spirometry, because of its important contribution in determining whether a patient with OSA develops daytime hypoxaemia, hypercapnia, and cor pulmonale.[74,75,373,731]

5.2 Consequences

These are shown in Table 5.1. Usually the stimulus of the interview with a doctor will prevent the patient appearing sleepy. However, he may have nodded off in the waiting room (one excuse for longer waiting times in outpatients!?).

The signs of respiratory failure may be present with cyanosis (better measured with an oximeter), polycythaemia (very injected sclera and eyelid vessels), and rarely the asterixis of CO_2 retention. The presence of ankle swelling and possibly a raised jugular venous pressure (JVP) will indicate the onset of cor pulmonale. The blood pressure should be measured as a matter of routine although there is no good evidence that OSA provokes daytime hypertension in excess of that expected from the usual obesity (see the section on systemic circulation in Chapter 3, p. 57).

It has been suggested that because the history and examination are not adequately predictive of the presence of OSA in a referred sleep clinic population, that they could be dispensed with until after the sleep study. There is some logic in this if a proper history and examination *is* done afterwards to go with the sleep study result. However, this approach will result in unnecessary sleep studies when the history clearly points to some other cause of the patient's symptoms. Pre-selection by postal questionnaire is used in some centres and may be necessary if demand for sleep clinic services continues to grow at the rate it has done over the last 5 years.

5.3 Outpatient investigations

Investigations to consider performing in outpatients are shown in Table 5.2. These are by no means mandatory of course, but are a guide to what may be useful if they seem clinically indicated. The T_4 is perhaps the test that

Table 5.2 Outpatient investigations to consider in OSA

Test	Abnormality sought
Haemoglobin	Polycythaemia
Thyroid function	Hypothyroid
Blood gases	Respiratory failure
(not usually necessary if	
$S_{aO_2} > 95\%$)	
Pulmonary function	Airflow obstruction
ECG	Left ventricular hypertrophy (LVH)
	from any hypertension
Blood sugar	Diabetes, as usually obese
Growth hormone	Acromegaly

ought to be routine over about 45 years of age due to the ease with which the diagnosis is missed, particularly when some of the features of the history in myxoedema are similar to OSA anyway.

6 The sleep study, recording and analysis

It will have been apparent from the section on definitions in Chapter 3 (p. 42) that the investigation of OSA with sleep studies is a most controversial area. This essentially arises from our ignorance as to what exactly constitutes a problem worth treating.

Sleep studies on patients with OSA began in laboratories interested in looking at classical sleep problems. This meant depression, insomnia, sleep deprivation effects, and drug effects. As a result much emphasis was put on sleep architecture as analysed according to the then current wisdom—fixed sleep stages in 20–60 s epochs.[554] Total sleep time, REM sleep latency, sleep state changes, amount of REM sleep, amount of SWS, and wakefulness after sleep onset were the routine measurements. Sleep apnoea was grafted onto this and because the problem appeared to be due to stopping breathing, breathing was measured and categorized in the same rigid way sleep had been. This was the era when apnoeas had to be over 10 s and there had to be more than a fixed number to be abnormal. Clinicians followed the lead from these research-based laboratories convinced that they needed to know *everything* about a patient's sleep physiology to properly assess his condition and choose treatment. Thus, polysomnography became the gold standard with measurements of EEG, EOG, EMG, rib-cage plus abdominal movements, oronasal airflow, ECG, snoring (sometimes), oxygen saturation, leg movements, and posture (sometimes).[443,528,728]

As discussed in the section on definitions in Chapter 3 (p. 42), this approach has been gradually superseded by laboratories who realized that what really needs to be measured is (1) the root respiratory cause of the problem and (2) the most important consequence, the sleep disruption that produces the symptom (sleepiness) that drives the requirement for treatment. Ultimately all successful sleep and breathing investigation techniques need to measure, either directly or indirectly, breathing and whether it is irregular or requires extra effort and the correlation between this and measures of sleep continuity. This then allows one to say that there is a certain amount of sleep disruption from a known respiratory cause (breathing-disordered sleep rather than sleep-disordered breathing) and that this is or is not commensurate with the patient's symptoms, and then whether a trial of nasal CPAP seems indicated.

In Chapter 3 we argued that the main problem was the occurrence of an increase in upper airways obstruction (pharyngeal collapse) producing a difficulty in maintaining adequate ventilation, leading to arousal. Sometimes this upper airway collapse causes complete apnoea, sometimes hypopnoea,[238] and sometimes just increased inspiratory effort producing arousal.[224,225,264,297] Thus, the ideal monitor would measure respiratory regularity and effort and cross-correlate it with a measure of sleep continuity of sufficient resolution to document the brief arousals seen in many patients with sleep and breathing disorders, for example, pleural pressure swings with a suitable continuous high resolution analysis of the EEG, probably by computer.

Conventional polysomnography, if analysed properly, certainly goes a long way to fulfilling these requirements by using both indirect and direct measurements of the main physiological problems, but with considerable duplication and signal redundancy. Table 6.1 shows the polysomnographic signals and the primary physiological changes that can be inferred from them. The use of polysomnography versus simpler alternatives is discussed later in this chapter (p. 105).

Table 6.1 Polysomnographic information

Signal	Information obtained
EEG EOG EMG	(a) Gross sleep architecture (b) Micro-arousals only if suitably analysed
Oronasal airflow	Apnoea–hypopnoea
Rib-cage and abdominal movements	Respiratory effort. Paradox may suggest upper airway obstruction
Calibrated rib-cage and abdominal movements (rarely accurate)	Apnoea–hypopnoea
ECG	Cardioacceleration of arousal Bradycardia of apnoea Arrhythmias
Snoring	Upper airway obstruction
Oxygen saturation	Respiratory adequacy, (indirectly apnoeas–hypopnoeas)
Posture	Links between posture and degree of upper airway obstruction
Leg movements	Detects periodic movements of the legs during sleep

6.1 Polysomnography

Polysomnography (or somnopolygraphy to the classical purists) really just means recording many signals during sleep. Conventionally it means measuring EEG, EOG, and EMG plus some measures of respiration. Different laboratories measure different signals but again the usual convention is to add airflow, rib-cage plus abdominal movements, ECG, and pulse oximetry. These signals are recorded either onto paper at speeds between 10 and 15 mm/s (which produces nearly 400 m of paper), onto magnetic tape, or digitized for computer storage. Subsequently, the sleep channels are analysed by hand, epoch by epoch (20 or 30 s) with the sleep stage noted. Thus, there will be about 1000 epochs over 8 h of sleep even at this coarse resolution. A good description of sleep staging can be found in several articles.[67,102,198,311,554] Even a skilled technician will take over 2 h to do this and many more hours if transient arousals (according to current definitions[60]) are added. All this work will provide a hypnogram (see Fig. 2.4, p. 9) that fails to convey the essence of the sleep disturbance in sleep apnoea: the recurrent arousals. This classic sleep staging is a rule-based system (see the section on sleep states in Chapter 2, p. 5) which is extremely difficult to computerize. Several attempts have been made to implement the rules on computer but this has not been very successful, except when sleep is relatively normal.[708] The disturbed sleep of sleep apnoea can be very difficult to score, even by hand, but the skilled scorer will make many subtle adjustments to the rules, that are difficult to include in computer algorithms, to produce a 'sensible' hypnogram. The most successful systems make an attempt at scoring and then allow interaction between the technician and the scoring process to 'clean it up'. This process can still take a long time and may not be much more time- and cost-effective than hand scoring.[49] The approach we take is to allow a computer system (Oxford Medical 9200) to make its best assessment of the sleep and then to check manually the areas of clinical importance, for example, (1) were there really long periods of undisturbed SWS? (2) was the sleep really as bad as the hypnogram suggests? (3) was there really REM sleep within the first hour of sleep? These kinds of assessments do not have to be very accurate since great accuracy does not produce clinical benefit.

Other approaches to computerizing EEG analysis are being developed. Schulz and colleagues[281] designed a system that produced a single derivative based on both frequency and amplitude of the EEG. Essentially the EEG is filtered into six frequency bands and eight amplitude bands. Over 10 s epochs the 6 × 8 matrix is processed to produce a single derivative that follows the descent of a subject into SWS in a continuous way. Thus, non-REM sleep is described as a 'continuous parameter' from wakefulness

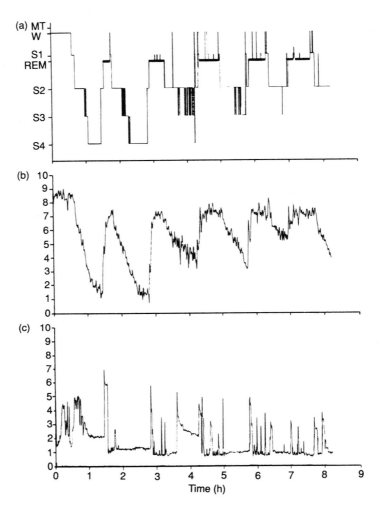

Fig. 6.1 (a) A conventional all night hypnogram from one normal subject. MT, movement time; W, wake; S1–S4, non-REM sleep stages. (b) The output from a computerized continuous EEG analysis system with a resolution of approximately 10 s (arbitrary units on the vertical axis). Note the gradual waxing and waning which the hypnogram can only partially represent. This system cannot differentiate REM sleep from stage 1 so that an EMG (c) is also used in order to further differentiate these two states. With permission from Haustein *et al.* (1986).[281]

down to the deepest stage 4. The activity of the EMG is then added to this
to differentiate light sleep from REM sleep, which has a 'continuous
parameter' value similar to conventional stage 1 (Fig. 6.1). However, even
this approach still only provided a resolution of 10 s, hence, transient
arousals were not necessarily measured. The problem with improving the
resolution to only a few seconds or less is that of separating true lightening
of the EEG from other brief changes that do not represent a move towards
arousal. Another approach that has been used is spectral analysis. Identification of slow wave activity (or Δ activity) in the region of 0.5–2 Hz by fast
Fourier transform is possible to a resolution of approximately 1 s. Even in
stage 2 there is low frequency activity (short bursts of slow waves and K
complexes). In stage 1 there is very little and it is probably not possible to
differentiate wakefulness and the lighter stages of sleep just from Δ activity.
However, there are commercial systems that extract Δ activity and other
frequency bands (for example, α activity from the 8–12 Hz band) for
display. This allows the interpreter a much better feel for the evolution and
fragmentation of the sleep (Fig. 6.2).

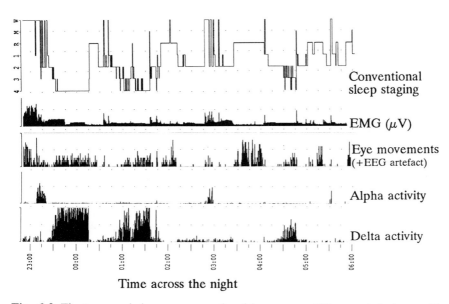

Fig. 6.2 The top panel shows a conventional hypnogram (20 s epochs) along with
computer derived continuous estimates of four of the components of classic sleep
staging: chin EMG, eye movements (which are contaminated by delta wave
activity), alpha activity, and delta activity. From an Oxford Medical 9200 system.

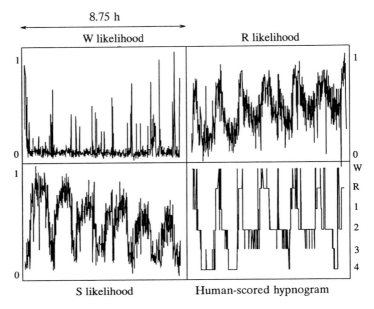

Fig. 6.3 The three outputs from a neural network based approach to EEG analysis in a normal subject. W, R, and S represent three competing processes that closely equate to conventional wakefulness, REM or stage 1 sleep, and slow wave sleep. The sum of the three always adds up to one. The fourth box contains a conventionally scored hypnogram for comparison. Although not discernible at the resolution displayed here, these three derivatives are available on a second to second basis. Tracings courtesy of Dr S. Roberts, University of Oxford.

However, the spectral analysis approach only uses a small amount of the information contained in the EEG. A major advance in this area has come from the availability of more powerful computers and a process called neural networking. Neural networking is essentially an empirical pattern recognition system. Given a complex signal, such a system will 'learn' to describe it in a certain way, making no assumptions about its character. When applied to the EEG, using no specific rules about frequency and amplitude, Roberts and Tarassenko[575] showed that the neural network could break the signal down into three competing processes, which on conventional analysis corresponded most closely to wakefulness, SWS, and REM sleep or stage 1/2. Figure 6.3 shows a sleep tracing of these three derivatives and the conventional hypnogram. The advantage of this system is that it can provide a resolution down to 1 s and, from the wakefulness likelihood tracing, brief transient arousals can be clearly seen and counted.

The use of computers in this sophisticated way has taken EEG analysis forward by several orders of magnitude. It should now be possible to measure sleep continuity and discontinuity in such a way that will allow us to work out what aspects are important in providing refreshing sleep and what aspects lead to daytime sleepiness. This in turn will allow us to identify in a clinical sleep study whether an abnormality is likely to be the explanation for a patient's symptoms. This is something we currently do very crudely and that is satisfactory only at the extremes of normality at one end and marked sleep disturbance from severe sleep apnoea at the other.

6.2 Respiratory signals

Monitoring respiratory signals gives a considerable amount of information about different aspects of breathing. Oronasal flow measurements really only give a crude qualitative statement as to whether there is flow or not. There is no way they can be quantitative unless a thermocouple is mounted at the single orifice of a face mask, well sealed on the face. The usual device consists of three thermistors, wired in series, one under each nostril and one in front of the mouth. Assuming the device has not been displaced, then a marked reduction in signal implies little airflow through the nose or mouth. Both nostrils need monitoring because of the centrally induced cycling of nasal resistance from side to side.[175] Nasal expiratory flow can also be monitored with a CO_2 device sampling air from both nostrils.

Respiratory effort can be monitored in a variety of ways. The most direct way, which is used routinely in a few laboratories, is via oesophageal pressures either with a balloon system or with pressure tipped catheters. Although this is undoubtedly the most accurate way, the accumulated problems of extra cost, time to set up, patient discomfort, and disturbed sleep greatly limit its use. More indirect measures of pleural pressure swings have been tried, for example, based on deformation of the supraclavicular fossa. Although this works in thin subjects in fixed postures, it has failed to be of value in the sleep laboratory.

A more promising approach to the non-invasive measurement of pleural pressure swings is to derive it indirectly from the systolic blood pressure. There are methods of measuring[587] beat to beat systolic blood pressure in a finger (for example, the Finapres device from Ohmeda) that demonstrate 'pulsus paradoxus'. The swing in systolic blood pressure with each breath is due to the fall in intrathoracic and intracardiac pressure being transmitted via the arterial fluid column to the periphery. The correlation between pleural pressure swings and the systolic BP swings with respiration are probably good enough for clinical purposes in a sleep laboratory.[404]

Movement of the rib-cage and abdomen can be used to imply respiratory effort whether or not there is accompanying nasal flow. Both compartments need to be measured to imply changes in volume inhaled or exhaled because of the changes in relative contribution that occur with sleep state[658] and under conditions of resistive loading. In the classic division of apnoeas into central or obstructive, chest wall monitoring is essential (Fig. 6.4). Some laboratories attempt to calibrate their rib-cage and abdomen movement transducers to give absolute measures of volume displacement, that is, a certain voltage output on the rib-cage transducer represents the same volume of air displaced in or out of the lungs as a similar voltage change on the abdomen transducer. This calibration can be achieved in essentially three ways (linear regression, two position, or isovolume), but such calibrations fail to be maintained if there is a change in posture, particularly if it involves changes in spinal angle.[657] The sum of the two channels is supposed to be tidal volume and to replace oronasal airflow. Particularly in obese patients moving around in bed, the results are really only qualitative or at best semi-quantitative.

The currently favoured device for measuring rib-cage and abdominal movement is the inductance plethysmograph. This device gives a signal proportional to the circumference squared and thus volume. It is probably slightly better than mercury/capillary strain gauges, mainly because of its better artefact rejection and questions over the safety of using mercury. Other devices based on pressure capsules, solid state force transducers, and piezo devices have advantages in terms of cost and robustness but may not perform as well.

In addition to registering overall effort, rib-cage and abdomen movement sensors can be used to imply resistive loading. Under conditions of increased inspiratory resistance (for example, snoring) either the rib-cage or the abdominal movement proves the stronger. In its extreme form this, of course, results in complete paradoxical movement of one compartment during obstructive apnoeas (Fig. 6.4). During heavy snoring there may be reduced outward movement of one channel compared to the other (it may

---

Fig. 6.4 Obstructive and central apnoeas. (a) An obstructive apnoea lasting approximately 35 s (whole trace is 60 s). Initially during the apnoea, when the respiratory efforts are small, the rib-cage and abdomen move together. As the effort increases across the apnoea, paradoxical movement of the two compartments occurs which reverts to normal again with the end of the apnoea. (b) Two short central apnoeas lasting 12 and 18 s (whole trace 60 seconds). Note absence of respiratory effort during the apnoea. The gain on the airflow signal is very high and shows the return of ventilation a breath or so before either the rib-cage or abdominal sensors. This patient has myotonic dystrophy.

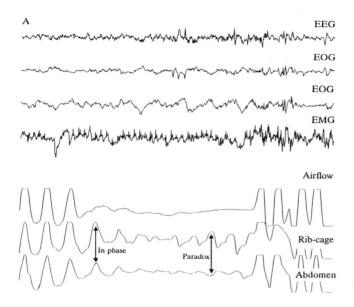

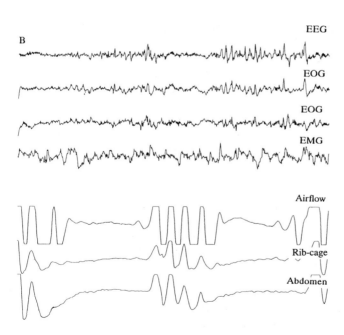

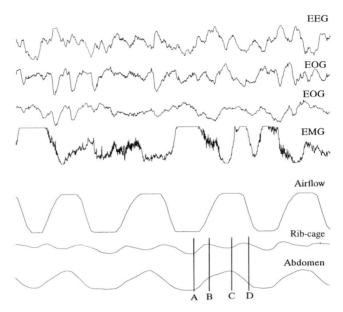

Fig. 6.5 Sixteen second tracing from a heavy snorer in stage 4 sleep. At A the rib-cage and abdomen begin to move outwards. Because of the upper airway obstruction the pleural pressures developed mainly by the stronger diaphragm are well below atmospheric (perhaps -30 to -40 cm H_2O) and thus prevents the rib-cage further expanding (and even pulls it back in) despite the action of the intercostals (point B). At point C the inspiratory effort falls allowing the rib-cage to spring out a bit and at point D the two compartments are passively relaxing together. The large swings in the EMG trace are respiratory artefact due to the increased respiratory movements.

even appear not to move) with transient springing out at the end of inspiration when the intrathoracic pressure rises back towards atmospheric (Fig. 6.5). Thus, heavy snoring can sometimes be inferred (with limited reliability) from the rib-cage and abdominal signals.

Manual analysis and a count of these respiratory events is very time-consuming, particularly if hypopnoeas as well as apnoeas are to be documented. It is questionable whether an accurate count is necessary and computers can make an *estimate* of what is going on. Unfortunately the respiratory signals are particularly prone to artefact, especially in obese patients, so that computer analyses should be viewed as a 'first impression' with manual checking of clinically important results.

There are likely to be advances soon in the analysis of respiratory signals similar to those occurring in EEG analysis. It may be better to analyse respiration as one might any other physiological signal, for example, with spectral analysis and neural networks. One advantage of such approaches would be to get away from analyses relying on thresholds, that is, > 10 s apnoeas, 50 per cent reductions in ventilation, and actually to measure what is occurring in order to allow proper correlations with both the EEG analysis and tests of daytime functioning.

6.3 Oximetry

The ability to continuously measure S_{aO_2} revolutionized the study of sleep and breathing disorders. By providing a measure of the adequacy of respiration many of the problems of trying to quantify the respiratory signals were solved. The original instruments commercially available and applied to the ear lobe (Waters oximeter) were based on two wavelength transmittance spectrometry. Oxygenated haemoglobin transmits 660 nm wavelength light (red) more than deoxygenated, whereas 940 nm light (near infrared) is transmitted equally by oxygenated and deoxygenated blood. Thus, the ratio of oxygenated to total haemoglobin is calculable. The contribution to colour absorption by the ear pigments was partially solved by measuring them first with the blood expelled, by inflating a balloon against the lobe. To register arterial blood colours required arterialization of the ear lobe, either by heat, rubbing, or vasodilator cream. These devices worked, but slight movements of the probe produced large artefacts in the S_{aO_2}. The second development, by Hewlett-Packard, was to use six further wavelengths to enable factoring out of the ear pigments using empirically derived algorithms. The eight different wavelengths were generated using a revolving wheel with eight colour filters and were shone sequentially through the ear via a fibre optic cable. This produced good accuracy above 50 per cent S_{aO_2} (95 per cent CI, 3 per cent S_{aO_2}) but the probe was cumbersome, disturbed sleep and displaced frequently.[165,653] Again the ear needed good arterialization to ensure that only arterial blood was in the light path.

The next major advance was to realize that the arterial contribution to the colour change could be singled out by only looking at *fluctuating* light intensities. In this way only the spectroscopic changes in pulsatile, that is, arterial, blood were assessed. This clever approach has led to a plethora of different pulse oximeters becoming available. These devices can be made accurate[723] and robust, as well as being able to work on non-arterialized ears, fingers, toes, and other suitable pieces of anatomy.

There are many different types of pulse oximeters, of varying accuracy.[26,490,613] The main stimulus for their development has been their use in operating theatres and the intensive care units. Although they may not be perfectly accurate for absolute S_{aO_2}, (best above 70 per cent) they measure change well and are more than adequate for clinical sleep work.[723] There is some debate over the sampling frequency for oximetry signals during sleep studies, but every 5 s is certainly adequate. The sampling algorithm used by the Ohmeda series of oximeters (when storing the data for later downloading) is the lowest S_{aO_2} value that occurred in the last 12 s, stored at the end of each 12 s: this can reasonably recreate the oscillating S_{aO_2} waveforms seen in clinical practice.[723]

In neonatal work there may be a requirement for a faster response time and more rapid sampling frequencies as it appears that babies can change their S_{aO_2} values faster than adults can.

What is more important with these pulse oximeters is their ability to reject artefact. If perfusion is low to the probe site, then there is very little pulsatile blood available for the spectroscopic analysis, which forces the oximeter to turn up its amplification of the signals. Any limb movement will change blood volume in a digit by transiently changing venous return and when arterial pulsations are weak, the consequent change in venous volume will be 'seen' as the pulsatile change and its oxygen saturation measured, and inevitably will be lower than real arterial. Thus, if the subject has a low cardiac output or lies on the relevant arm, then the oximeter will read a falsely low S_{aO_2}. The best oximeters monitor the signal quality and are able to reject data under these circumstances, but there can still be errors. Sometimes the pattern of artefact is recognizable, in association with an unlikely and variable pulse rate (since the arterial pulse is no longer locked onto), but particularly in children this may not be so obvious. In our experience the artefact rejection of the Ohmeda series has been satisfactory in subjects over two years of age.

To what extent the measurement of falls in S_{aO_2} can substitute for actually measuring ventilation is not clear. There have been several papers looking at the relationship between hypoxic dips and apnoeas (or apnoeas and hypopnoeas). Any assessment of this work is complicated by different definitions of hypoxic dipping and of apnoeas or hypopnoeas. For example, the algorithm used to detect hypoxic dips may use different degrees of dipping (3 per cent, >3 per cent, 4 per cent, >4 per cent, etc.) as well as different starting S_{aO_2} values from which to begin measuring a dip. Some authors have used a fixed baseline throughout the night (which may miss many dips), some use a running baseline (which may vary widely in the presence of OSA), and others use a running maximum which is able to take account of wildly fluctuating S_{aO_2} values. The analysis of apnoeas and hypopnoeas is equally variable, as some units require concurrent hypoxia to label a fall in the ventilation tracing as a hypopnoea, while others do not.[423] The actual percentage fall in the ventilation tracing defined as a hypopnoea may vary as well. Thus, it is not surprising that attempts to correlate hypoxic dipping with an apnoea—hypopnoea score have met with varying success.

Most authors have found good correlations,[185,218,375,551,650,755] but not all[167] and it has been suggested that the oximetry-derived events might actually correlate *better* with the consequences that matter, that is, arousals, than the apnoea–hypopnoea index, although recent evidence would argue against this.[114] The oximeter will, however, miss arousals due to heavy snoring, which of course the ventilatory data would also fail to identify and this is explained by the ability of some patients to compensate fully for their increased upper airway resistance.[264,297] They then wake up in response to the increased effort before hypoventilation or hypoxaemia can develop to any significant extent.[224,225] If there are characteristic S_{aO_2} dips from a normal starting baseline then there is no argument but if there are not, then abnormalities may be missed (see Fig. 3.16, p. 45).

A further complication is that a fixed fall in S_{aO_2} of say 4 per cent represents a big fall in P_{aO_2} and ventilation, if the starting S_{aO_2} is above 94 per cent. When the baseline starting S_{aO_2} is low then a 4 per cent fall can occur easily with very small fall in P_{aO_2} and ventilation. This makes counts of say 4 per cent S_{aO_2} dips quite unreliable as a substitute for apnoeas or hypopnoeas in patients with resting hypoxaemia, for example, due to chronic lung disease (see the later section on sleep and chronic lung disease, p. 207). It might be better to convert S_{aO_2} falls to theoretical P_{aO_2} falls to improve the usefulness of oximetry, but this appears not to have been done.

Rather than counting hypoxic dips of a fixed size, it may be better simply to inspect oximetry tracings and make an overall assessment. Certainly most physicians using oximetry become skilled at interpreting such tracings, as long as they are always displayed in the same format with sufficient resolution to see individual dips. An experienced physician's classification of a tracing is probably better than using computer-derived numbers.[167,673] A little used part of oximetry is the pulse rate that is also obtained: the use of this as a marker of arousal was mentioned on p. 49 and will be discussed further in the section on polysomnography versus simpler alternatives later in this chapter (p. 105).

6.4 Snoring

Snoring must be measured in some way. It is important as an indirect measure of upper airway narrowing. An absence of snoring virtually excludes significant OSA except under the circumstances discussed in the section on nocturnal symptoms in Chapter 4 (p. 74), particularly after a uvulopalatopharyngoplasty. Snoring will usually be recorded onto the audio channel of a video recorder but can also be recorded on a polygraph as the raw microphone signal, integrated, (see Fig. 4.5, p. 75), or only registered

if above a certain threshold. The audio bandwidth of interest is 40–
~150 Hz, but there are higher harmonics present too, between 300 and
1000 Hz.[413,517] The microphone can be mounted above the subject or fixed
over the pharynx laterally: in this latter case very low frequency movement
artefact (<40 Hz) can be filtered out if the microphone couples to the skin
via a small air chamber with a small leak.[519,650]

6.5 Electrocardiogram

During polysomnography the recording of the ECG is not helpful in the
diagnosis of OSA, when much better information is obviously available
from other signals. Its use in simpler studies is discussed on page 105. Its
value is in detecting potentially dangerous cardiac dysrhythmias. However,
most laboratories do not look assiduously for such dysrhythmias during
clinical studies. If clinical decisions are to be based on the ECG findings
(that is, the more urgent provision of nasal CPAP) then a conventional 24 h
Holter monitor system is more appropriate.

6.6 Blood pressure

In the section on blood pressure and pleural pressure swings in Chapter 3
(p. 51) the changes in beat to beat blood pressure in OSA were discussed.
The two essential features were the recurrent *falls* in systolic blood pressure
with each inspiration (pulsus paradoxus), greater as respiratory effort
increases progressively during an apnoea and the big *rises* after each apnoea
ends (see Fig. 3.17, p. 47). This pattern is very characteristic and it should
be possible to use such tracings to diagnose obstructive sleep apnoea. In
theory, embedded in the beat to beat blood pressure tracing are indirect
measures of the two physiological events most important in symptomatic
OSA—upper airway obstruction and arousals.
  Attempts have been made to validate these assumptions and to assess if
computer-derived indices from an all night beat to beat blood pressure trace
could reliably diagnose sleep apnoea. This kind of work has been made
possible through the invention of a non-invasive device to measure beat to
beat blood pressure.
  This device (Ohmeda 2300, 'Finapres', Englewood Co., USA) measures
blood pressure continuously and produces a tracing similar to an intra-
arterial line. It is based on the volume clamp method of Peñáz and also
developed by Wesseling and colleagues[477] in the Netherlands. The method

uses a circumferential balloon inside a restricting cuff on a finger. This balloon is inflatable and can compress the digital artery. The pressure inside the balloon is controlled on a continuous basis by a servo-controlled motor. If the digital artery is compressed from the outside, with a pressure equal to the arterial pressure inside, by a system that can adjust this pressure 40 times per second, then the pressure in the compressing balloon can track the intra-arterial pressure. If the pressure in the balloon were too high it would of course simply obliterate the arterial lumen and if too low not apply any pressure at all. The pressure in the balloon is kept at the point of 'arterial unloading', which is where the arterial wall is neither stretched or shrunk but at its neutral position. This is found by gradually increasing the pressure in the balloon and looking at the arterial pulsation (with a beam of infrared light that 'reads' the arterial volume): the pulsations get gradually bigger and are greatest at the point when the artery is unloaded and the walls can stretch and shrink maximally. As the external pressure rises further the pulsations reduce again and finally disappear when the artery is flattened. Once the unloaded position of the artery has been determined then the pressure in the balloon is controlled by the servo system to keep the volume of the artery constant. This again uses the infrared light path. As long as the infrared transmittance is kept constant at the unloaded point, then the pressure in the balloon must be the same as the arterial pressure because there is no pressure gradient across the unloaded arterial wall. This device has been shown to track arterial blood pressure extremely well even when there is peripheral vasoconstriction.[162,510,735] The main problem is that digital arterial pressure is not quite the same as systemic: the hand position alters BP by the height that it is above or below the heart and the finger cuff has to be carefully applied to get good results. Although the device may not record absolute BP precisely, it is able to follow *changes* in BP very accurately. Continuous use is uncomfortable and the cuff should be deflated for approximately 5 min every 30 min.

By using the Finapres device it was shown that the swings in systolic BP tracked the swings in pleural pressure during obstructed inspirations simulating OSA.[404] Figure 6.6 shows systolic BP (SBP) tracking mouth pressure and pleural pressure in a normal subject during simulated OSA. Also shown is the correlation between swings in SBP and swings in mouth pressure (virtually equivalent to pleural pressure during obstructed inspirations) (Fig. 6.7).

The response of the SBP to arousal was discussed in the section on blood pressure and pleural pressure changes in Chapter 3 (p. 51). In particular it was pointed out that SBP rises were very sensitive as a marker of arousal[146] and did not seem to adapt as a subject received repetitive stimuli, in the same way that cortical arousal does.[172,335] This may indeed mean it is too sensitive a marker of arousal.

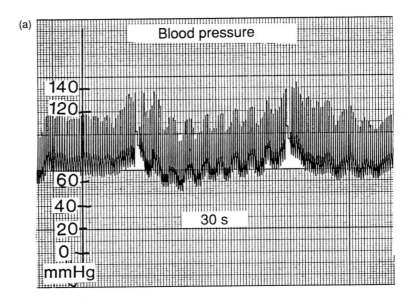

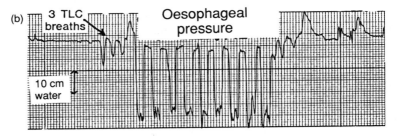

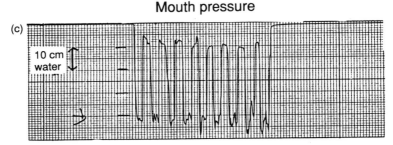

Fig. 6.6 (a) The arterial blood pressure tracing obtained non-invasively from the Ohmeda Finapres device. During the middle minute of the tracing this normal subject repeatedly inspired against a blocked airway, simulating obstructive apnoea. (b) and (c) Records of the pressure swings generated at the mouth behind the block and via an oesophageal balloon. Note the way the systolic blood pressure tracing follows the oesophageal pressure demonstrating pulsus paradoxus.

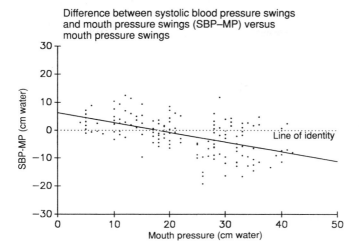

Fig. 6.7 This plot shows in one subject simulating OSA the difference between pressure swings at the mouth (MP) and swings of the systolic blood pressure (SBP) against the level of inspiratory effort from the mouth pressure. Note the broad equivalence, but a tendency of the blood pressure swings to overestimate at low pressure swings and underestimate during higher pressure swings.

Figures 6.8 and 6.9 show the results of a study looking at SBP falls (of respiratory frequency) and rises (occurring over 10–15 s) in patients undergoing sleep studies. Work on this device is in its infancy but it does appear that non-invasive beat to beat SBP measurement may be a useful investigative tool for sleep apnoea in the future.

6.7 Leg movements

Periodic movements of the legs during sleep is a recognized abnormality and in some cases causes daytime sleepiness, due to sleep disturbance.[126] In this condition, one or both legs move briefly as often as every 30 s throughout non-REM sleep. The movement is not a twitch (thus, the alternative name nocturnal myoclonus is uninformative) but more a semi-purposeful extension and flexion of all the joints in the leg. Each movement lasts approximately 1–2 s and is similar to the previous one and is best appreciated by fast forwarding a video recording of such a patient. The cause of this condition is unknown but often occurs in association with other problems and may also occur in isolation, particularly in the elderly. For

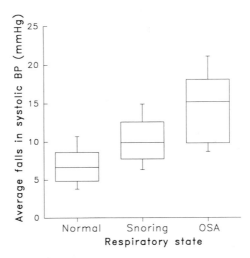

Fig. 6.8 This graph shows the size of the systolic blood pressure swings due to respiration (pulsus paradoxus) in three groups of subjects: normal subjects, proven snorers (whilst snoring) and patients with proven obstructive sleep apnoea (during periods of obstruction).

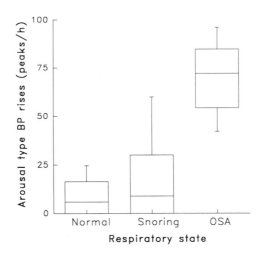

Fig. 6.9 This graph shows the number per hour of transient rises in blood pressure (>18 mmHg) occurring over a time frame of 10–30 s in three groups of subjects: normal subjects, proven snorers (some with EEG arousal, some without), and patients with obstructive sleep apnoea (OSA). Not surprisingly the patients with OSA have many more surges in blood pressure due to their recurrent arousals.

example, it sometimes occurs with OSA and may take some weeks to disappear after successful treatment with CPAP.

Because it is an alternative cause of hypersomnolence, it needs to be considered if OSA seems unlikely or has been excluded, thus, monitoring of leg movements during a sleep study is often necessary.

The techniques for this vary, but the usual approach is to put an EMG-type surface electrode on the anterior tibialis muscle of each leg and feed these into two spare EEG channels on the polygraph. One recording channel can be saved by putting one input of a differential amplifier on each leg, thus, movement of either leg will give a signal. Alternatively any device measuring movement can be used, such as a piezo device or other form of actigraph, on each leg.

6.8 Polysomnography versus simpler alternatives

Some of the background to the current arguments about whether full polysomnography is really necessary have been aired earlier in this chapter. It was pointed out that because respiratory sleep studies arose from laboratories interested primarily in sleep architecture, considerable emphasis was inevitably placed on the neurophysiological monitoring. This, and the benefits of an expensive investigation,[256] until recently delayed a reassessment of what is really required from a respiratory sleep study. The adequacy of a sleep study should be judged on its ability to separate patients with sleep apnoea and its variants who will respond to treatment, from those who are normal or would not benefit from treatment. When comparisons between polysomnography and simpler studies have been made it was assumed that polysomnography was the 'gold standard'. It was mentioned earlier that the definitions of pathological respiratory events are very inconsistent between laboratories[423] (thus there are different 'gold standards') and also that conventional polysomnography may not pick up all pathological events, for example, snoring-induced arousals.[264,297] Thus, the use of polysomnography as the reference with which to compare newer, simpler techniques is fundamentally flawed. As with all other areas of medicine, clinical outcome is the true gold standard and the value of a test should be judged according to whether it identifies patients who will benefit from treatment. At present no studies have compared polysomnography with simpler techniques according to their ability to pick out patients who are sleepy enough due to upper airway problems, to benefit from nasal CPAP, currently the definitive treatment for OSA. Until this approach is adopted, it is not correct to say that a simpler approach to sleep studies is not as good as polysomnography just because it does not count the same numbers of apnoeas or other events. For example, a device that measured increases in upper airway resistance and correlated these with sleep fragmentation would be able to document the *relevant* obstructive apnoeas, hypopnoeas, and snoring induced arousals, but it is unlikely that a count of these events would correlate well with the apnoea–hypopnoea count from polysomnography in a cross-section of patients with all grades of disease severity from simple snoring through to severe OSA. This point has been laboured because potentially good ideas have tended to be dismissed when they have not correlated particularly well with polysomnography.[271,537,551,688,753]

Many laboratories now employ simpler studies on a routine clinical basis. A recent review of clinical practice in EEC countries revealed that each laboratory was using different combinations of signals for the full study and a range of techniques for simplified studies.[656] These simplified studies are variously referred to as screening, pre-selection, ambulatory, or limited studies.

The various EEC laboratories were all able to assess respiratory effort, respiratory success (or adequacy, for example, S_{aO_2} levels), and some aspect of sleep fragmentation. Sleep fragmentation was sometimes measured from body movements or pulse rate changes rather than EEG. The conclusion from this is that if a clinician understands the conditions he is treating and the limitations imposed by his diagnostic tools, then a variety of approaches to sleep studies are satisfactory: what is important is the physician's understanding of the problem, not how many channels he has on his polygraph. Table 6.2 shows the variation in approaches taken for both full studies and limited studies in 10 different centres in Europe.

Respiratory effort and regularity can be assessed not only from rib-cage and abdominal movement sensors, but also from surface diaphragm EMG signals, inferred from snoring, by tracheal sounds, by direct observation of video recordings, and from the pulsus paradoxus observed on a beat to beat arterial blood pressure tracing (for example, from the non-invasive Finapres device). Respiratory adequacy or success, can be assessed from oximeter recordings and to some extent from calibrated rib-cage with abdominal movement signals. Sleep fragmentation can be inferred from an EEG, pulse rate or blood pressure rises (in the absence of an autonomic neuropathy or β blockade), and from body movement. Movement can be measured in a variety of ways, including radar, infrared, video-derived, static charge sensitive bed, piezo devices, and accelerometer/vibration detectors. The sensitivity of the movement detector will determine how sensitive the device is at measuring sleep disturbance. Wrist movement has been extensively assessed for its ability to define sleep and sleep disruption.[30,125,376,481,555,593,594,671] A system using the video signal to derive movement was shown to be capable of defining sleep times and arousals in excess of 2 s with sufficient accuracy for clinical purposes.[669,715] It should come as no surprise that plots of body movement

Table 6.2 Combinations of signals used by European sleep centres in the evaluation of sleep and breathing disorders

	Full studies	Limited studies or pre-selection, precise use depending on patient group
Centre 1	*Classical polysomnography + snoring + movement arousals	Actigraphy Oximetry (only for follow-up)
Centre 2	*Classical polysomnography	Oximetry + observation (strong suspicion of OSA)
Centre 3	*Classical polysomnography + video (posture)	None
Centre 4 (mainly paediatric)	*Classical polysomnography + EMG activity from diaphragm using surface electrodes + sound + ECG + Finapres	(a) Vitalog system (for CPAP review) (b) Oximetry + observation
Centre 5	Rarely used	(a) Vitalog system (respiratory effort, airflow, oximetry rate, body movements, posture) (b) Oximetry alone
Centre 6	*Classical polysomnography + video (posture) + ECG	Same as full studies but during afternoon nap
Centre 7	*Classical polysomnography + movement arousals + ECG	Oximetry
Centre 8	*Classical polysomnography + ECG + transcutaneous P_{O_2} and P_{CO_2} + snoring + video (posture)	Somnolog system (documenting α and Δ activity, EMG level, EOG, actigraphy, sound, heart rate, and respiration)
Centre 9	*Classical polysomnography	MESAM IV system (snoring, heart rate, oximetry, and posture)
Centre 10	**Classical polysomnography + video (posture, snoring)	Oximetry and video Oximetry alone (pulse included in analysis)

*Classical polysomnography is EEG, EOG, EMG, oronasal airflow, and one or two respiratory movement transducers, oximetry. Sleep staging by 20 s or longer epochs.
**Not formally scored, except manually by computer, reviewed for evidence of sleep fragmentation and presence of REM sleep.

Table 6.3 Categories of patients for sleep studies

---

1.   Patients with a *low* probability of having a sleep and breathing disorder, for example, snorers with no other relevant symptoms and an atypical physiognomy

2.   Patients with a *high* probability of having obstructive sleep apnoea, that is, with typical symptoms and physiognomy. Only need a confirmatory and severity-assessing study

3.   Patients in whom the diagnosis of obstructive sleep apnoea is *already known* and in whom the response to treatment is being followed

4.   Patients with *unexplained sleep—wake disorders* where full information is required to make a diagnosis. An unclear screening study would also put a patient in this group

5.   Assessment of *nocturnal hypoventilation* syndromes, for example, scoliosis. Hypoxaemia is the dominant signal of interest

---

can be used to define sleep since the degree of movement is very heavily dependent on sleep state and movement virtually always implies arousal, except in REM sleep.[529,749]

Part of the intelligent use of the limited systems detailed in Table 6.2 is the appreciation that not all patients needing sleep studies for sleep apnoea and its variants present the same diagnostic difficulties. The EEC group mentioned above also agreed that such patients could be divided into five main categories which could be used to determine which sleep studies would be appropriate. Table 6.3 shows these five categories.

The first category includes patients whom the clinician feels are unlikely to have a sleep and breathing problem and thus sleep apnoea needs to be *excluded*. There are an increasing number of such patients including, for example, snorers who are not sleepy but who may be worried, hypertensive, or have other unusual symptoms. This sort of patient is being studied just to be sure that there is no significant sleep apnoea.

The second category includes patients with what appears to be very obvious sleep apnoea. There will be a history of sleepiness, snoring, witnessed apnoeas, and on examination the patient will be overweight with a big neck and a small wrinkly pharynx. This sort of patient needs only a confirmatory sleep study and perhaps also a severity assessing study to rate their priority on any waiting list for treatment.

The third category includes patients who seem less likely to have a sleep and breathing problem, have significant sleepiness, but may not have all the usual features, perhaps being thin with a normal looking pharynx. This type of patient needs a full study as he is less likely to be as obvious a case as in category 2 and because he has symptoms to explain. This category also includes patients from any other category who have had limited studies which have been uninterpretable or unhelpful for some reason.

Category 4 patients are those who have already had diagnostic studies and in whom repeat studies are needed to assess response to treatment. For example, a patient with known OSA and hypoxic dipping may only need oximetry or actigraphy subsequently to determine whether his CPAP is functioning correctly.

Category 5 patients are different and their problem has not been discussed yet. They consist of patients with non-obstructive nocturnal hypoventilation syndromes such as scoliosis, post-polio syndrome, and other neuromuscular disorders. Here nocturnal hypoxaemia *is* the key event to measure initially. If there is no hypoxaemia (with the patient breathing air of course) then there is no problem.

These categories do not cover all patients arriving at a general sleep clinic, but do cover virtually all those arriving at clinics dealing mostly with sleep-related breathing problems.

At present the third category needs comprehensive monitoring which in most centres means full polysomnography. Some centres feel they can assess these patients in other ways, for example, with oximetry and video recordings (suitably analysed) or full respiratory monitoring and a move-ment detector. The other categories may well be adequately dealt with using limited studies. For example, in category 1 patients, a system that excluded any snoring, sleep disruption, or hypoxaemia in the supine posture would have a very low false-negative rate and thus prevent a significant sleep and breathing problem from going undiagnosed. The MESAM IV ambulatory system (Fig. 6.10) can do this by recording oximetry, pulse rate (mainly for arousals), snoring, and posture.[650] An earlier version recorded only heart rate and snoring.[519] Depending on the exact thresholds used to define normality this device is very unlikely to miss abnormal patients, but as a consequence has a high false-positive rate. This may of course negate any financial savings if polysomnography is often required subsequently. Oximetry (preferably with pulse rate) combined with actigraphy is useful in category 1: a normal oximetry, pulse and overnight movement tracing should virtually exclude significant sleep apnoea,[30] but the false-positive and false-negative rates have not been properly assessed. Oximetry and video record-ings are particularly useful, especially if the analysis is partly automatic. All night records of S_{aO_2}, pulse rate, snoring, and movement can be derived from oximetry and video recordings. If all these are normal, then it is almost inconceivable that the patient has a sleep-related breathing problem.

Category 2 patients (obvious cases of sleep apnoea) could have almost any of the already mentioned physiological signals monitored and they would confirm a significant problem. For example, observation (directly or

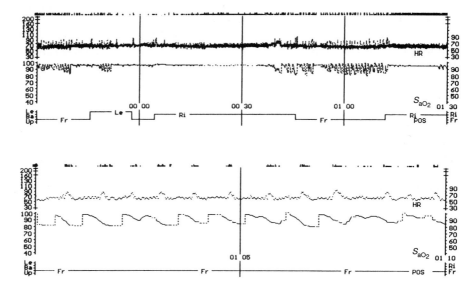

Fig. 6.10 Examples of two tracings from a MESAM IV system. Each tracing has four channels: first line, snoring (three levels); second line, heart rate; third line, S_{aO_2} (per cent); fourth line, body position (left, Le; right, Ri; back, Ba; front, Fr; sitting up, Up). The top tracing 2 h in length, showing almost continuous snoring with two periods of episodic hypoxaemia and heart rate oscillations. The bottom tracing is 10 min in length from a period of obstructive sleep apnoea: note the episodic S_{aO_2} dips, pulse rate rises, and the snore/silence/snore pattern. The heart rate rises and snoring are at the points of arousal, but the S_{aO_2} recovery is about 30 s later due to the circulation time delay between lungs and the finger oximeter probe.

via a video) could be enough and oximetry or MESAM IV would be virtually diagnostic. There is sometimes concern that central sleep apnoea looks like OSA on oximetry, but assuming the patient is coming in for institution of nasal CPAP then the obstructive nature of his problem can be confirmed then.

Category 4 patients (follow-up cases) can have a variety of physiological signals monitored to confirm satisfactory treatment. For example, patients on CPAP may only require oximetry, monitoring of mask pressure (pressure swings indicate breathing, no pressure swings mean apnoea or major leaks), respiration, or some aspect of sleep disturbance.

Category 5 patients (to be discussed in Chapter 11) only require oximetry to exclude a nocturnal hypoventilation problem. If the patient is on added inspired oxygen then something else needs to be used, transcutaneous CO_2 probably being the best. If there is nocturnal hypoxaemia then the cause may need to be elucidated with a full study, particularly if additional upper airway obstruction is suspected. Polysomnography may fail to detect additional upper airway obstruction in patients with weak inspiratory muscles because, in the face of upper airway obstruction, inspiration may be too weak to produce detectable movement of the rib-cage or abdominal movement transducers.

This breakdown of patients into certain categories, and the description of the many alternative approaches to monitoring them has, I hope, impressed upon the reader that there is no one right way to do a sleep study. What is required is a clear understanding of the conditions being studied and an appreciation that most of the signals one can monitor are *indirect* measures of the primary problems in OSA (upper airway obstruction and sleep disturbance) and, thus, have limitations. This approach and a good understanding of the problem is infinitely more important than insisting on having the full polysomnographic kit used on all patients, as if this alone guarantees diagnostic excellence.

6.9 Aspects of analysis and interpretation

In the early days of understanding hypertension there were attempts to define normal versus abnormal blood pressure. It was George Pickering who convinced everyone that such arguments were sterile and that blood pressure in a population was a continuous variable. Attached to this continuous distribution of blood pressures was an increasing risk of complications; the higher the BP, the higher the risk. Many disorders in medicine are like this, for example, type II diabetes, atheroma, and hypercholesterolaemia, whereas some disorders clearly do not exhibit a continuous spectrum such as cancer or myocardial infarction. There has always been a tendency to want to decide if someone has a condition or not, because uncertainty is difficult to deal with. However, the problem in hypertension was solved by thinking of both the risks associated with certain BP levels, the risks associated with treatment, and then trying to balance one against the other to establish risk/benefit ratios for different treatments in different circumstances.

Hopefully we are now moving away from viewing obstructive sleep apnoea as a condition which you either do or do not have. However, units still talk about cut-off levels for abnormality at either 10 or 15 apnoeas or hypopnoeas per hour of sleep. These cut-offs may be appropriate for research work to define populations under study, but are wholly inappropriate in clinical practice. To suggest that a patient with 14 apnoeas per hour is different from a patient with 16 apnoeas per hour is clearly nonsense, particularly when the night to night variation of an apnoea–hypopnoea index (AHI) in this range is enormous.[3,479,668] In one European country reimbursement for CPAP is only allowed if the AHI is over 15, leading to the absurd situation of severely sleepy patients having studies repeated until they reach the magic threshold.

Upper airway problems during sleep behave as a continuum as has been emphasized earlier. The precise risk to the patient as the severity worsens is not really known, nor is the best way to quantify properly this spectrum (cf. the argument over one-off blood pressures and 24 h BP monitoring). The clinical description of this spectrum starts with people who snore only with alcohol when supine, moving to supine snorers without alcohol, to snorers with arousals when supine only with perhaps non-arousing snoring in other postures, to obstructive events when supine only, to full blown obstructive sleep apnoea in any posture. A description of where a patient lies on this spectrum is useful, but an apnoea–hypopnoea index does not provide this information adequately.

A patient with OSA in all postures will have an AHI in excess of 30 because the cycle time rarely exceeds 2 min and is usually approximately 1 min giving AHI values of approximately 60. A patient with OSA only when supine can potentially have an AHI anywhere between zero and 60 or so depending on how long he happens to spend supine on the study night (Fig. 6.11). A patient with snoring induced arousals throughout the night may only have a few classic obstructive events and have a 'normal' AHI.

All this leads to the conclusion that the patient's breathing during sleep needs to be characterized into broad categories. For example, these might be normal; mild, moderate, or severe OSA; mild, moderate, or severe snoring with or without arousals. Great accuracy is not required, but these descriptions are *combined with the history* to make decisions about treatment. If a patient is sleepy and has no evidence of upper airway problems producing sleep disruption then it is probably inappropriate to try CPAP. If he is only mildly sleepy then NCPAP might not be worth trying unless the OSA is very severe, conversely, if he is severely sleepy then even if the sleep disruption due to upper airway problems is apparently mild one might try CPAP. These are 'grey' decisions and, in our current state of knowledge, so they should be.

How then can one gain the information required to run a sleep and breathing service if there are no clear guidelines? The answer is that, as with any other branch of medicine, an apprenticeship is required. One cannot, for example, learn how to do and interpret a bronchoscopy or an echocardiographic examination of the heart from a book, although the principles and foundations necessary to make rapid use of subsequent practical experience may be so gained.

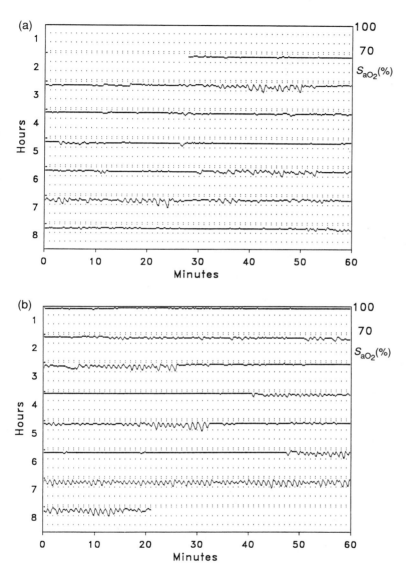

Fig. 6.11 Two separate overnight tracings of arterial oxygen saturation from the same subject with obstructive sleep apnoea only when supine. (a) The >4 per cent S_{aO_2} dip rate is 2.9 per hour on the first occasion and (b) higher at 10.8 per hour on the second because a greater proportion of the night was spent supine. The >4 per cent S_{aO_2} dip rate whilst supine is actually approximately 55 per hour.

6.10 The Oxford approach

The systems used in the three sleep laboratories in the Oxford Sleep Unit have evolved over several years as our understanding of sleep-related breathing conditions has evolved (Fig. 6.12). This process will of course continue and the drive is to establish an ambulatory approach that will be similar to the 24 h Holter monitoring approach to ECG recording. Specific *numbers* for apnoeas, hypoxic events, etc., have never been used to determine treatment options, but the study results are interpreted taking account of the patient's symptoms. The essential question is 'does this person have a sleep study result that could explain his symptoms and would he therefore be likely to respond to a particular treatment?'

Following outpatient assessment, the patient is allocated to the categories outlined earlier in this chapter (p. 108). Patients in categories 1 and 2 are studied in laboratories set up for oximetry and video recordings. The data are automatically processed to produce tracings of movement, snoring, S_{aO_2}, and pulse rate. Visual analysis of these tracings allows an assessment of sleep quality and will suggest possible causes of sleep disruption such as sleep apnoea or periodic leg movements. Areas of interest are reviewed on the video recording which verifies if the patient is awake or asleep, obstructing or snoring, or having periodic leg movements. If it seems that the patient is having events commensurate with his symptoms then appropriate treatment is offered.

Patients with unclear histories, or requiring further studies (category 3), are admitted for full polysomnography with oximetry and video. Often the oximetry and video recordings are still more useful than the polysomnography, particularly in picking up subtle problems of upper airway obstruction leading to recurrent arousals.

The problems of category 4 patients may be solved with home oximetry recordings, but sometimes it is not clear why, for example, a patient on CPAP suddenly gets a return of OSA halfway through the night. Thus, oximetry and video together are useful since the video can be inspected at the point where OSA returns. This will reveal, for example, that the patient dislodged the mask, rolled onto his back, his mouth fell open, or there were no apparent changes. This would allow the appropriate advice or perhaps a chin support or reassessment of the CPAP pressure required.

Category 5 patients just need oximetry in the first instance. Since these patients are often disabled in other ways, this makes home (or other hospital) recordings very useful. If the tracing is normal then, assuming the patient slept, there is no problem. If the tracing is abnormal it may be interpretable or may require a full study.

Oxford approach to the use of sleep studies

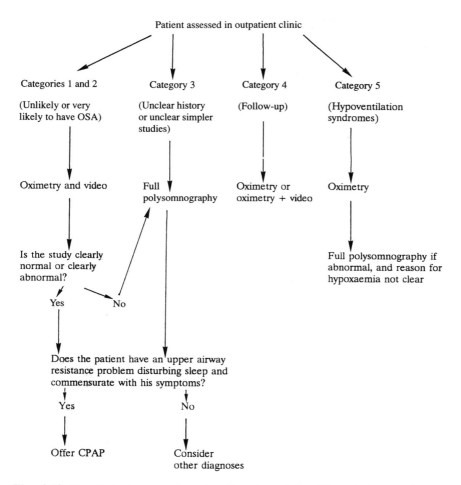

Fig. 6.12 The Oxford approach to the allocation of the different sleep studies to different patient categories.

In all studies not using classical sleep staging the question of whether the patient slept is usually raised. All the patients answer a post-study question on sleep quality. If the patient says they slept much less than usual then the study may need repeating. Patients may *under*estimate their sleep, but in our experience they do not *over*estimate. Even if they say they slept much less than normal it may be clear from the video that they slept for long periods. The available data on the usefulness of full *conventional* sleep staging suggest that it adds nothing to a respiratory sleep study for clinical purposes.[167]

7 Treatment of obstructive sleep apnoea

Treatment for obstructive sleep apnoea has to be appropriate to the severity of the symptoms. It is inappropriate to put a young man with minor sleepiness and mild sleep disruption on nasal continuous positive airway pressure (CPAP), he simply will not tolerate it. Therefore, a graded approach, with the aggressiveness of therapy tailored to the symptoms, is the best approach. The dominant symptom is of course daytime sleepiness. The problems of assessing this were discussed in the sections on daytime sleepiness and its measurement (pp. 65 and 68). On the whole the patient will make the decision for the clinician. Following the sleep study, where perhaps it was decided CPAP might be a good idea, the patient discusses the results and possible treatment with the clinician. CPAP and its potential benefits and problems are described and either the patient feels this is a potential solution commensurate with his symptoms or that it is not. Discussion with the patient is absolutely vital in order to gain the co-operation necessary to institute a therapy like CPAP. The rest of this chapter describes each of the various treatments and their suitability, but all along it is assumed that they are being assessed in the light of the patient's symptoms.

There are two caveats to the above paragraph. First, as mentioned before, the degree of sleepiness may not be fully appreciated by the patient himself and one is thus using the family's description of the sleepiness more than the patient's. In this circumstance the patient may need a little persuasion to try a treatment (see below). Second, although sleepiness is the dominant symptom guiding therapy there are others that sometimes need to be taken into account. For example, if a patient has associated lower airways obstruction and is in ventilatory failure (see p. 56) then CPAP will improve this failure bringing the P_{aCO_2} down and the P_{aO_2} up. In the presence of ischaemic heart disease marked hypoxaemia and blood pressure surges may initiate angina or malignant arrhythmias, making urgent treatment necessary.

7.1 Simple approaches

If obstructive sleep apnoea is mild or only minimally symptomatic then the patient is unlikely to want surgery or nasal CPAP. The mild to moderate group usually only have sleep disruption from OSA or heavy snoring whilst lying supine (see Fig. 6.11, p. 113). If an apnoea index is calculated it would usually be somewhere between five and 25 events per hour (that is, some sleep hours normal whilst lying decubitus and some sleep hours with apnoea indices nearer 60). These patients have upper airways that can sometimes remain open at night if they are in the right posture. It is interesting that in the Oxford epidemiology study[661] there were symptomless subjects with very short periods of supine OSA (perhaps 20 min in total) who would roll over onto their backs, have a few apnoeas and be woken enough to roll back onto their sides. It seems that some patients do not respond to their supine obstructions appropriately and simply lie there, repeatedly awakening after each apnoea, for long periods. It may be that there comes a critical time in the evolution of OSA when there is enough sleep disruption and consequent sleepiness to prevent the appropriate avoidance manoeuvre (that is, turning over) from occurring. This then ensures its continuation. We have had histories suggesting that symptoms began to be significant following some other event that disturbed sleep and made the patient more sleepy, for example, a long time shift on a west to east air flight. This is of course speculation, but it is curious that some people respond to their supine apnoeas appropriately (and unconsciously) whereas others do not. Cartwright and colleagues[103] have shown that posture training in this group can be successful. Although there are electronic posture alarms, the age-old remedy of a tennis ball in a pocket sewn onto the back of a tightish T-shirt seems to work well. The pocket is necessary to allow removal of the tennis ball(s) whilst washing the T-shirt, soggy tennis balls taking a long time to dry.

Other important advice in this mild to moderate group is shown in Table 7.1. Alcohol reduces muscle tone and encourages upper airway collapse (see the section on alcohol in Chapter 3, p. 39)[63,324,576,609,690] as do all the sedatives such as diazepam (Chapter 3, p. 40).[64,406] Snoring can be converted into obstructive sleep apnoea with quite small amounts of alcohol (Fig. 7.1).

Achieving adequate weight loss is a big problem. The results of weight loss programmes are very disappointing and only marginally better when an anorectic drug is used as well.[268] Even if a patient can be persuaded to lose weight, most gradually return to their original degree of obesity.[333] In mild cases, quite small amounts of weight loss can be effective and thus this approach is worth persevering with. There is the feeling that patients with OSA find it particularly difficult to lose weight. This could be for several

Table 7.1 Advice for patients with mild to moderate OSA, usually due to postural dependence

Learn to sleep on your side and avoid sleeping on your back
No alcohol after 18.00 hours
No sedatives
Lose weight
Stop smoking
Keep the nose as clear as possible

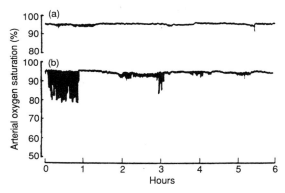

Fig. 7.1 The effect of alcohol on the overnight oxygen tracing of a snorer: (a) no alcohol, (b) with alcohol. Note the generation of worse hypoxaemia early on in the night when alcohol levels were at their highest. With permission from Issa and Sullivan (1982).[324]

reasons. First, sleep deprivation reduces the will-power necessary to stick to a diet, second, sleep deprivation may increase appetite, third, the sleepiness reduces daytime activity and, thus, the metabolic rate, and, fourth, the decreased growth hormone levels these patients have[242] may encourage the conversion of excess calories into fat at the expense of muscle bulk.[588] However, it has not been the experience of most units that many patients magically lose weight after successful treatment of their OSA, so the above mechanisms are unlikely to be very significant. One of our patients put on more weight after treatment, claiming we had increased his enthusiasm once again for sampling the culinary delights of yet more restaurants.

It has not been shown that stopping smoking helps to reduce OSA, but it is a known risk factor for snoring.[57] This may be through nasal congestion or by producing a degree of pharyngeal oedema. Since stopping smoking can lead to weight gain, it may not be appropriate to advise stopping smoking initially.

The relevance of the nose to sleep apnoea was discussed earlier (see the section on nasal blockage in Chapter 3, p. 41). It is unlikely that in severe OSA clearing a semi-blocked nose will help, but in mild OSA and perhaps snoring-induced arousals, it can help. This may require surgery, but nasal steroids (aqueous preparations instilled head down) and anticholinergics work quite well in our experience. For the small percentage with anterior nasal valve collapse, a nasal splint may help (for example, the Nosovent; see Plate 2).

For a long time there has been an interest in various prosthetic devices to try and keep the upper airway clear during sleep, usually by keeping the jaw and/or the tongue forward. There is some preliminary evidence that these devices can help in mild cases but seem unlikely to be of use in severe cases.[23,103,421,458,606,610] There may also be side-effects in the form of temporomandibular joint pain and tooth loosening.[247]

Only very limited surgery will be appropriate in this mild to moderate group. Surgery for a blocked nose, such as polypectomy or septal straightening, may in fact be accepted more for its possible benefits on snoring than daytime sleepiness. If there is an obvious anatomical abnormality in the pharynx, usually persisting enlarged tonsils, then tonsillectomy would seem appropriate and does work.[652] More extensive surgery, such as uvulopalatopharyngoplasty (see the following section) would not in our view be indicated unless the degree of obstruction with arousals was minimal and the pressure from the patient was more to treat the noise of snoring.

Various drugs have been tried in OSA, but have been very disappointing. They are mentioned at this stage because if they do have a place, it is only in the mildly affected patient. Tricyclic antidepressants have the best record and have been shown to improve symptoms,[89,121] and perhaps reduce the degree of upper airway obstruction during sleep, although well controlled studies have found no benefit.[743] The mechanism of action is not clear. By greatly reducing the amount of REM sleep, the time when OSA is leading to most hypoxaemia may be reduced, thus improving apparent overall severity. Protriptyline also increases upper airway muscle activity relative to diaphragmatic drive,[64] but whether this is of value in OSA, when these muscles are working harder with each inspiration already,[466,686,739] is not known. Protriptyline may also improve symptoms without actually improving the degree of sleep apnoea[540] but how it might do this is extremely unclear.

Medroxyprogesterone acetate has been shown to have a small effect, mainly in CO_2 retaining patients, where its mild stimulant activity on ventilation is appropriate.[687] An alternative explanation for any action could be a redistribution of fat to a more female pattern and thus away from the neck. Other ventilatory stimulants (for example, almitrine) actually make classic OSA worse, probably by increasing ventilatory effort and provoking faster (and therefore more) arousals.[371] Strychnine in theory might help OSA by reducing the degree of muscle hypotonia and in one limited trial it seemed to help,[559] but toxicity is clearly a problem here. Nicotine may have a similar action and again has been shown to have a small effect, but side-effects and a short half-life have so far precluded its use.[236]

Some units have used theophylline and claim benefits, but reported trials have not shown significant benefits,[44,253] despite a stimulating action on upper airway muscles similar to protriptyline.[386] Acetazolamide has also been tried in OSA with no useful effect.[743]

Finally, added oxygen has been tried. The main effect of this is to slightly lengthen the apnoea and therefore lessen the overall number of arousals per hour as well as tending to convert apparent central apnoeas and mixed apnoeas to more obviously obstructive apnoeas. There are small[227] improvements in symptoms in a small number of patients[444,638] but it is likely that there will be a greater nocturnal CO_2 retention, with the theoretical consequences of accelerating the onset of diurnal CO_2 retention. Given the expense of providing overnight oxygen there seems no good reason to use this therapy when there are better approaches.

7.2 Medical treatment—nasal continuous positive airway pressure therapy

7.2.1 Evolution of CPAP and how it works

Nasal continuous positive airway pressure therapy (NCPAP) is in theory a beautifully simple and appropriate treatment for OSA. Just as OSA is essentially a mechanical problem, NCPAP is a mechanical solution. The cause of OSA is the predominance of collapsing forces around the pharynx overcoming dilator forces: NCPAP provides an internal dilator force by raising intraluminal pressures and literally blowing open the pharynx so it no longer obstructs. There was initially some debate as to whether CPAP might also work by stimulating upper airway muscles, but in fact these muscles 'go silent' during therapy.[676] There was also the suggestion that the inevitable rise in functional residual capacity (FRC) was helping, but there is no good evidence for this theory either.[2] This remarkable development of CPAP in the treatment of OSA was made by Colin Sullivan[326,680] in Sydney, Australia. Figure 7.2 is from two of his original papers and shows how he originally applied this increased pressure to his patients during sleep. It involved the use of a small, close-fitting, nasal mask that

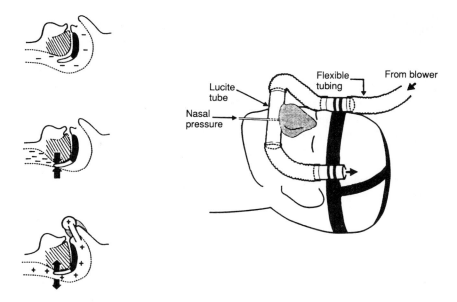

Fig. 7.2 Diagrams from the first papers on nasal continuous positive airway pressure from the originators showing the mechanism of action and the mask system in use then. With permission from Sullivan *et al*. (1981)[680] and Issa and Sullivan (1984).[326]

was sealed on the nose each night with medical grade silicone adhesive. This made fitting patients with a system fairly labour intensive, as did the custom-made masks that came a little later. In addition, most sleep laboratories had to have the pumps specially manufactured. This approach was tolerable whilst numbers remained low, but within a few years there were thousands of people on NCPAP. The next advance was the appearance on the commercial scene of CPAP units that could simply be bought 'off the shelf' with comfortable masks that fitted most patients with no customization (Fig. 7.3). Respironics were one of the first companies to enter this market with others following suit. A range of machines have appeared over the last few years, with increasing sophistication (Plate 4).

The secret of the masks was to design a shape that sealed with minimal pressure on the face. This was achieved with a skirt and buttress arrangement (Fig. 7.3). The buttresses give under pressure, with little deformation and much of the sealing is provided by the internal air pressure acting on the skirt. This design has stood the test of time for several years and been copied by other companies. There are a range of sizes to suit different shaped faces, but most people are happy with either a small or medium size.

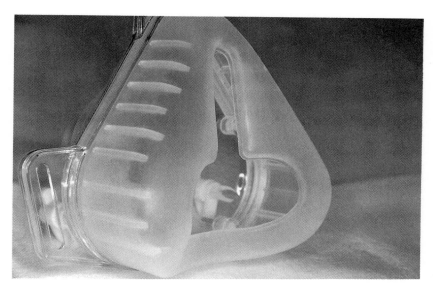

Fig. 7.3 Respironics nasal mask showing the skirt and buttress design that allowed a few sizes of mask to fit and seal well over most noses.

A recent development of this type of mask using a thinner skirt ('bubble' mask) appears to be a significant improvement.

The only other different development in this area of mask design has been the 'Adams circuit' (Fig. 7.4). This uses two soft cushions that plug into the nasal entrance. These are mounted on a bridge and, because they are corrugated, under inflation they elongate a little and help to seal against the nasal entrance. The idea is excellent, but the success of the system is limited by the poor strap arrangement holding the bridge and cushions in place. For odd shaped faces, patients with a mask phobia or persistent nasal bridge ulceration (Plate 5) it can be very useful. It can be used with any pump.

Because of commercial pressures new models with extra bells and whistles are being produced. However, a basic system that provides as constant a pressure as possible across inspiration and expiration is all that is really required. Some of the new developments in this area are described later (p. 132).

The essential requirement of a CPAP system is to provide a constant pressure at the nose and to prevent reinhalation of expired CO_2. The pump used should be able to keep its pressure constant at different flow rates so that a higher pressure is not met by the patient during expiration, as this is uncomfortable. Early systems began by using a blower with as flat pressure–flow characteristics as possible and used a blow-off valve set at

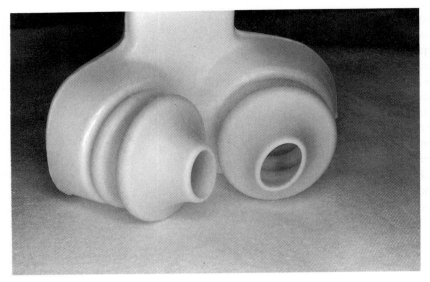

Fig. 7.4 The Adams' circuit nasal cushions, an alternative to the mask system.

the required pressure. The alternative was to use a much more powerful blower with a big bypass blow-off at the mask. This meant that the amount of air removed and added to the overall flow rate (about 200 l/min) was so small that the pressure did not change much. More recently blowers with better pressure—flow characteristics and feedback controls have allowed a return to lower flows and a quieter, reduced blow-off at the mask without increasing the inspiratory—expiratory pressure swings. In these systems the pressure is controlled by altering the motor speed rather than by a valve or by the degree of blow-off.

Additional requirements of these simple systems are that they should be reliable, quiet, portable, dual or triple (12 V DC) voltage, and not too 'medical' in their appearance.

7.2.2 Starting CPAP

Assuming the situation is not urgent, patients assessed as likely to benefit from CPAP are seen after their sleep study in the outpatient department to discuss this treatment. Because CPAP at first seems so bizarre, a careful explanation of what is wrong and why this therapy will work is required. If patients are reluctant to accept they have a problem and a little extra pressure is required (perhaps the wife recognizes how disabling the sleepiness is better than the patient) then we show the patient his video recording. A short section showing good OSA is selected. The patient is usually so astonished that further persuasion is not usually required! If the patient has impotence, then the fact that one can be fairly hopeful this will improve is a useful point to make. A date is booked and he is asked to use a nasal aqueous steroid preparation (instilled head down) twice a day for the week prior to coming in. This reduces the reactivity of the nose and the problem of rapid onset nasal blockage after commencing CPAP. In addition, an anticholinergic spray is provided (Rinatec) for use just at night. This is mainly of value on the trial night to help prevent any reactive congestion and reduce the rhinitis that sometimes occurs. These preparations can usually be dispensed with after the first week but may be required long-term, with perhaps 10 per cent of patients[678] having continuing nasal problems, but only about one or two per cent severe enough to prevent CPAP use. Anticholinergic or sympathomimetic sprays are also useful for nasal blockage during a cold.

In the outpatients department the patient is given a leaflet on CPAP and what to expect. They are encouraged to ring beforehand if there are any worries prior to admission. It is stressed that *trying* the treatment does not commit them to long-term use, that a trial period is usual after the first night in hospital, and that if after two weeks the benefits do not outweigh the inconvenience then they can return the machine with nothing lost.

We feel that the first night should be done in hospital for several reasons, although some other units do not do this. Part of convincing the patient that this bizarre therapy is appropriate is a fully successful first night. The patient needs to wake the following morning with a 'road to Damascus' feeling about CPAP. Sometimes the patients are highly emotional about the whole experience, just because they do feel so vastly better even after one night. If the first night has not gone well, then the enthusiasm is much less. Thus, it is important to get the right mask and make it comfortable with the correct tension on the headgear, problems of leakage need attending to, acute nasal congestion may need more aggressive decongestants (ephedrine or xylo-metazoline), and of course the minimum pressure required to overcome the OSA needs establishing. When the patient comes in during the evening he is shown the system and a mask size is chosen. He is then allowed to try it with the minimum pressure for a while. Our practice is then to let the patient fall asleep without the system for approximately 30 min, wake them up, and then put the system on with minimum pressure. Following the return to sleep, which may be lengthy but is usually less if they have had a *short* sleep just beforehand, the CPAP pressure is raised to abolish the apnoeas. We tend to increase it suddenly during an apnoea and to try and break that apnoea prior to the next arousal, thus the patient never wakes with the new higher pressure present. Should he wake, the pressure is dropped rapidly and the next good apnoea is used again to try and establish the pressure required. When the correct pressure is found, by altering the pressure up and down slightly while observing the effects, the patient is left with that pressure for the rest of the night. The pressure required varies between approximately 7 and 16 cm H_2O being higher in the heavier patients.[698]

The best feedback allowing one to acutely establish the pressure correctly is direct observation of the obstructive events by the bedside or on video. Alternatively, the swings of pressure in the mask can be as sensitive. Because of the delay in the S_{aO_2} at the ear or finger, oximetry is less useful here, although as an overnight device to assess therapy it is ideal.

The following morning, if the response has been less than satisfactory and the oximetry tracing shows periods of OSA, then the video recording is inspected for the explanation. The patient may know this was because of nasal blockage or that he took the mask off. On the video recordings mouth leaks, inadvertent removal, or a change in posture may be identified. If no apparent cause is seen then the OSA periods may well be during REM sleep when slightly higher pressures may be required. We tend to encourage the supine posture so we know that period, when the pressures need to be highest, is covered.

The following morning, if the patient agrees, which they almost always do, a new system is set to the pressure established the previous night and he takes this home for two weeks and reports back at that time to discuss if he wants to keep it. If one night has been a success it is extremely rare to fail thereafter.

This is not the only way to institute CPAP of course. Much of the above could be done in the outpatient department and some of the niceties could be abandoned. One unit shows patients a video about CPAP the night after their diagnostic study and then gives them a machine set at the commonest pressure, 10 cm H_2O, to take home. Two weeks later they come in for fine adjustment of the pressure. There will be many other ways to save time and the balance has to be struck between the benefits of a successful first night and labour intensiveness plus cost. Each unit will evolve the practice that suits their set-up, but simply providing a system set at 10 cm H_2O and leaving the patient to struggle with the complexities and problems himself will not achieve as good a success rate.

Compliance rates vary enormously between units and this may depend on the effort expended and the severity of symptoms deemed worthy of a trial of CPAP. In our experience the compliance falls off when CPAP is given to patients without considerable sleepiness and this has also been demonstrated in other units.[580] This is not surprising there needs to be considerable motivation to sleep every night with a piece of machinery that makes you resemble an elephant. The low compliance reported by some units[346,491,721] probably reflects their selection of patients (based more on sleep study results rather than symptoms) and their method of induction. In addition, previous palatal surgery is associated with poorer compliance,[721] as is a higher pressure requirement.

Patients will stop their treatment from time to time and the symptoms inevitably return after a day or so. On average the first night off treatment (following several weeks on) will not be as bad as pre-treatment, but by the third night it will be as bad. The explanation for this 'carry-over' effect is not clear, but may be due to the removal of sleep deprivation (which improves upper airway activity[405]) or an improvement in pharyngeal volume through a reduction in mucosal oedema.[592] Patients need to experiment so that if they are going away for a night or two they know if they are able to do without their CPAP. If alcohol is to be consumed on this night away, then we would recommend taking the machine. Some patients regularly have one or two nights off a week which gives them a feeling of less dependency on a machine.

7.2.3 Getting off CPAP

There are three ways a patient may be able to get off CPAP, weight loss, correction of a medical cause, and surgery (or all three). It is unusual for a patient to lose enough weight to cure himself although gastric restriction surgery may allow this.[685] Weight loss from the neck is most important and it is our experience that patients have to reduce their neck circumference for a reduction in CPAP pressure to be possible. Occasionally there will be a reversible reason, such as acromegaly or myxoedema that is successfully treated. Some of our patients have had large tonsils which have subsequently been removed. We would advise putting a patient with severe OSA on CPAP before and immediately after surgery, even if the surgery is thought to be potentially curative. This is because anaesthesia and opiates are potentially fatal for patients with OSA due to both a further reduction in upper airway tone and a suppression of their arousal response to obstruction. In addition, pharyngeal surgery can lead to acute further narrowing of the lumen from oedema and haematoma.[211,280,547]

If it seems likely that a patient has reduced his risk factors then he is readmitted overnight for oximetry and video recording following two nights at home off CPAP. It may be possible simply to ask the patient's spouse about return of snoring when off CPAP to establish whether a trial in hospital is indicated.

After getting off CPAP successfully the patient and their spouse are warned to watch for a return of symptoms. Routine monitoring is only done in response to symptom recurrence.

7.2.4 Results of treatment

In severe OSA the response to CPAP is like the response to penicillin. It is dramatic and gratifying, the biggest subjective response is usually after the first and second night, but improvement probably continues for at least two weeks.[388] The first night's sleep is much improved objectively with much more SWS and sometimes rebound REM sleep (with occasional particularly vivid nightmares).[8] Formal long-term controlled trials compared to placebos are unlikely to be done in view of the obvious benefits, but some short-term controlled trials have been performed. As stated above, patients would not go on using nasal CPAP if it were not beneficial. The family of the patient are often startled to see the return of a bright personality not seen for many years.[562] The improvement in any impotence is usually appreciated as well.

There have been some short-term objective studies looking at improvements in vigilance,[388] driving simulator performance,[189] sleepiness,[212,598] and mood.[159,206]

For example, in a simulated monotonous drive of 30 min where nearly 800 avoidance manoeuvres were required, on average normal control subjects hit nine obstacles, untreated patients with OSA hit 44 and in a treated group this fell to 13 hits ($P < 0.05$).[189] The multiple sleep latency test (MSLT) has shown[598] that pre-treatment patients with OSA fall asleep when left alone in under 3 min and that this improves to about 8 min after treatment (still in the slightly sleepy range). Other groups have also found that although the MSLT and maintenance of wakefulness test improve, they do not go back to normal.[212,614]

It is not clear whether failure of the measured sleepiness to fully return to normal is real, or due to the failure of the tests to really describe what is going on. It is possible that the CPAP mask itself is a little disturbing and prevents a return to completely normal sleep. On the other hand the MSLT measures ability to fall asleep rather than true sleepiness[489] and after years of short sleep latencies these patients may retain the ability to fall asleep quickly through behavioural adaptation, without necessarily being involuntarily sleepy.

Other consequences of CPAP therapy are on body physiology and long-term survival. The abolition of the upper airway obstruction removes all the immediate consequences. The hypoxic episodes disappear and the mean S_{aO_2} level rises (Fig. 7.5). Interestingly the rise in mean S_{aO_2} may not be very marked because the tracings during OSA may have had recurrent post-apnoeic ventilatory overshoots (with elevated S_{aO_2}) as well as apnoeas with hypoxaemia. The pulse rate stabilizes, partly because there are no arousals (tachycardia) and partly because the diving

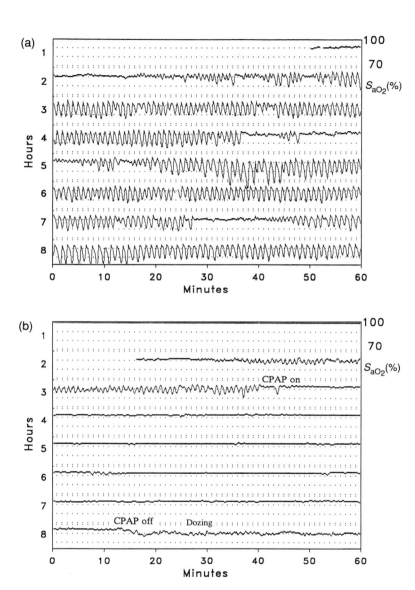

Fig. 7.5 Two separate overnight tracings of arterial oxygen saturation from the same patient with severe obstructive sleep apnoea. The top panel is before treatment and the second panel is on the first night of the nasal continuous positive airway pressure. Once an adequate pressure has been established the apnoeas are completely abolished.

reflex is no longer activated (bradycardia) (see the section on pulse rate, p. 49).

The swings in blood pressure are dampened out and this includes both the recurrent falls due to the increased pleural pressure swings, and the rise after the termination of each apnoea.[13] Figure 7.6 shows the dramatic effect of CPAP removal and reapplication on the arterial blood pressure tracing of a patient with OSA.

The true polyuria during sleep, discussed in the section on hormonal changes (p. 54), is abolished on the first night of CPAP (see Fig. 3.21, p. 55). This is often commented on by patients and the subsequent return of nocturia can indicate failure of nasal CPAP for some reason. This usually develops with the sleepiness, but occasionally appears to antedate it. The acute effects of OSA on hormones such as growth hormone also appear to rapidly reverse.[242]

Thus, it appears that all the acute effects of OSA on the body during sleep are reversed by nasal CPAP. Sometimes the ventilation does not fully return to normal immediately, but takes a few weeks with persistence of irregularity apparently central in origin.[732] This may be due to changes in brainstem control that take longer to readapt, for example, if there is a degree of CO_2 retention then the removal of upper airway loading during sleep may destabilize control due to relative hypocapnia and alkalosis. Readjustment of brainstem bicarbonate would be expected to take a few days and this is commensurate with the time course of the increase in CO_2 sensitivity observed following the commencement of CPAP.[48] These post-treatment irregularities of ventilation were much more common after tracheostomy[732] than after NCPAP[441,597] presumably indicating the importance of upper airway reflexes to respiratory stability or the stabilizing effect of a constant added respiratory load. Persisting central ventilatory irregularities after CPAP implies an additional diagnosis such as heart failure.[441]

We have also observed the appearance of periodic movements of the legs during nasal CPAP therapy with a similar periodicity to the original apnoeas. Whether the arousals due to the OSA originally obscured the periodic movements or whether this abnormality truly appeared after CPAP is not clear. They tend to disappear over approximately a month and may represent some longer term effect of sleep disruption on brain function. The practical consequence is that sleep may not be as dramatically improved as expected due to the sleep disruption of the periodic leg movements (see the section on leg movements in Chapter 6, p. 103).

There is very little information about the long-term effects of CPAP, particularly on mortality. He et al.[282] have published the only data. They followed 25 patients on CPAP for up to five years and compared the survival with a control group consisting of 104 untreated patients. There was a

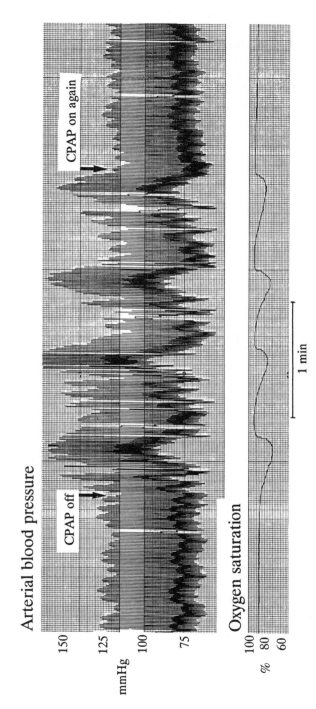

Fig. 7.6 The effect of obstructive sleep apnoea and continuous positive airway pressure (CPAP) treatment on the blood pressure oscillations. Note that instantly the CPAP is reduced the obstructions return with pulsus paradoxus and arousal-related blood pressure surges.

significant reduction in mortality by two years that had improved further at six years. This improvement in survival was not seen in a group of 60 patients treated with uvulopalatopharyngoplasty (UPPP) (Fig. 7.9, p. 138). The limitations of these studies were discussed previously (p. 57) and although matching of the groups was a problem, the conclusion that nasal CPAP reduces mortality is probably true.

7.2.5 *Future developments in CPAP equipment*

Several new developments in CPAP machines are appearing. Some machines have a period after being switched on before they come up to pressure. This allows the patient to fall asleep with a very low pressure and may aid compliance although it is not known how significant this is. New mask designs are appearing, although most are copies of the original Respironics design. The most significant change in mask design is the 'bubble' mask from Australia. This is similar to a standard mask, but with an ever-thinning skirt with a small hole as the nasal entrance (Fig. 7.7). The air pressure in the mask blows the soft skirt onto the skin with a better seal, requiring less added pressure through the attachment straps. More side to side movement of the mask is possible without air leakages.

Advances are also being made towards an 'intelligent' CPAP machine that determines the patient's pressure requirement automatically.[470] The simplest is a system that varies the pressure up and down throughout the night so that a plot of pressure versus apnoeas is available the following morning. From this the minimum pressure required to abolish apnoeas can be read off. Unfortunately, with this approach the patient may not get full benefit from his first night on CPAP and this may reduce his enthusiasm to try it further at home. The next stage is to have a system that adjusts the pressure automatically to find a level that abolishes the apnoeas. The problem here is what feedback signal to use to indicate the presence or absence of respiratory problems. Clearly S_{aO_2} is unlikely to be useful because of the delay between apnoea onset and subsequent hypoxia. Such a system would be constantly hunting around the correct set point. An alternative would be to use the mask pressure: as long as apnoeas (no pressure swings) were occurring then the pressure would continue to rise at a certain rate. Once continuous respiratory oscillations in pressure were present, then presumably the pressure would be high enough. The pressure could then be reduced slightly, followed by an increase once more to make sure the real set point had been reached. Such a system would be 'happy' with snoring, as long as pressure swings in the mask were occurring. Thus, it would be likely to settle at too low a pressure. Snoring and flow patterns could be monitored as well and such intelligent CPAP systems may have to

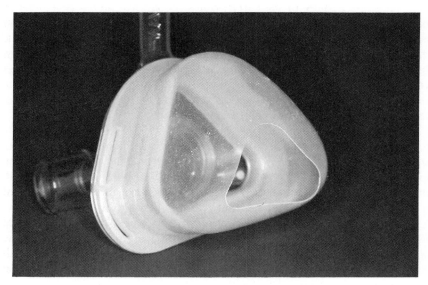

Fig. 7.7 A ResCare bubble mask showing an alternative skirt system that reduces further the chances of any points of localized pressure on the nasal bridge and face.

monitor a range of variables and build them into an algorithm before they would be safe to use.

The enormous advantages of such a sophisticated CPAP system would be on the first night in the laboratory or at home, allowing unattended CPAP titration. If such machines cost little more than the conventional ones, then they could be used by patients at home. This would allow night to night adjustment of pressure depending on posture, alcohol consumption, and weight changes. Whether such systems will sufficiently affect patient compliance compared to basic machines to be worth the extra expense is, of course, not yet known.

7.3 Surgical treatment of OSA

The use of a surgical approach to the treatment of OSA arouses hot debate. Nasal CPAP therapy is unpleasant and the thought of spending years and possibly the rest of one's life, needing nightly connection to a machine is clearly a major driving force to seek an alternative, one-off, solution. Thus, despite the excellent results of nasal CPAP, a less satisfactory result from a surgical approach may be acceptable. This also means that there will be a strong placebo effect of any operation if it means the possibility of coming off nasal CPAP. Many of the early studies on surgical approaches did not take a placebo effect into account, using only symptoms to claim success[294] and none had any control groups. There is certainly a poor correlation between symptomatic improvement and the improvement in the sleep study post-UPPP.[608] Although throughout this book we have stressed that symptoms should dictate therapy, we would *not* argue that apparent resolution of symptoms automatically means an adequate response to therapy, because of this powerful placebo effect.

The justification for a surgical approach to OSA is that there is an anatomical cause that can be corrected. In the case of markedly enlarged tonsils this is clearly true.[652] In the majority of patients with OSA, apart from obesity, it is difficult to be convinced that there is a true causal anatomical problem. In the section on causes of OSA the problem of whether an abnormality *causes* OSA or *results* from it, was discussed (p. 37). Cephalometric studies have shown many differences between patients with OSA and control subjects.[258,330,422,674] The dominant abnormality is subtle shortening and repositioning of the mandible and possibly the maxilla, thus reducing the retroglossal space. The second dominant finding is a large and elongated soft palate. The problem is that the enlarged soft palate may *result* from the presence of OSA[143,427,592] rather than be a cause. This may also be true of the third commonly found difference in OSA patients, that of a low and retropositioned hyoid bone (see Fig. 3.13, p. 38). Lugaresi *et al.*[427] first suggested that the enormous inspiratory effort made during actual obstruction could have secondary remodelling consequences, for example, pulling down palatal tissue, hypertrophy of genioglossus, and a drawing down of the root of the tongue out of the pharynx, through its attachment to the hyoid, this latter movement being seen after mandibular reduction surgery and interpreted as a normal response to pharyngeal crowding.[744]

This leads to the possibility that surgical approaches to 'correct' these abnormalities may be inappropriate. All this, coupled with the fact that obesity is by far and away the dominant risk factor for OSA, makes it clear that good evidence of an adequate and long-term response to a surgical technique should be sought before its widespread acceptance. This did not happen in the case of UPPP.

7.3.1 *Tracheostomy*

Tracheostomy was the first surgical treatment for OSA, tried in 1969, and is highly effective.[380] The tracheostomy is kept closed during the day and open at night, thus effectively bypassing the pharyngeal obstruction.

Many tracheostomies were done for OSA prior to the introduction of UPPP and nasal CPAP.[262,628,732] There are of course many problems associated with tracheostomy, particularly psychosocial. There are the problems of keeping the stoma clean and odour-free, bleeding, granulation tissue, infection, embarrassment, and in obese subjects one of their multiple chins can obstruct the entrance during sleep with return of sleep apnoea. These problems have led to the virtual abandonment of tracheostomy for OSA, but it should still be considered in very selected cases. Absolute refusal to consider nasal CPAP in the presence of severe OSA would be an example although this has only been appropriate in one of our patients. Tracheostomy has been used to 'cover' other interventions that may make matters temporarily worse (such as UPPP), but nasal CPAP should be a better alternative to this as long as the post-operative oedema is not so severe as to obliterate the pharyngeal lumen completely.

The precise construction of a tracheostomy varies between surgeons and there are a variety of tracheostomy tubes available. The most appropriate is a small (1 cm outer diameter), fenestrated, uncuffed tube with an inner tube (to allow the easiest cleaning) with a secure plug for daytime use. A minitracheostomy has been tried, but the airflow available is not adequate. Although in theory a small hole in the trachea might lessen the vacuum generated in the pharynx and prevent collapse, this does not seem to be significant enough to prevent pharyngeal obstruction.

7.3.2 Nasal surgery

These operations were discussed in the section on simple approaches earlier in this chapter (p. 120) when considering treatment for mild OSA. In severe OSA, with complete collapse of the pharynx, altering nasal resistance should not *in theory* help. This is because the pharynx probably behaves like a Starling resistor (see Fig. 3.15, p. 42). During inspiration, through a semi-blocked nose, the intrapharyngeal pressures will be well below atmospheric and draw in the pharyngeal walls. Once *complete* collapse occurs then there is no longer any flow and no longer any generation of a subatmospheric pressure, so the pharynx springs open again. With flow resumption it will again be sucked in, thus *snoring* will be provoked by a high nasal resistance, but not in theory *full continuing obstruction*. Therefore, nasal surgery may help snoring and perhaps snoring-induced arousals, but not OSA. However, there may be considerable hysteresis in the pressure–volume characteristics of the pharynx such that it is not a perfect Starling resistor. This would mean that if the pharynx could be stopped from collapsing in the first place there would be some benefit. An alternative explanation is based on the finding that nasal 'flow' receptors can influence the activity of pharyngeal dilator muscles.[449] Thus, nasal obstruction can induce a few obstructive events during sleep in normal subjects,[401,402,457,769] a phenomenon also noted after nasal packing for epistaxis or following nasal surgery.[183,691,737] There is little evidence for these mechanisms being important in severe OSA, but there are a few isolated reports of benefit from nasal surgery, including anterior nasal reconstruction,[152] septal straightening, and polyp removal.[290,585]

7.3.3 *Uvulopalatopharyngoplasty*

Uvulopalatopharyngoplasty (UPPP) is an operation designed to increase the volume of the pharynx (and possibly reduce its compliance) by resecting pharyngeal wall tissue and the soft palate. There are many different ways to perform this operation and in practice range from little more than an uvulectomy to radical resection of most of the soft palate, tonsillar fauces, and other mucosal folds in the pharynx (Fig. 7.8). Some of these differences are described by Fairbanks *et al.*[184] Ikematsu[321] is credited with introducing this operation for snoring, first trying it in 1952, and his first report of this method appeared in Japanese in 1964. It was Fujita *et al.*[209] who first published in English and tried it for OSA. Although initial reports did include some caution as to the universal applicability of this operation,[184] it soon became routine in the USA for the treatment of OSA. More recently there has been a waning of enthusiasm and an admission that UPPP is too infrequently curative[247] and does not improve long-term survival as does CPAP or tracheostomy[282] (Fig. 7.9, see also Figs 3.23 and 24, pp. 59 and 60).

Early on it was realized that not all patients were cured by UPPP, although most improved to some extent. In 1985 Fujita *et al.*[210] published a post-operative evaluation on 66 patients showing that 76 per cent claimed improvement in daytime sleepiness, but only 50 per cent had a reduction to less than half their previous apnoea index at six weeks post-surgery. A longer term (one year) study of the same patients[129] showed similar results; 50 per cent had a 50 per cent reduction in apnoea index compared to the pre-operative evaluation.

This response rate has been reproduced by other centres[93,153,210,221,347,357,629] although some seem to have done better[623] while others somewhat worse.[722] Table 7.2 is a breakdown of the results from some studies. Differences in the severity of the starting population make direct comparisons difficult. Many centres claiming a good response rate do not do repeat studies, but assume that improved symptoms mean a cure. One group has shown that although the apnoeas may be lessened, many are replaced by hypopnoeas instead[536] with, therefore, much less improvement in sleep quality than is suggested by the improved apnoea index. Nor can the disappearance of snoring be taken as evidence of cure since the patient may continue obstructing just as badly, but with little or very different, upper

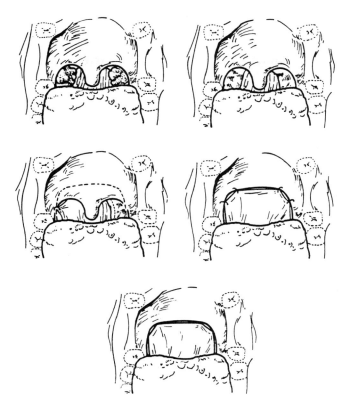

Fig. 7.8 Diagrammatic representation of the technique of uvulopalatopharyngo-plasty. With permission from Thawley and Shepard (1985).[702]

airway noise. Some patients post-UPPP have an unpleasant inspiratory sucking noise in place of snoring.

Because of the variable response to UPPP it was sensible to try and find a predictor of surgical success so as to operate only on those likely to benefit. There have been several such studies often with very different conclusions.

Table 7.2 shows the response to UPPP and also tabulates some of the features thought to influence the outcome. It should be stressed at this point that none of the predictors were by any means absolute, only relative, so that in an individual patient one could not guarantee success or failure, but only change the odds a little. The disappointing aspect of this work is that there is no agreement. For example, Simmons et al.[629] and Fujita et al.[210] found an opposite effect of body weight although most people feel that excessive obesity lessens the chances of success.[221] Riley[566] found that in UPPP

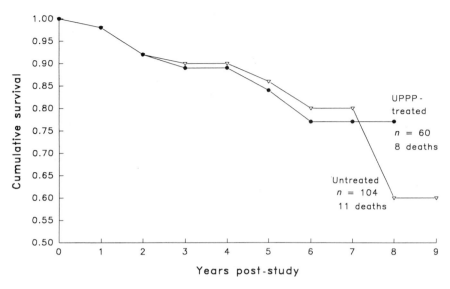

Fig. 7.9 This survival graph shows the failure of uvulopalatopharyngoplasty to alter the increased mortality associated with obstructive sleep apnoea. Redrawn with permission from He *et al.* (1988).[282]

failures there tended to be a narrower retroglossal space whereas Ryan *et al.*[589,591] effectively found the opposite. The site of collapse visualized by fibre optic endoscopy during a Müeller manoeuvre initially looked promising[623] but others could not repeat this.[137,208] Visualization during benzodiazepine-induced sleep has been tried, but in our experience this produces *more* upper airway collapse and obstruction than does sleep itself. Direct measurement of the site of obstruction during a normal sleep study, using a pressure catheter technique, has also failed to predict a good outcome from UPPP.[464] Even a recent optimistic review felt that careful selection could only increase the 'success' rate from 50 to 66 per cent.[621] Thus, it is impossible at present to give confident guidance on selection procedures to improve the response of OSA to UPPP so that one is left with an operation that, on average, half improves half the patients; not a particularly good outcome. Our current practice is only to consider UPPP for OSA in non-obese patients with big soft palates, no obvious retrognathia, who really cannot tolerate nasal CPAP. This approach is very conservative and may well be denying certain patients a successful operation, but in the absence of better data it is not possible to be more discriminating. If a UPPP is performed for OSA then a follow-up study is clearly important.

If UPPP was a harmless operation then perhaps failures might not be such a significant problem. However, there is a significant morbidity and occasional mortality.[259,280] The acute post-operative problems consist of acute upper airway obstruction[211,280,334] and haemorrhage. Some centres use either a covering tracheostomy or nasal CPAP to prevent problems of obstruction. Severe pain is very common, with a reluctance to use opiate analgesia because of the detrimental effect on obstructive sleep apnoea itself. Regurgitation of fluids back through the nose is common initially, but usually subsides. Aspiration pneumonia can occasionally be precipitated. Occasional nasopharyngeal stenosis is seen.[345] There has been concern that loss of the soft palate would prevent subsequent use of CPAP because there would be a failure to seal the oral cavity with mouth leakage of air. Should mouth leakage occur, then a chin support can help, but is likely to lessen the acceptability of the system.[721]

Another long-term consequence, apart from persisting regurgitation, is a change in the voice.[482,545,596] This is usually very slight, but may be important in a patient whose voice is important for his job.

7.3.4 Experimental surgical treatments

Some of these can be seen in Fig. 7.10. Because of the relative failure of UPPP, other surgical approaches have been tried alone, or in combination with UPPP.

A variety of operations on the mandible and maxilla have been tried, particularly by the Stanford group.[546,568,569] Maxilla and mandibular advancement is a major operation that brings forward both the mandible and the maxilla to preserve teeth alignment. This operation has been done for many years for cosmetic reasons, as has the reverse operation (which can provoke OSA[570]). It is appropriate to consider this approach if there is a considerable degree of retrognathia with a very narrow retroglossal space.[40,381,718] Again it is probably only appropriate to go to these lengths in patients unable to tolerate nasal CPAP.[546]

The hyoid bone links the mandible and the anterior wall of the hypoglossal pharynx. In theory, if it could be moved forward it should enlarge the retroglossal space. The limitation of this would be that the tongue would also be brought forward, but without there being extra space for it to move into. Attempts to move the hyoid forward have involved expansion hyoidoplasty and mandibular osteotomy. Although mandibular osteotomy clearly moves the hyoid forward and can relieve OSA, there is considerable doubt about the long-term outcome of this approach and it is likely that the hyoid will return to some extent to its previous position. The hyoid's position is plastic and will move in response to alterations in upper airway anatomy.[744]

Table 7.2 Results of UPPP and predictors of success/failure

Reference	Sample size	% of original sample	Length of follow-up	% with >50% improvement in PSG findings	Factors improving UPPP response rate	Apnoea–hypopnoea index (mean)	
						Pre-op	Post-op
Simmons et al. (1983)[629]	20	–	3 months	45	Thinner	45	29
Zorick et al. (1983)[766b]	31	–	6 weeks	52		62	30
Fujita et al. (1985)[210]	66	55	6 weeks	50	Fatter	61	7
Conway et al. (1985)[129]	20	<20	1 year	–		61	9
Norman et al. (1985)[357]	43	–	9 months	44	Less severe apnoea	53	41
Kimmelman et al. (1985)[357]	20	100	4 months	60	More radical palate resection	43	28
Walker et al. (1989)[722]	11	–	1 year	9	Presence of large tonsils and their removal	70	60
Sher et al. (1985)[623]	30	18	6 months	87	Oropharyngeal collapse during Müeller manoeuvre	82	33

de Berry-Borowiecki et al. (1985)[153]	30	100	3 months	47	Narrowing at level of soft palate and less severe disease	57	38
Riley et al. (1985)[566]	9	Selected as UPPP failure			Smaller retroglossal space and inferiorly placed hyoid bone compared to successful UPPP	60	67
Caldarelli et al. (1986)[93]	22	100	8 weeks	50	Worse sleep apnoea	70	35
Katsantonis et al. (1986)[347]	26	100	6 weeks	42	Narrowing at level of soft palate demonstrated during sleep	N/A	N/A
Gislason et al. (1988)[221]	34	100	6 weeks	65	Less severe sleep apnoea and thinner	50	21
Fujita (1990)[208]	64	Classified according to Müeller manoeuvre result on area of collapse			No predictive value	73	38
Ryan et al. (1990)[589]	60	100	3 months	83	Narrowing at retroglossal level, larger tongue	27 (AI)	6 (AI)
Ryan et al. (1991)[591]					Smaller pharyngeal volume, larger tongue		

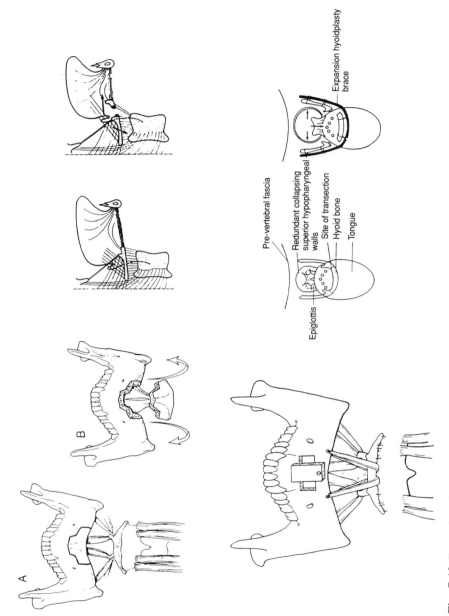

Fig. 7.10 Examples of some experimental operations to try and draw forward the root of the tongue. With permission from Cohn (1986),[124] Patton *et al.* (1983)[518] and Powell (1990).[546]

Labels in figure:

Pre-vertebral fascia

Redundant collapsing superior hypopharyngeal walls

Site of transection

Hyoid bone

Tongue

Epiglottis

Expansion hyoidplasty brace

A

B

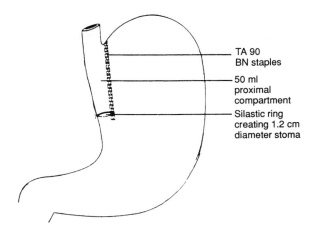

TA 90
BN staples

50 ml
proximal
compartment

Silastic ring
creating 1.2 cm
diameter stoma

Fig. 7.11 Technique of silastic ring gastroplasty that creates an non-enlargeable 50 ml compartment at the top of the stomach and implants a small inextensible ring through which food has to pass. With permission from Summers *et al.* (1990).[685]

Preliminary data show a good response to this very extensive combined surgical approach of hyoid, maxillary, and mandibular advancement in highly selected patients.[567,568] The criteria for operation included gross obesity, failed UPPP, failed CPAP, and significant retrognathia. In our experience this would represent an extremely small percentage of the OSA population.

Because the effect of being overweight on OSA seems to be mainly through neck obesity, direct removal of this fat has been tried.[259] In our experience (unpublished) it was difficult to remove enough fat from this area without risking vital structures: although chin numbers decreased there was little effect on the findings during a sleep study.

7.3.5 Gastric surgery

Attempts by obese patients to lose weight are not often successful, particularly in the long-term.[333] Since obesity is the dominant risk factor, it is reasonable to consider trying to bring about weight loss by other means.

The early surgical approaches for inducing weight loss, such as gastro-jejunal bypass, were hazardous due to metabolic disturbances. More recently gastroplasty or (gastroplexy) has become popular.[445] This operation (Fig. 7.11) produces a 50 ml pouch at the top of the stomach, above an inextensible orifice to the rest of the stomach. Thus, food will only pass at a certain rate, rather as in achalasia of the cardia. Overeating leads to regurgitation and a reversal of the operation is possible if weight loss becomes excessive. However, some patients seem to go on finding ways to consume enough calories to maintain their weight! The effect on OSA can be dramatic.[182,382,611,685] Operating on extremely obese patients is of course hazardous, but the risks will be greatly reduced when this operation can be performed laparoscopically.

8 Snoring

In earlier sections it has been stressed that snoring and OSA are essentially similar.[428,430] Snoring alone is really a 'forme fruste' of OSA and of course once OSA has developed, snoring is an important marker. The reasons for discussing snoring separately in this section are (1) because of recent evidence suggesting that snoring, even without apnoeas, may be harmful and (2) an increasing number of patients are coming to sleep clinics desperate for help with their snoring.

8.1 Is snoring alone harmful?

Early on in the history of OSA only apnoeas alone were recognized as abnormal obstructive events leading to arousal and sleep disturbance.[265] Then it was realized that hypopnoeas due to upper airway obstruction could lead to hypoxaemia and arousal, with consequences similar to classical OSA.[238] Hence, the apnoea index (AI, apnoeas per hour of sleep) became the apnoea–hypopnoea index (AHI). This broadening of the definition of the pathological events certainly brought more people into the diagnostic category 'OSA' and they derived benefit from effective treatment such as nasal CPAP. Some of these patients with shorter apnoeas and hypopnoeas did not necessarily get significant hypoxaemia and their symptoms could only be ascribed to the sleep disruption.

Various pieces of evidence began to suggest that even measuring hypopnoeas and apnoeas might not be identifying all patients with sleep disrupting upper airway narrowing during sleep (identified by a history of snoring) and the daytime consequences of hypersomnolence. Sleep clinics who saw sleepy snorers and performed sleep studies, found only a proportion to have an AHI apparently high enough to account for their sleepiness. For example, Crocker et al.[134] studied 100 patients, referred primarily with snoring, for the possibility of OSA. When comparing those who turned out to have OSA (AHI > 15 was their definition) with those who did not (AHI < 15), there was no difference in the prevalence of excessive daytime sleepiness. In 1986, Berry et al.[43] studied 46 snorers recruited via newspaper advertisements and found that there was no difference in the self-rated sleepiness of three subgroups, AHI = 0, AHI > 0–< 5, and

AHI $\geq$ 5. Whyte *et al.*[742] also found that the degree of hypersomnolence did not depend on the presence of classically defined OSA (by AHI) or its severity. Viner *et al.*[712] found that in 410 patients referred to a sleep clinic for possible sleep apnoea the presence or absence of OSA (defined as AI > 10) could not be predicted from symptoms of daytime sleepiness. Our group had also found that daytime sleepiness did not predict the presence of OSA in a group of sleep clinic patients.[145] However, sleep clinic patients are highly selected and of course sleepiness will be present in a large number anyway, thereby reducing the chances of finding differences based on the presence of OSA.

Other evidence to suggest that apnoeas and hypopnoeas were not the whole story came from epidemiological data. For example, Schmidt-Nowara *et al.*[607] found that reported daytime sleepiness correlated with a history of snoring. We also found that sleepiness and snoring were correlated in 900 randomly selected men aged 35–65 years, even when allowance was made for confounding variables and any nocturnal hypoxic dipping.[662] This study showed that the number of middle-aged men who could have significant daytime sleepiness due to snoring might be more than that due to frank sleep apnoea (defined by >4 per cent S_{aO_2} dipping). Figure 8.1 shows that the odds ratios for a variety of questions related to sleepiness and the effects of being a snorer. For example, nearly 10 per cent of 'often' snorers (about 17 per cent of the total men studied) (Fig. 8.2) admitted to almost having two or more accidents whilst driving due to sleepiness, compared to only 2 per cent of 'sometimes', 'rarely', or 'never' snorers. This effect of snoring could not be ascribed to a possible covariable such as obesity, alcohol consumption, hypnotic usage, shift work, or other illnesses.[662]

More evidence came from a big study of 580 patients referred to a sleep clinic with 'heavy snoring'.[297] Only 217 were classified as having OSA and 363 were labelled as snorers without OSA. There were differences in the symptom scores of the two groups, but with considerable overlap. Some of the 'simple snorers' had severe daytime sleepiness, as socially disabling as the patients with the worst OSA.

Our own work using the multiple unprepared reaction time as a crude measure of vigilance also showed that snorers without classical apnoeas or hypopnoeas could have as severely reduced vigilance as patients with OSA (Fig. 8.3).

It was tracings like that in Fig. 8.4 that alerted us to the phenomenon of snoring induced arousals. A typical polysomnographic tracing could appear normal apart from recurrent brief arousals. Without apnoeas, hypopnoeas, or episodes of hypoxaemia it was difficult to define or recognize a 'respiratory event'. However, on video it was easily recognizable that these patients were waking in response to increased snoring. The pattern, we

	Snoring status		Odds ratio and 95% CI	
	'Often' snorers	The rest	Before allowance for other variables	After allowance for other variables
Do you get chronic sleepiness, fatigue or weariness that you cannot explain?				
Never/Rarely	86.5	93.1	2.1	1.7
Sometimes/Often	13.5	6.9	1.2–3.7	1.0–3.1
Do you fall asleep during the day, particularly when not busy?				
Never/Rarely	46	56	1.5	1.4
Sometimes/Often	54	44	1.1–2.1	0.9–2.0
Do you fall asleep reading or watching television?				
Never/Rarely	36	50	1.7	1.5
Sometimes/Often	64	50	1.2–2.5	1.0–2.2
Do you fall asleep during the day against your will?				
Never/Rarely	92.9	98.5	4.9	4.9
Sometimes/Often	7.1	1.5	2.0–11.7	2.0–11.7
Have you almost had an accident whilst driving due to sleepiness?				
Once or less	90.1	97.9	5.1	5.8
Twice or more	9.9	2.1	2.4–10.9	2.7–12.5
Do you have to pull off the road whilst driving due to sleepiness?				
Never/Rarely	87.9	95.0	2.6	2.1
Sometimes/Often	12.1	5.0	1.4–4.8	1.1–4.0
Do you get morning fatigue, fogginess, or wake up feeling unrefreshed?				
Never/Rarely	60.0	72.0	1.7	1.5
Sometimes/Often	40.0	28.0	1.2–2.5	1.0–2.2

Fig. 8.1 Examples of the effect of being a snorer on the likelihood of being sleepy. 'Often' snorers are compared to the rest of a middle-aged male population (35–65 years). For example, 9.9 per cent of snorers admit to almost having had an accident whilst driving due to sleepiness on two or more occasions, whereas only 2.1 per cent of the rest of the population admit this. This produces an odds ratio of 5.8 after allowance for confounding variables such as alcohol consumption. Data from Stradling *et al*. (1991).[662]

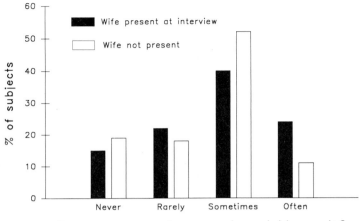

Fig. 8.2 Prevalence of snoring in 35–65 year old men (nearly 900 subjects) depending whether the wife or partner was present at the interview. Data from Stradling and Crosby (1991).[661]

termed crescendo snoring, was of increasing loudness of snoring with each inspiration (over a period of approximately 20–120 s) terminated by an arousal and repeated over and over again as in classical OSA. Without a record of snoring or the video to study, such a polysomnographic recording might well have been incorrectly scored as periodic movements of the legs with arousals, particularly if the leg(s) moved early on in the arousal.[549]

Guilleminault's group[264,648,649] at Stanford have published their observations on what they call the 'upper airway resistance syndrome'. Figure 8.5 shows increasing respiratory effort to overcome increasing upper airway resistance resulting in louder and louder snoring and is clearly the same phenomenon as that we called crescendo snoring. Their term is probably more accurate than ours because this increasing upper airway resistance during sleep may very occasionally not generate snoring. The abolition of snoring, but not the obstruction, is well recognized after UPPP, but Guilleminault believes that this syndrome of increasing upper airway obstruction with detectable arousals can occur in patients presenting with sleepiness and no history of snoring (particularly in obese women).[263] This totally new group of patients with potentially treatable sleepiness has not so far been recognized by any other sleep laboratory.

In addition to the recurrent brief EEG arousals seen in these 'snoring induced arousals', there are also the cardiovascular changes described in Chapter 3 (p. 49). There are falls in systolic blood pressure with each

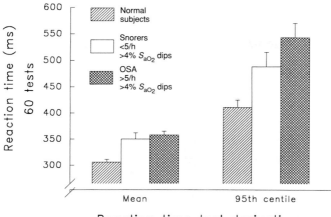

Reaction time test derivatives

Fig. 8.3 Results of the multiple unprepared reaction time test in three groups of subjects, normal control subjects, clinic snorers with less than five per hour of >4 per cent S_{aO_2} dips and patients with obstructive sleep apnoea with more than five per hour of >4 per cent S_{aO_2} dips. The columns labelled mean are the mean reaction times of the second 60 tests (out of a total of 120 lasting 14 min altogether) and the 95 centile column is the 95th centile of the results for the same period of the test. Each column is the mean and SEM of these derivatives for each group of subjects. Note that the snorers have significantly decreased vigilance as well as the patients with obstructive sleep apnoea.

increased respiratory effort as well as rises with each arousal (see Fig. 3.19, p. 52). Thus, if these blood pressure swings are part of the cause of the increased cardiovascular mortality in patients with OSA (see p. 57) then these heavy snorers may be at similar risk.[447] Our own data on snorers who rarely arouse (see Figs 3.25 and 3.26, pp. 62 and 63) shows that their overnight blood pressures behave similarly to non-snorers.[151] The epidemiological data on snoring as a risk factor for cardiovascular disease has been presented, but is as yet unconvincing. This may be because snorers with arousals are heavily diluted with snorers who do not awaken themselves or snore only occasionally.

The reason why heavy snorers might recurrently awaken despite no apnoea, hypoxaemia, or hypopnoea is probably because of the increasing respiratory effort they make to overcome the resistance. This was discussed in the section on sleep disruption in Chapter 3 (p. 49). Gleeson *et al.*[224,225] have shown that it is the degree of increased respiratory effort that wakes subjects in response to hypoxaemia, hypercapnia, increased inspiratory resistance, or an adenosine infusion, rather than the original stimulus (see

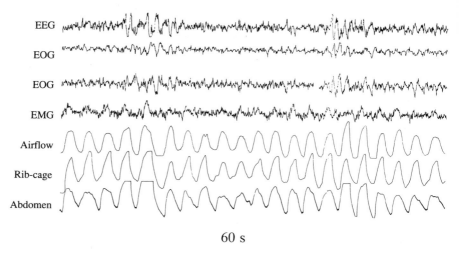

60 s

Fig. 8.4 Tracings from a patient with snoring-induced arousals showing the recurrent arousals, but no hypopnoea or apnoea. A slight waxing and waning of the three respiratory traces is evident though.

Fig. 3.18, p. 50). Normal subjects awake at levels of inspiratory effort (-10 to -20 cm H_2O) far less than those that can be seen in heavy snorers (up to -80 cm H_2O or so).[426]

The final proof that it is indeed the increased upper airway resistance (with or without snoring) that is provoking the recurrent arousals and daytime hypersomnolence is provided by the dramatic response to CPAP that we and others have seen. As discussed in the section on the interpretation of sleep studies in Chapter 6 (p. 111), it is impossible to draw up criteria for diagnosing 'sleep apnoea' when the spectrum of upper airway problems leading to sleep disruption is broadening all the time. The pragmatic approach of having to offer a trial of CPAP to anyone with disabling sleepiness and a history of snoring is rapidly appearing over the horizon, unless we can find the correct variables to measure.

Uvulopalatopharyngoplasty, when used for snoring alone, has been shown to improve vigilance in a driving simulator, a result that at first appears bizarre, but may be explained by a reduction in the number of snoring-induced arousals.[278]

8.2 Management of 'benign' snoring

This section describes a simple graded approach to helping someone deal with their snoring. The causes are broadly similar to those of OSA itself of

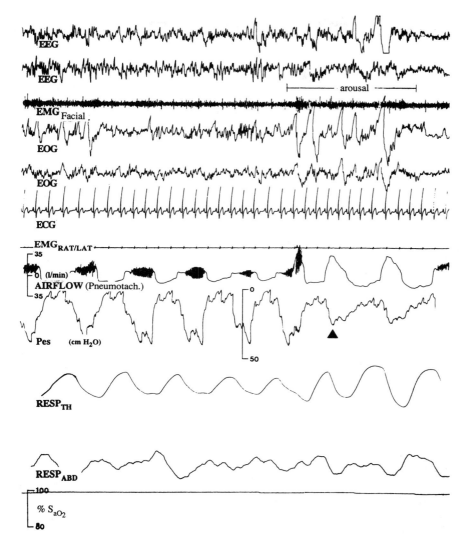

Fig. 8.5 Tracings of one snoring-induced arousal. Note the snoring being picked up on the flow limited AIRFLOW tracing, and the big inspiratory efforts shown on the oesophageal pressure tracing (Pes) falling as low as -40 cm H_2O. Just before the triangle (Pes tracing) the snorer wakes with a sudden increase in inspiratory flow and a reduction of the oesophageal pressure swings. There is very little hypoventilation and no hypoxaemia. $EMG_{RAT/LAT}$, leg electrodes; $RESP_{TH}$, rib-cage movement; $RESP_{ABD}$, abdominal movement. With permission from Guilleminault et al. (1991).[264]

course and were discussed in detail in the section on upper airway function in Chapter 3 (p. 23).

8.2.1 *Usual causes of snoring*

Various studies have shown that the dominant risk factors for snoring are obesity, male gender, increasing age (up to 65), smoking, increased nasal resistance (or nasal stuffiness), and alcohol or hypnotic use prior to sleep.[57,350,465,661] The strongest risk factor is obesity or, more specifically, neck obesity as estimated by neck circumference.[661] All these factors together only explain a small proportion of the variance of self-reported snoring. This means that there must be other important factors not measured or that self-reported snoring is not a very 'quantitative' measure of actual snoring (see p. 154). Although craniofacial abnormalities have been extensively studied in OSA this approach in assessing the cause of snoring has been limited. One has to assume that the same factors operate in simple snoring as in OSA and thus a degree of micrognathia or retrognathia is likely to be important: clinically this appears so.

If help is to be offered to snorers then it is important to try and estimate the contribution from the above factors in each individual patient. Our approach is very simple and consists of first asking about smoking, alcohol, sedative usage, and problems of nasal stuffiness, particularly at night. The effect on snoring of posture, alcohol, and colds is also asked about. The nasal patency is assessed, neck circumference measured, and the pharynx inspected for obvious abnormalities such as residual tonsils. A clinical assessment of possible hypothyroidism is made.

8.2.2 *Treatment of snoring*

On the basis of the information obtained from this assessment, simple advice can be given. Some of what follows was discussed in the section on the treatment of mild OSA (p. 118). It is important to point out to the patient that it is unlikely that their snoring is due to a single cause and that several lines of attack together may be necessary (Table 8.1). It is easy to take advantage of snorers as they are often desperate for a cure. Any 'new' approach receives instant publicity but new treatments, particularly surgical, should be properly assessed with controlled trials. Very few controlled and objective studies of antisnoring advice and treatments have been done and most of our advice is based on our and others' experience: what follows is therefore largely anecdotal.

Sympathomimetic nasal decongestants may be appropriate for occasional use or as a diagnostic trial to prove that the nose is the cause of the snoring. Nasal ipratropium appears to be a safe long-term decongestant although less

Table 8.1 Simple advice to snorers

Stop alcohol after 18.00 hours
Stop sedatives/hypnotics
Lose weight
Stop smoking
Sleep on sides only
Improve nasal patency
   Nasal decongestants (ipratropium)
   Hayfever therapy (steroids)
   Elevate bed head
   Nozovent device (see Plate 2)
Ear plugs for the partner

---

powerful than the sympathomimetic preparations. Elevating the bed head (but not with extra pillows which tend to flex the neck and worsen snoring) can prevent the increased nasal congestion that some people get on lying flat. We recommend pillows or a foam wedge under the head end of the mattress. Nasal steroids are worth trying even in those without a good history of hayfever. High doses of aqueous preparations instilled head down are useful initially to provoke shrinkage of the turbinate mucosa.

The Nozovent (see Plate 2) is a simple plastic splint that holds open the anterior nares. In our experience about 5−10 per cent of snorers get some benefit from this device although it tends to fall out during the night. During the examination the effect of splinting open the anterior nares on inspiratory nasal flow is assessed and, if it appears substantial, then it is suggested that the patient tries a Nozovent. They cost approximately £6 and are now widely available in chemist shops.

Posture training is helpful for supine snorers and ranges from digs in the ribs to sophisticated sound-actuated electric shock devices that wake the snorer up and make him roll over onto his side. The age-old remedy of a tennis ball in a pocket sewn on the back of a tightish T-shirt does work, but patients often will not try this simple approach because it does not seem 'scientific enough', although they will buy one of the electric shock devices!

Very occasionally a patient will be prepared to try nasal CPAP for snoring, even in the absence of daytime symptoms. This, in our experience, is very uncommon and if the patient can persist with nasal CPAP then it is because there has been relief of daytime symptoms which were previously unappreciated.

Ear plugs for the spouse can work quite well, but have to be either the compressible foam ones or the wax type. Industrial ear plugs are designed to filter out mainly high frequencies rather than the lower frequencies of snoring. Ear plugs are difficult to sleep with initially and take a few nights to get used to.

8.2.3 Surgery for snoring

The first surgical approach to snoring is to improve nasal patency when medical approaches have failed. Although both nasal passages may be patent it may still be worth making them clearer, particularly if a short trial of a sympathomimetic nasal decongestant (for example, xylometazoline, Otrivine) produced some improvement. The various approaches available include turbinate reduction, polypectomy, and straightening of the nasal septum.

We regard a uvulopalatopharyngoplasty (UPPP) for snoring as very much a last resort, but it is appropriate when all else fails. Because of the data on its efficacy in OSA, we tend to only offer it to non-obese snorers. In addition, a sleep study has to have ruled out significant obstructive episodes.

When offered in this very limited way it is usually successful and appreciated by the patients. In a recent follow-up audit of 30 Oxford patients who had had UPPP for snoring after trying various medical approaches, 26 said their snoring was better or much better and that they would recommend it to a friend when all else had failed. However, 17 had continuing problems of occasional nasal escape of fluids and 11 thought their voice had changed noticeably.

Other surgical approaches have been tried for snoring, but before any other procedure can be recommended it should be submitted to a controlled trial with objective measures of snoring before and after.

8.2.4 Verification of snoring

It may seem curious to have a separate section on proving that snoring is actually occurring, but read on. We originally took the history of snoring at its face value and assumed that if snoring had brought a patient (or couple) to the clinic then it must be a significant problem. Early on it was apparent that supposedly heroic snorers were silent in the sleep laboratory. We put this down to the different environment (although we did not know what factors might be important, for example, bedding, temperature, anxiety, etc.) or perhaps a lower pre-sleep alcohol intake.

It was also apparent that sometimes there was considerable animosity between a couple, often with the offending partner only present under great duress. Considerable snoring can definitely produce marital disharmony through lost sleep and the adoption of separate bedrooms. The relationship with alcohol also had the potential for arguments when a wife tries to limit her husband's drinking, knowing it will produce a noisy and disturbed night for her.

However, it sometimes seemed that the complaint of snoring and the retreat to a separate bedroom was a result of marital disharmony rather than the cause. It is difficult for the alleged snorer to deny that he (or she) was responsible for their partner's disturbed night and this provides a potentially powerful weapon to be used to justify various actions. If this were true in a particular case, then major efforts to help the snoring, perhaps leading to surgery, would almost certainly be inappropriate and marriage guidance more useful.

There is some preliminary evidence to back up the anecdotal impressions that the complaint of snoring may sometimes be considerably overstated. The failure to snore during a sleep study, when this is the primary complaint, correlates to some extent with a simple score of marital disharmony (C. Croft, personal communication). Comparisons between the amount of snoring measured in the laboratory and at home (with identical audio recording systems) only occasionally show significant differences (F. Series, personal communication), thus laboratory recordings may not be too unfair a representation of what happens at home after all.

If a partner is woken or kept awake by snoring, then it may seem as if the snoring is much longer than it really is, if they are actually asleep the rest of the time when there is no snoring.

Because of this uncertainty about what reported snoring actually meant, we have made audio recordings at home on two consecutive nights of subjects who, in our epidemiological survey of sleep apnoea and associations, had said they either 'never' snored or 'often' snored according to them or their partner.[651] We had already established that when the wife was present at the interview the prevalence of 'often' snoring was apparently higher than when the man was interviewed alone.[661] We used tape recorders with modified voice-actuated audio tape recorders, sensitive to sound down to 58 dB (and more recently 53 dB), which is equivalent to a very quiet snore. Snoring even quieter than this merges into noisy breathing and is easily blotted out with ear plugs if necessary. The operation of these 'snorometers', when placed on the bedside table, was verified in the sleep laboratory. Sound recorded on the tapes at home was also checked to ensure it really was snoring and not artefact.

The first surprise was that many of the 'often' snorers did not snore at all or only for a few minutes, on either of the two recording nights. However, there was some variation within the two nights, perhaps indicating that other nights could be a lot worse. In addition, some of the 'never' snorers had short periods of snoring (Fig. 8.6). This meant several things. First, questionnaire-defined categories of snoring are likely to be imprecise, leading to weaker associations (with either causes or consequences) than is

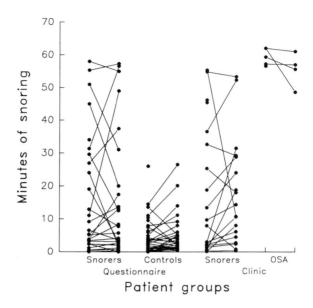

Fig. 8.6 Home measurements of snoring with sensitive voice-actuated tape recorders (maximum total record time is approximately 60 min). Most subjects monitored on two consecutive nights. Column one, subjects who on a questionnaire survey say they 'often' snore. Column two, subjects who on a questionnaire say they 'never' snore. Column three, patients presenting to the clinic with loud snoring who are contemplating surgical treatment. Column four, patients with obstructive sleep apnoea. Noise recorded is verified as snoring.

really the case and, second, that perhaps only a few minutes snoring is sometimes perceived and labelled by the partner as 'often' snoring. This led to repeating this exercise in patients referred to the sleep clinic. Snorers, who had got to the point of considering surgery (UPPP), having tried everything else, were asked to record their snoring over a minimum of two nights with the snorometer and for their partner to say whether during the night there had been a normal amount of snoring. Figure 8.6 shows that although many of the patients had the maximum amount of snoring recordable on the tape (60 min) on one or both nights, there were many with hardly any or none. In some of these latter patients the snoring had been described as similar to normal. Some of these patients went on to have up to six nights of recording, but no more than a few minutes of snoring was found.

This problem of not knowing just how bad snoring is, presents a significant problem when more than just simple therapy is being demanded by the patient or his spouse. It is surely bad practice to perform a UPPP on someone with only 10 min sleep-onset snoring (the commonest occasion for a short burst of snoring). Such surgery almost becomes ritualistic or sacrificial!

The best solution to this problem is not clear, but anyone assessing snorers needs to be aware of it. Sometimes discussing with the couple the sleep study and the home recordings, when they show minimal amounts of snoring, leads to a reduction in the demand for surgery by both parties.

To those not yet involved in assessing patients with snoring and sleep apnoea this section on the verification of snoring may seem a little bizarre, but the problem is not really any different to many other areas of medicine where symptoms (such as chest pain or headache) do not necessarily indicate the underlying pathology that is first expected, but are indicators of discontent.[38]

9 Epidemiology of adult sleep apnoea

The problems of investigating the epidemiology of OSA have already been mentioned. OSA is not a condition you have, or do not have, but there exists a continuum from no upper airway problems at night, right through to complete obstruction whenever asleep in any posture. Thus, the prevalence of sleep-related upper airway obstruction depends on the threshold level at which you arbitrarily choose to define it. In addition, in the mid-range of severity, there is considerable night to night variation[668] which means that individuals may cross a particular threshold depending on the night of study (Fig. 9.1).

It may therefore be better to look at symptoms, since these are what concerns the patient. But sleepiness is very hard to measure and can of course be due to many other problems, not just OSA.

This situation is exactly analogous to hypertension. Here is a condition with a continuum, variability in the measurement, moderate correlation between the measured abnormality and the physiological consequences, uncertainty over the best way to measure it (one-off versus 24 h monitoring), and finally some of the target organ damage looked for may not be due to just hypertension (for example, atheroma).

In terms of treatment the similarity continues. Decisions about the treatment for hypertension involve weighing drug side-effects against reduction of hypertensive consequences. In the same way the unpleasantness of nasal CPAP has to be weighed against the reduction in sleepiness.

A considerable amount of confusion about the epidemiology of OSA would be resolved if the continuum approach to thinking about the condition was adopted, rather than the use of arbitrary thresholds.

9.1 What to measure

In a condition with low prevalence it is necessary to study a large number of apparently normal subjects to obtain an unbiased value with reasonable confidence intervals. It has been prohibitively expensive (as well as having a high refusal rate) to do polysomnography on thousands of apparently normal people. There are essentially two ways in which this problem has been tackled. The first approach is to sample by an initial questionnaire, then to withdraw from a big population certain subgroups based on symptoms

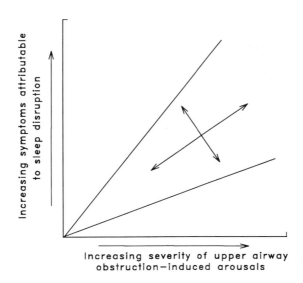

Fig. 9.1 Diagrammatic representation of the wide relationship between the severity of upper airway obstruction at night and the severity of symptoms. The exact position of an individual on this graph will depend on a great variety of factors. For example, (1) alcohol and sleeping posture, (2) individual response to sleep disturbance, (3) degree of arousal provoked by each respiratory event, and (4) opportunity to prolong the sleep period to partially compensate, as well as many others.

and to study them intensively with polysomnography. This leads to sampling biases and the inability to extrapolate confidently back to the unstudied population. For example, to what extent did the questions used stratify effectively on the basis of the physiological abnormality under study? The second approach is to study the whole population of interest, but to use a much simpler investigative tool to measure the degree of OSA, accepting a reduction in precision in exchange for bigger numbers and no bias. There are studies using both approaches and at some time in the future the results will be available from a very expensive survey where every subject is being studied with laboratory-based polysomnography.[765]

If the simplified sleep study approach is being used, then there is a choice of physiological signals that could be measured. The arguments about what to measure are, of course, the same as were discussed when assessing the place of limited screening sleep studies in clinical practice (Chapter 6, p. 105). The difference is that in clinical practice one cannot afford false-negatives, so one tolerates false-positives, whereas in epidemiology if the false-positives and -negatives are known to balance out the prevalence estimate will be correct, the absence of a bias being more important than high precision.

Table 9.1 lists some of the simpler techniques one could try and apply to a large population and their potential limitations. Combinations of limited signals could of course be used, but subject acceptability falls with increasing complexity of the instrumentation. The next section describes the available studies on prevalence which have used these approaches.

9.2 Prevalence data

Prevalence data are shown in Table 9.2. The first attempt at a prevalence study was from Italy in 1982. Franceschi and colleagues[204] prospectively evaluated all patients admitted to a general hospital in Milan over one year. Psychiatric, neurological, or specific sleep disorders patients were not included. A sleep questionnaire was administered to all. On the basis of this questionnaire, 87 (3.4 per cent) out of the original 2518 patients (1347 female, 1171 male) were selected as suffering from excessive daytime sleepiness. Although this questionnaire was based on their experience in the sleep clinic, no validation was offered, nor was a control group (selected for no sleepiness) studied. The mean age of their patients was 55.2 (range 6–92) years. Further study of these 87 patients (clinical examination and polysomnography) found 28 (1.1 per cent) with 'true' sleepiness. Of these 28, 25 had sleep apnoea syndrome defined as more than 10 apnoeas per hour of sleep of more than 10 s each. In fact only one patient had an apnoea index (AI) of more than 21 per hour and he had Prader–Willi syndrome (AI = 60). The other three patients with excessive sleepiness were thought to have either narcolepsy or idiopathic CNS hypersomnia. Thus, their approximate prevalence of sleep apnoea, defined by an AI of more than 10, was about 1 per cent. This population was clearly not representative of a randomly selected one, but subsequent studies have come up with broadly similar prevalences.

The study by Lavie[396] in Israel started with a questionnaire returned by 1502 industrial workers. At one point they are described as 'presumably healthy working men' and at another point as 84 per cent male and 16 per cent female. From these 1502 subjects, 300 men were selected, in proportions equal to the percentages of three different sleep complaint groups (8.1 per cent sleepy, 20.1 per cent insomnia, and 71.8 per cent no complaints) for possible hospital polysomnography. Eighty per cent of the selected 'sleepy' group agreed to be studied, but only 19 per cent of the 'no complaint' group agreed. Seven of the 20 in the 'sleepy' group, one of the 17 in the 'insomnia' group, and three of the 41 in the 'no complaint' group had AI values above 10. Thus, 11 out of the original randomly selected 300

Table 9.1 Limited monitoring techniques potentially appropriate for epidemiological studies on sleep apnoea

Measured signal	Device	Disadvantage
Body movement	Actigraph	Picks up any form of sleep disturbance and may miss micro-arousals
S_{aO_2}	Oximeter	Only registers events leading to hypoxia, some of which may not be arousing. Artefact can be a problem
Air flow	Thermistor CO$_2$ monitor	Picks up much respiratory irregularity which may not arouse and may be occurring while awake. May miss short arousing events
Chest wall monitoring	Movement transducers	As above and big problem with movement artefact
Snoring	Pharyngeal or room microphone	Difficult to differentiate arousing from non-arousing upper airway obstructive noises

had AI values above 10, but three had symptomless central apnoeas and probably should not really be regarded as subjects with significant OSA. Thus, eight out of 300 (2.7 per cent) is an estimate of overall prevalence for an AI of 10. There are problems of bias here which make it difficult to extrapolate back to the original population. In addition, it was not recorded if these apnoeas led to either hypoxaemia or arousal.

Berry et al.[43] recruited 46 heavy snorers by newspaper advertisements (men over 30 years) and studied them in the laboratory. It is impossible to know what proportion of a randomly selected population they were but perhaps 10 per cent of men are heavy snorers. Six out of the 30 men had AI values over five per hour which gives an approximate prevalence of 1.3 per cent.

Telakivi et al.[700] investigated men aged 40–50 years recruited from a Finnish twin study. Two subgroups had laboratory studies; 25 were 'always' or 'almost always' snorers (9 per cent of total population) and 27 were 'occasional' or 'never' snorers. On the basis of a sleep study with the Bio-Matt (records body and breathing movements) and oximetry, four were thought possibly to have a sleep and breathing disorder. Subsequently, only one had an AI > 10 on polysomnography.

Gislason et al.[220] sent a postal questionnaire to 4064 randomly selected men aged 30–69 years and achieved an 80 per cent return rate (3201). Of

Table 9.2 Prevalence data on sleep apnoea

Reference	Country	Population	Age range	Method	Criteria	Estimated whole population prevalence
Franceschi et al. (1982)[204]	Italy	2518 consecutive hospital admissions ♂ and ♀	6–92	(1) Questionnaire (2) Polysomnography on subgroup of 87 (no oximetry)	AI > 10/h	1%
Lavie (1983)[396]	Israel	1262 ♂	Working age	(1) Questionnaire (2) Polysomnography on 78 (no oximetry)	AI > 10/h AI > 20/h	2.7% 0.7%
Berry et al. (1986)[43]	US	60 heavy snorers	30–?	(1) Newspaper advert recruitment (2) Polysomnography on 46	AHI > 5/h	?1.3%
Telakivi et al. (1987)[700]	Finland	Approximately 278 ♂	41–50	(1) Part of a twin study (2) 25 snorers and 27 non-snorers had polysomnography	AHI > 20/h >10/h >4% S_{aO_2} dips	0.4% 1.4%

Study	Country	N	Age	Method	Criteria	Prevalence
Gislason et al. (1988)[220]	Sweden	3100 ♂	30–69	(1) Questionnaire (2) 61 sleepy snorers had polysomnography	AHI >10/h AHI >5/h	0.9% 1.4%
Cirignotta et al. (1989)[118,119]	Italy	1170	30–69	(1) Questionnaire (2) 40 heavy snorers had polysomnography	Severe and symptomatic AHI >10/h AHI >5/h	0.5% 3.3% 5.1%
Stradling and Crosby (1991)[659]	UK	1001 ♂	35–65	Oximetry on 893	Severe, symptomatic and >20/h >4% S_{aO_2} dips >10/h >4% S_{aO_2} dips >5/h >4% S_{aO_2} dips	0.3% 1% 4.6%
Gleadhill et al. (1991)[222]	Northern Ireland	920 ♂	40–64	(1) Questionnaire (2) Oximetry on 138 'symptomatic', 164 'controls'	>10/h >3% S_{aO_2} dips + symptoms	0.8%
Approximate average					**>20 events/h** **>10 events/h** **>5 events/h**	**0.3–0.7%** **0.8–3%** **1.5–5%**

these, 3100 men answered questions on snoring and sleepiness, from which the 166 with the highest scores for these two symptoms were selected. Sixty-one of these 166 came for laboratory polysomnography. Apnoea and hypopnoea indices were measured, there being 16 with an AHI over five and 10 with an AHI over 10. Extrapolating backwards and assuming the 166 are the appropriate population containing all the subjects with AHI values over five, then the prevalences for AHI values of five and 10 are 1.4 and 0.9 per cent respectively. The major assumption here is that all the abnormal subjects are selected by their questionnaire; if this is not so, then these prevalences are a minimum estimate.

Cirignotta et al.[118] sent questionnaires to 3479 men aged 30–69 years. Of these, 1170 returned the questionnaire (34 per cent) and about 119 admitted to 'every-night' snoring. From these 119 snorers, 40 were admitted for polysomnography. Thirteen subjects had an AI over 10 and 20 subjects over five, thus approximately 3.3 per cent of the original population had an AI over 10 and 5.1 per cent over five. Severe symptomatic OSA was actually only present in the two with the highest AI, thus making the prevalence of OSA probably requiring treatment about 0.5 per cent.

Our study[661] attempted to avoid bias by doing a limited sleep study on all subjects selected. If the symptoms are not well correlated with sleep study findings, then just studying an apparently symptomatic group will underestimate the prevalence of the physiological abnormality, because it will be present in some apparently normal people. Certainly in the clinic there are patients with severe OSA who deny symptoms initially and who have usually only come to the clinic at the insistence of their wives. Initially 1001 men, aged 35–65 years, were selected from one group general practice. Nine hundred agreed to be seen and questioned at home, 893 of whom agreed to have overnight oximetry at home. Forty-six subjects (4.6 per cent) had >4 per cent S_{aO_2} dip rates of over five per hour, 10 (1 per cent) over 10 per hour and three (0.3 per cent) over 20 per hour (Fig. 9.2). Thirty-one of the 46 with dip rates over five per hour were studied in a sleep laboratory: the three subjects (0.3 per cent) with dip rates over 20 per hour had severe symptomatic OSA and the rest who slept adequately in the laboratory had postural (supine only) obstructive sleep apnoea which accounted for their lower number of desaturations (Fig. 9.3).

The last study described here, from Northern Ireland[222] involved analysing 920 questionnaires received back from men aged 40–64 years. Of these, 163 (17.7 per cent) had 'symptoms suggestive of sleep apnoea'. Home oximetry studies were performed on 138 of these symptomatic subjects and on 164 control subjects. Seven of the study group (0.8 per cent of the total) had over 10 per hour of >3 per cent S_{aO_2} dips. The desaturation rates of the two groups were different, suggesting that the questionnaire had

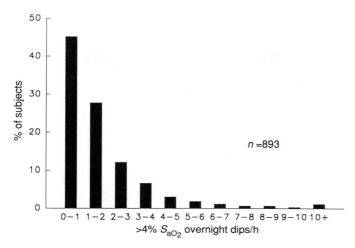

Fig. 9.2 Prevalence of different rates of nocturnal hypoxaemic dipping in men aged 35–65 years. Note the smooth fall off in prevalence towards the higher dipping rates with no suggestion of a bimodal distribution.

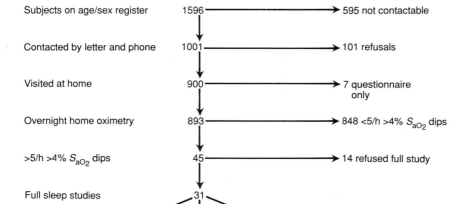

Fig. 9.3 Results of the Oxford community survey of nocturnal hypoxic events showing the starting population and the numbers selected at each stage for further study.

managed to select a higher risk subgroup. Snoring was the best predictor of S_{aO_2} dipping.

If all these studies are put together and an average prevalence of different levels of 'sleep apnoea activity' estimated, then it appears that approximately 0.3—0.7 per cent of the adult male population (under 70 years) have symptomatic sleep apnoea with 'apnoea rates' over 20 per hour. Apnoea rates over 10 per hour occur in approximately 0.8—3 per cent of adult males and rates over five per hour in approximately 1.5—5 per cent. These are extremely rough estimates because of the different techniques used by the different groups and therefore like is not being compared exactly with like. Having said that, there is broad agreement considering the different approaches.

The problem only partially addressed by any of the studies is whether the so-called symptoms of sleep apnoea bore any relation to the apnoea activity subsequently discovered. There were many subjects, selected by questionnaire for likely sleep apnoea, who did *not* have it on further study. In our study, where everyone had oximetry, it was very hard to show that the group with desaturation rates between five and 20 per hour were any different from the rest. They claimed to be a little more sleepy in the questionnaire (mostly so in relation to driving) but, on subsequent formal testing with the Wilkinson multiple unprepared reaction time test,[752] they were no different from a control group, despite this vigilance test being abnormal in most clinic patients with OSA.[659] As was also discussed earlier (see the section on definitions in Chapter 3, p. 42), snoring alone may disrupt sleep and produce similar symptoms to classic OSA, but without apnoeas, hypopnoeas, or hypoxic dips, none of the above studies would have identified such subjects. On the other hand a recent study,[523] looking at an older group of 92 healthy men (50—80 years), found a higher prevalence of 'sleep-disordered breathing' than in any of the studies described above. This group found that 15 per cent apparently had five or more apnoeas/hypopnoeas per hour (mostly obstructive), but this 15 per cent were no worse on a range of daytime function tests (including the multiple sleep latency test) than the rest. This higher prevalence in the elderly will be discussed in the following section. Thus, one is left with considerable uncertainty as to whether any of the studies will have accurately estimated the true prevalence of significant, symptomatic upper airway problems during sleep.

At an anecdotal level, from the amalgamated data above, there ought to be approximately one or two adult male patients with severe OSA in each general practice of 2000—3000 patients. In our experience when a general practice has had one such patient diagnosed they tend to find at least one or two others, thus this prevalence appears approximately right and is certainly not an overestimate.

If the prevalence of severe OSA of approximately three per 1000 in adult men is approximately right, then there should be approximately 36 000 in the UK (95 per cent confidence intervals 8 400–108 000). This would produce approximately 100 patients per chest physician who probably require nasal CPAP. This is a prevalence greater than sarcoidosis and fibrosing alveolitis combined, which therefore has important resource implications.[164,661]

9.3 Predictive correlates of sleep apnoea in epidemiological surveys

Some of the epidemiological surveys assumed that some aspect of a questionnaire would predict a high probability of OSA, but only a proportion contained a control group to prove this point. Thus, this section looks at possible predictors of OSA in those epidemiological studies that have control groups and those studies where all subjects were monitored.

In the study of Lavie[396] three groups were studied; sleepy, insomnia, and normal. The prevalence of AI > 10 in the sleepy group was 29 per cent and 2.7 per cent in the whole group. Thus, on the basis of their questionnaire about sleepiness alone, there was a 10-fold increase in the degree of OSA. The other factors predicting a higher degree of OSA were age, heavy snoring, restless sleep, frequent headaches, ENT abnormalities, and hypertension. No predictive effect was seen from body weight, smoking, alcohol, sedative use, or presence of lung disease.

In our study[661] several factors were investigated to see if they were related to an increased risk of sleep apnoea. One problem is that many of the possible risk factors are themselves related (for example, alcohol, snoring, weight, and age). Thus, it is necessary to use multivariate statistical approaches, such as multiple linear (or logistic) regression, to try and tease out the true independent predictors. Using this approach[661] we found that the following were *not* independent predictors of the severity of OSA, although they may have been correlated to some extent on single regression: cigarette consumption, nasal obstruction, ENT surgery (including tonsillectomy), sedative use, or use of other drugs. The factors that *were* independent predictors were: measures of obesity, snoring history, age, questions on sleepiness, and alcohol consumption (for example, Figs 9.4–9.8).

The association with obesity (Fig. 9.4) was expected and 'explained' approximately 6 per cent of the variance in desaturation rates. However, the neck circumference (measured with a tape measure at the level of the cricothyroid membrane) was slightly more predictive; 8 per cent of variance was explained (Fig. 9.5), particularly when a small correction for height was made.[661] Inspection of Figs 9.4 and 9.5 shows the small increase in

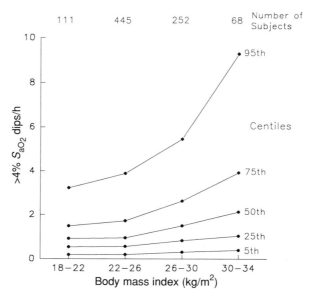

Fig. 9.4 Relationships between body mass index and hypoxic dipping overnight in the Oxford community survey. At the larger levels of obesity there is a tail of higher rates of hypoxic dipping (the 95th centile of the dip rate data almost trebling across the weight range). Numbers of subjects in each group are shown at top of graph.

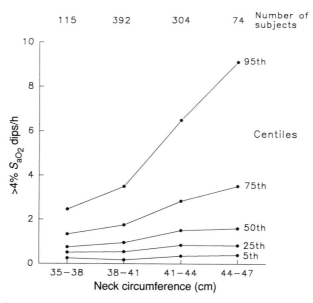

Fig. 9.5 Relationship between neck circumference and hypoxic dipping overnight in the Oxford community survey. The 95th centile of the dip rate data almost quadruples across the neck circumference range.

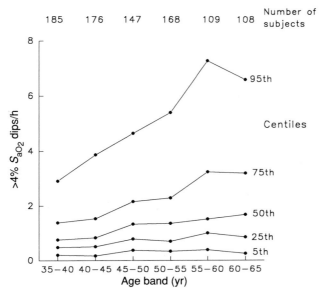

Fig. 9.6 Relationship between age and hypoxic dipping overnight in the Oxford community survey. There is a slight suggestion of a reduction in hypoxic dipping in the highest age group, a similar finding to others.

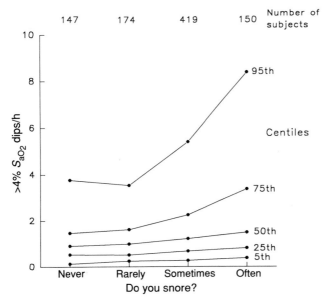

Fig. 9.7 Relationship between reported snoring and hypoxic dipping overnight in the Oxford community survey.

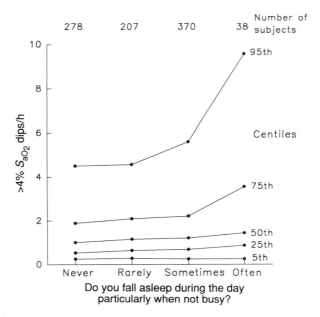

Fig. 9.8 Relationship between daytime sleepiness and hypoxic dipping in the Oxford community survey. Again, an effect of snoring is seen best as a tail of higher dip rates (95th centile) in the often sleepy group.

desaturation rate with increasing weight or neck circumference, but also reveals that only some individuals are affected, hence, the marked rise in the 95th centile line indicating that the higher desaturation rate individuals are concentrated at the obese end of the spectrum. The reason for neck obesity provoking OSA was discussed in the section on anatomical abnormalities in Chapter 3 (p. 32) and this association has been observed in clinic populations[143,145,348] as well as in this and other epidemiological surveys.

The effect of age has been observed by most groups. The possible slight decline in the oldest group may be real (Fig. 9.6). Gislason et al.[220] found most of their cases of OSA in the age band 50–59 years, with less in the 60–69 years band. In addition, the prevalence of snoring seems to rise up to about 60 years and then fall.[425,607] This conflicts with other data suggesting a progressive rise in AHI with increasing age[18,53,523] and sometimes very high prevalence rates of AHI > 5 of 25–50 per cent.[17,435] The explanation for this discrepancy could be that although AHI rises with age it may be due mainly to short obstructive episodes without hypoxaemia or snoring, resulting from the respiratory instability of light sleep, rather than classical OSA.[360,507,626] Any correlation between AHI and symptoms in the elderly is extremely poor, which also perhaps suggests a different aetiology.[374,435,523]

The explanation for a rise in OSA prevalence with age is not clear. Although part of it will be the gradual rise in body weight that most people experience with age, there is an independent effect of age. Structural changes in the pharynx or weaker pharyngeal dilators, as well as changes in ventilatory control have all been postulated, but no satisfactory explanation has been given. In a demented subgroup of elderly subjects the AHI was much higher compared to non-demented subjects,[16,434,539] suggesting brain damage as a possible mechanism.

Alcohol consumption is a significant predictor of the level of overnight hypoxic dipping, although the effect is small (about 2 per cent of variance explained by self-reported alcohol intake). The immediate effect of alcohol is to decrease upper airway tone[63,576] and provokes snoring and OSA,[324,609] but there may also be longer term effects on respiratory control, the explanation for which is not clear.[110]

As one would expect, snoring was a predictor of the presence of sleep hypoxaemia (Fig. 9.7) although it was really only in the 'often snoring' group that there was a subset of subjects with higher desaturation rates. Other groups have found snoring to be an important marker for OSA and approximately 5−10 per cent of 'often' snorers seem to have an AHI of over 10 per hour.

As mentioned earlier, sleepiness is a marker for OSA, but the results from different groups have been variable. How sleepiness is asked about is also important and simple questions such as 'do you fall asleep during the day, particularly when not busy?' may not be very specific for truly abnormal hypersomnolence (Fig. 9.8). Lavie et al.[396] found a 10-fold increase in the prevalence of AHI values over 10 per hour in their 'sleepy' group, but none of our questions increased the prevalence by more than four-fold. The problem of assessing sleepiness was discussed in the section on measuring daytime sleepiness in Chapter 4 (p. 68) and there are probably better scales now than were used in our survey.[332]

Thus, symptoms in a questionnaire can probably select out most of the subjects with significant OSA, but do not catch them all. This means that epidemiological studies pre-selecting on the basis of symptoms will slightly underestimate the prevalence. However, many of the subjects selected in this way (approximately 75−85 per cent) will turn out *not* to have significant OSA and therefore the questionnaire method is not a very efficient way to find cases.

10 Paediatric aspects of obstructive sleep apnoea

This section covers some aspects of OSA that are different in children. The condition is still essentially the same as in adults; increased upper airway resistance during sleep leads to sleep disruption and sometimes hypoxaemia. However, the commonest cause and some of the consequences, are different. This section does not cover the sleep and breathing problems of very young children, such as apnoea of prematurity or sudden infant death syndrome (if indeed this is a sleep apnoea syndrome). The reader is referred to recent reviews on these topics for further information.[358,475,641]

10.1 Aetiology and definitions

The problem of defining what is abnormal during sleep in children is just as difficult as in adults. Again there is a spectrum from completely quiet, undisturbed, sleep through to loud snoring, recurrent pharyngeal obstruction, and repetitive arousals with disorganized sleep. Although early on a significant problem was only defined if complete obstruction was found during polysomnography,[255] it was soon realized that lesser degrees of obstruction could produce symptoms (somewhat earlier in fact than this was recognized in adults).[84,267]

Early reports of bad sleep apnoea in children described the daytime respiratory failure, cor pulmonale, and upper airway obstruction, but failed initially to appreciate that the obstruction was very much worse during sleep.[460,495] Diurnal cardiorespiratory failure as a late presentation of obstructive sleep apnoea in children mercifully is very rare, most cases being recognized and treated much earlier.[542] The definition of 'obstructive sleep apnoea' in children is now essentially based on a combination of symptoms and some evidence that sleep is being disturbed by upper airway narrowing, usually evident as snoring.[85,97,542,543,689] This imprecise definition presents problems with epidemiological studies (see p. 158) but is the best possible at present.

The usual cause of pharyngeal narrowing and OSA in children is tonsillar enlargement (Plate 6). It is not clear whether adenoidal enlargement is as important, but clinically it seems that the tonsils have to be removed adequately to relieve the OSA, rather than the adenoids. Adenoidal size does not correlate with sleep apnoea severity although tonsillar size does.[135] No proper trial has been done to assess this point. Tonsillar enlargement alone is not the whole story, because some children with large tonsils do not even snore and some children with OSA have only small tonsils (but will still usually respond to tonsillectomy). It appears that a narrow pharynx from side to side (measured intraoperatively) is also important,[79,80] but pre-operative head radiographs do not seem to help predict which child will have significant upper airway obstruction and sleep disturbance[395,432] except where tonsillar size is being estimated. Sometimes children are not completely cured by tonsillectomy[544,670] and one assumes these are the ones with the congenitally narrowest pharynges.

Tonsillar hypertrophy usually begins from the age of two years (but can be much earlier), peaks at about four to five years and then there is atrophy at a very variable rate thereafter. In some children there is little atrophy with the lymphoid tissue replaced by scar tissue.

Much less commonly, OSA in children is due to other anatomical abnormalities involving the upper airway. These range from micrognathia (or Pierre Robin syndrome) to disorders of craniofacial development (craniosynostosis) such as Creuzon's and Apert's syndromes (Plate 7). Deposition disorders such as the mucopolysaccharidoses (particularly Hunter's and Hurler's) can narrow the pharyngeal airway enough, even early in childhood, to precipitate OSA.[255,622]

Obesity is much less common a cause for sleep apnoea in children compared to adults, although it may be a contributory factor. Although sleep apnoea has been associated with the Prader—Willi syndrome,[615,710] it is likely that obesity and tonsillar hypertrophy are the causes rather than any other specific abnormality associated with this chromosomal deletion disorder.

In Down's syndrome the prevalence of OSA is extremely high (perhaps 30 per cent) and seems to be related to tongue enlargement as well as tonsillar enlargement (including the lingual tonsils).[161,411,437,524,584,627,642,646,701] The hypoxia that these children can get may contribute to their cardiovascular problems, particularly pulmonary hypertension.

Although very occasionally OSA may be due to a primary neurological problem, such as an Arnold—Chiari malformation with brain stem compression,[4,255,302] this is extremely rare and an upper airway anatomical explanation should always be assumed and sought first.

10.2 Epidemiology and consequences

Data on the epidemiology of sleep apnoea in children is extremely limited. Part of this stems from the difficulties of definition referred to above. Given that tonsillar hypertrophy is the dominant cause and that rates of tonsillectomy have fallen dramatically over the last 40 years,[291,452,541] it is possible that the prevalence of OSA has been steadily increasing over the same period.[113] For example, the tonsillectomy rate in the 1950s was approximately 40 per cent by the age of nine years, whereas a recent survey put the current rate at less than 1 per cent.[51,207] Because the symptoms of childhood sleep apnoea are fairly non-specific (for example, sleepiness, hyperactivity, poor school performance, bad behaviour—see p. 180) it is quite possible that any gradual rise in prevalence would go unnoticed.

It was against this background that we performed two studies to assess whether sleep apnoea was a common problem in children and was being missed. In the first instance we looked for sleep apnoea over a period of one year in a group of snoring children (aged 2–14 years) who were put on the waiting list for adenotonsillectomy.[670] Only one of these children had been referred for the possibility of sleep apnoea, the others because of recurrent tonsillitis. Although initially 89 such children were studied, only 61 had follow-up studies six months post-tonsillectomy. This represented 27 per cent of the tonsillectomies done that year. In order to make comparisons, 31 normal children, matched for age and sex, were also studied twice (six months apart) to provide control data.

The children were all visited at home and a symptom questionnaire completed with the parents. Height and weight were measured. A portable oximeter with internal memory (Ohmeda 3700) was left for overnight recording of S_{aO_2} levels,[723] using a toe probe, covered with a sock, to prevent problems of wire entanglement. The overnight hypoxaemia was quantified as the number of dips in S_{aO_2} of more than 4 per cent per hour of the study. In order to ensure that any S_{aO_2} dips found were indeed due to obstructive events and not artefact, we originally arranged to record on video some of the children during the overnight oximetry. This confirmed that hypoxic events were due to snoring or complete obstruction, but also revealed sleep disruption due to similar events, even when there was no hypoxaemia, that is, the children were waking and restoring adequate airflow prior to any fall in the S_{aO_2} levels. Thus, all the children were recorded on video (with sound) during their night study from that point onwards.

In order to try and quantify the sleep disturbance from the video recordings, we devised a simple movement detection system which measured, with photocells, the fluctuations in light intensity on the video screen over where

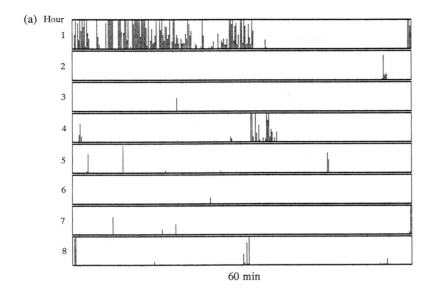

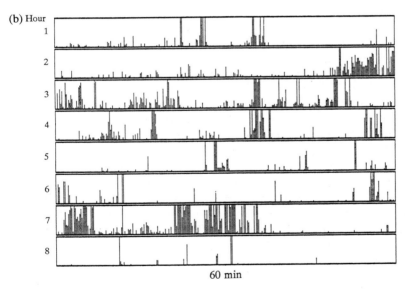

Fig. 10.1 Examples of two, all-night, tracings derived from a video recording (refer to the text for details). The tracings start top left, are eight sequential 1 h segments, and finish bottom right. A vertical line indicates movement has been detected and is semiquantitative. (a) A normal child falling asleep after approximately 30 min and having approximately 10 brief arousals during the night. (b) A child with sleep apnoea with repetitive movements throughout the night.

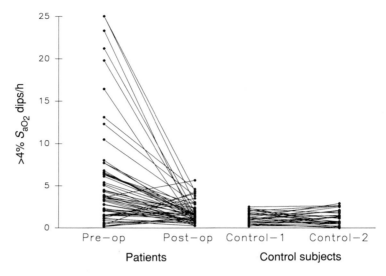

Fig. 10.2 Overnight hypoxaemic dipping rates in children pre- and post-adenotonsillectomy, in comparison to a control group of children studied twice. Note the high prevalence of abnormal degrees of hypoxaemic dipping pre-operatively, and the almost complete return to normal post-operatively.

the child lay.[669] Figure 10.1 is an example of two tracings, normal and abnormal, using this system. The movement was quantified as 'per cent of the study time spent moving', with periods of maintained wakefulness (> 1 min) excluded from the analysis, thus transient arousals only were documented. This approach to documenting short arousals in adults has recently been validated.[715]

Figure 10.2 shows the overnight hypoxic dipping data, Fig. 10.3 the overnight movement data. The striking observation was that, compared to controls, a large percentage of the pre-operative children had abnormal numbers of hypoxic dips, which had virtually recovered to normal six months post-operatively. The abnormal hypoxia was always due to obstructed breathing, often just snoring or short (< 10 s) apnoeas. Only the worst children had classic, long, complete apnoeas. In addition, the excessive movement was nearly always in association with snoring and obstruction. Before surgery 61 per cent of the children had more than three per hour of >4 per cent S_{aO_2} dips compared with 13 per cent post-operatively and none of the controls had this level of hypoxaemia. Before surgery, 65 per cent of the children spent >8 per cent of their sleep time moving compared to 4 per cent post-operatively: none of the control children were so disturbed.

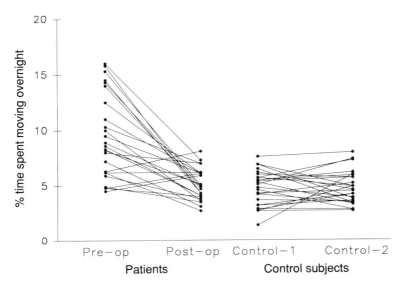

Fig. 10.3 Overnight sleep disturbance (quantified as per cent time spent moving) in children pre- and post-adenotonsillectomy, in comparison to a control group of children studied twice.

The pattern of answers to the questions asked about the children's behaviour were also very different to those of control children and greatly improved post-operatively (Fig. 10.4). Of course we had no proof that the different behaviour was due to the sleep disturbance, but these sorts of poor behaviour have been seen in all the reported series on children with sleep apnoea,[5,84,135,255,544,689] so it seems likely. It is perhaps of some concern that at six months post-operatively the behaviour patterns were still different to the control children. Learnt behaviour patterns may persist for much longer than the physiological cause for them, as may the parental attitudes to a child perceived as particularly difficult for a period of time.

Also of interest in this study was the significantly shorter stature of the snoring children and the significantly higher growth rate seen over the six months post-operatively compared to controls. The height velocities of the operated and control children being 9.7 cm per year and 7.5 cm per year respectively. There could be a variety of reasons for this growth spurt, but increased growth hormone production is one of them. In prepubertal children growth hormone is released almost exclusively during early undisturbed sleep when the deepest SWS is observed.[193] Thus, recurrent sleep disruption might well suppress the production of growth hormone. Increased growth following improved sleep has been observed by others,

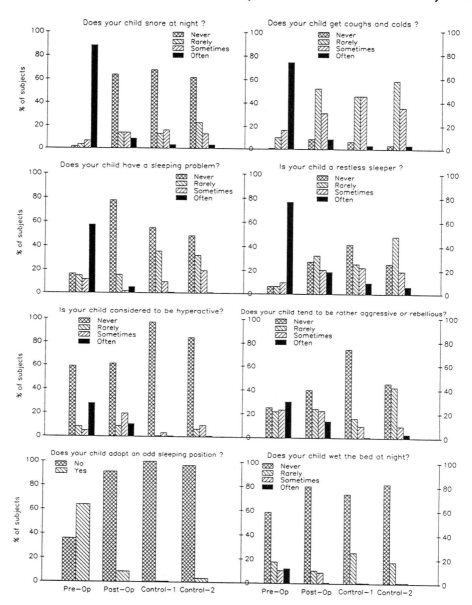

Fig. 10.4 The answers given to eight questions asked about children pre- and post-adenotonsillectomy (first and second sets of histograms in each graph) compared to a control group of children studied twice (third and fourth sets of histograms). Each set of four columns shows the distribution of the answers to the question above the graph, in the order never, rarely, sometimes, or often. The graph bottom left has only two options, no or yes. Note how the left set of histograms has a high percentage answering often (black column) to the questions, compared to post-operatively and the control subjects.

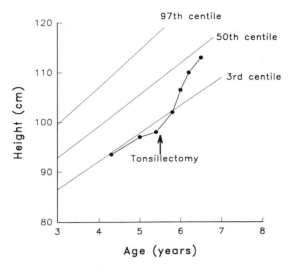

Fig. 10.5 Example of retarded growth before tonsillectomy and a growth spurt post-operatively. Redrawn with permission from Bate *et al.* (1984).[39]

some with growth hormone measurements[84,245,590,758] (Fig. 10.5), but this is better documented in adult sleep apnoea.[242]

Other reports on sleep apnoea in children[5,84,135,255,544,689] have found similar symptoms but with hypersomnolence being less dominant than it is in adults (Table 10.1). When children are sleep-deprived it appears they fight it with consequent overactive behaviour rather than sleep during the day. Other studies have stressed the falling standards at school, presumably due to inattention, but we did not see this problem using the very simple question on learning difficulties in our questionnaire.

The hypoxaemia seen in this study was not severe except in a few of the children. However, overnight pulse rate (10 bpm higher on average in the pre-operative group) correlated best with the >4 per cent S_{aO_2} dip rate, perhaps indicating some cardiac effect from the hypoxaemia. Considerably worse hypoxaemia has been seen in children referred to us with a prior clinical diagnosis of OSA. Wilkinson *et al.*[750] found three of 92 children to have right ventricular hypertrophy (RVH) on ECG prior to routine tonsillectomy which resolved post-operatively. Other studies using radionucleotide ventriculography have found right ventricular function to be depressed in children with obvious sleep apnoea, even in the absence of RVH on ECG.[29]

What would have happened to the children in our study if they had not had a tonsillectomy for recurrent tonsillitis? Presumably the majority would

Table 10.1 Symptoms of obstructive sleep apnoea in children

Daytime problems	Late complications	Nighttime problems
Excessive hyperactivitiy	Cor pulmonale, acute respiratory and cardiac failure	Increased sleep time
Increased aggressiveness		Disrupted and restless sleep
Excessive sleepiness		Continuous loud snoring
Delayed learning or language development		Apnoeas may be apparent to the parents
Under or over weight		Nocturnal enuresis
Recurrent tonsillitis, coughs and colds		Odd sleeping positions, e.g. head well extended
Difficulty arousing in the morning		
Dislike of going to bed		
Morning headaches		

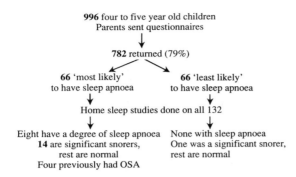

996 four to five year old children
Parents sent questionnaires

↓

782 returned (79%)

66 'most likely'   **66** 'least likely'
to have sleep apnoea   to have sleep apnoea

↓   ↓

Home sleep studies done on all 132

↓   ↓

Eight have a degree of sleep apnoea   None with sleep apnoea
14 are significant snorers,   One was a significant snorer,
rest are normal   rest are normal
Four previously had OSA

Therefore prevalence about **12/996 (1.2%)**

Fig. 10.6 Results of the Oxford community survey of sleep and breathing disorders in 4–5 year old children, showing the starting population and the numbers selected at each stage.

have had spontaneous atrophy of their tonsils with gradual resolution, perhaps over years, of sleep apnoea, leaving only a few (if any) with persistent problems.

Because of the extraordinarily high prevalence of apparently symptomatic abnormal sleep and breathing problems found in these children we went on to undertake a true prevalence study on randomly selected children in the age group with the highest prevalence found in the first study, that is, four to five years old.[15] The parents of 996 such children completed a simple questionnaire on the symptoms of sleep apnoea (snoring, sleep disturbance, etc.). On the basis of the answers, two groups (each of 66 children, 13.3 per cent of the original survey population) were chosen—those *most* likely to have sleep apnoea (high risk) and those *least* likely. These 132 children then had sleep studies, identical to those done in the earlier study (Fig. 10.6).

The 'high risk' group spent more time moving during sleep, had higher overnight pulse rates and >4 per cent S_{aO_2} dip rates compared to the controls. Twenty out of the 66 (30 per cent) had values above the 95th centile established for these indices in the previous study.[670] Review of video recordings revealed seven of these 20 children to have clear evidence of snoring and upper airway obstruction producing arousals and a further four who snored only. Four of the selected children in the high risk group had by chance been in the previous study when a little younger and had had obvious sleep apnoea, which had largely resolved post-operatively. Thus, assuming these four children would still have had a problem if they had not had a tonsillectomy, the prevalence in this study was approximately 12 per 996 (1.2 per cent, 95 per cent confidence intervals, 0.6–2.0 per cent). This of course also assumes that there were no further cases in the other 86.7 per cent not studied. Since there presumably were some, this is likely to be a slight underestimate. Thus, perhaps 1−2 per cent of four to five year old children have clear evidence of sleep disturbance due to snoring and upper airway obstruction on a one night sleep study. Since all the children in the 'high risk' group were said to be 'often' snorers (one of the selection criteria), it is curious that in only 11 out of the 66 did we demonstrate any snoring. Presumably snoring will vary with current upper respiratory tract infections (children with current infections were not studied until better) and perhaps parents were answering the questionnaire concentrating preferentially on the bad periods. One of the risk factors for childhood snoring was maternal smoking, a relationship observed by others.[132]

We also assessed whether there were any differences in the behaviour of the two selected groups.[14] Using Conners'[128] behaviour scale we found that the high risk group were significantly more likely to be rated as more aggressive and hyperactive by both their teachers and parents, compared to controls. This was an effect from the group as a whole and did not depend on the 11 with abnormal sleep studies. This also suggests that the parents' statements about snoring and sleep disruption were correct, even though we failed to demonstrate it on one night's study. Thus, it appears that there is an undiagnosed group of children with disturbed sleep due to snoring who have measurable deterioration in their daytime behaviour. We would stress that the behaviour patterns were not extremely poor and in some of them a tonsillectomy would not have been the appropriate response, when natural resolution would be expected in due course anyway.

Although this study provided some information on prevalence and consequences, it did not answer the important question: 'at what level of severity should a tonsillectomy be considered?' This will be extremely difficult to answer until a longer term follow-up study with control groups is done, as has been for the problem of glue ear and its developmental consequences.[108]

10.3 Examination

Most children with mild to moderate sleep apnoea will appear normal on examination. They are likely to have visibly large tonsils (although not necessarily) and be mouth breathers.[709] Micrognathia and any other predisposing cause such as a craniofacial disorder or mucopolysaccharidosis should be obvious or already known about prior to presentation. When marked obesity is present, the Prader−Willi syndrome should be thought of with its cardinal features of infantile hypotonia, early obesity due

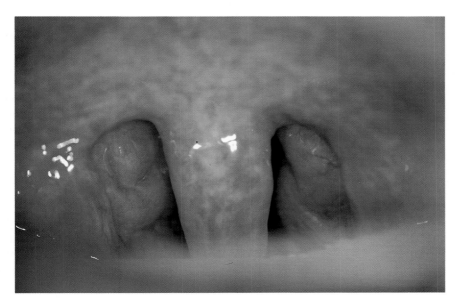

1 Large tonsils in an adult, the removal of which cured severe obstructive sleep apnoea.

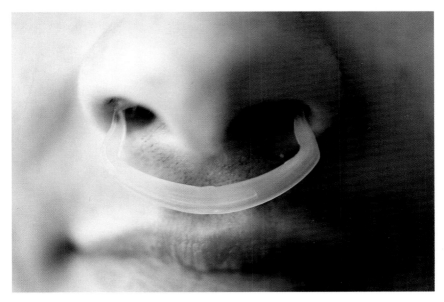

2 The Nosovent device is designed to be worn at night and dilates the anterior nasal valve. In a few snorers this is a site of considerable inspiratory resistance. Sometimes in this situation snoring is helped by this device.

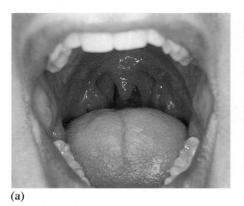
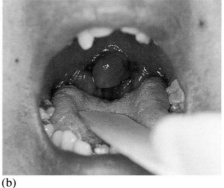

(a)   (b)

3 (a) A normal pharynx in a young male with residual tonsils, but an entirely normal sleep study and no history of snoring. (b) A middle-aged male with severe sleep apnoea and a long history of snoring. The tonsils are present but the most striking abnormality is pharyngeal crowding from all directions and a relatively enlarged uvula.

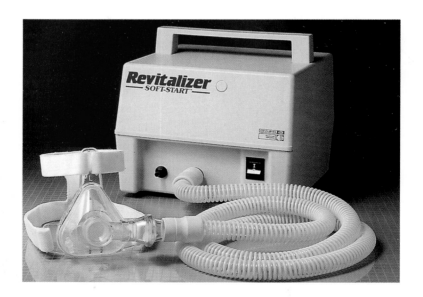

4 A DeVilbiss continuous positive airway pressure blower for the treatment of obstructive sleep apnoea. Courtesy of DeVilbiss Health Care UK Ltd.

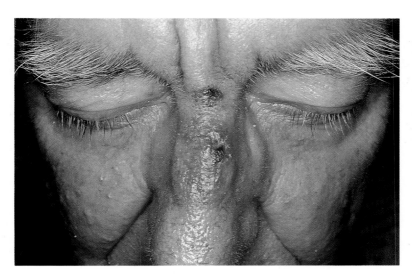

5 Nasal bridge ulceration from a nasal mask.

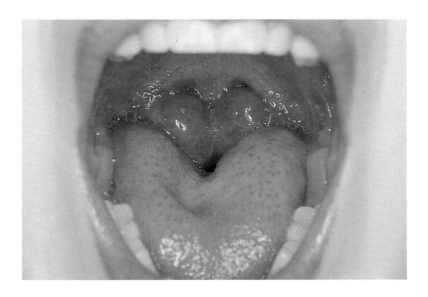

6 Example of large tonsils in a child producing considerable upper airway obstruction during sleep with hypoxaemia and sleep disturbance.

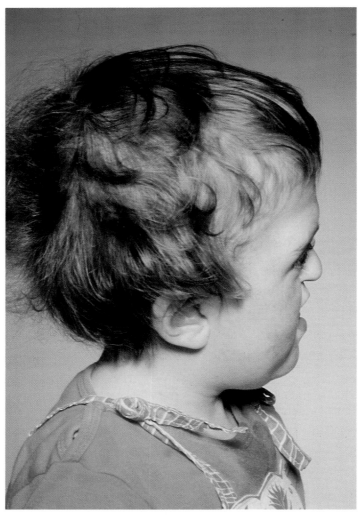

7 Apert's syndrome. One of the craniodysostoses. Retropositioning of the mandible and maxilla narrow the upper airway at several places.

to hyperphagia, mental deficiency, short stature, hypersomnolence, and hypogonadism.

In severe OSA the child may snore even whilst awake because the obstruction is so extensive (often with tonsils meeting in the midline). In the very advanced state the child will be floppy and only half awake most of the time, with perhaps evidence of cardiorespiratory failure.

10.4 Investigation

The problem of *what* to measure in these children is not resolved and we do not know *how much* of any abnormality measured requires treatment. As discussed earlier, the combination of appropriate symptoms and some evidence of obstructed breathing with arousals at night is currently the best recommendation.[542] This evidence may be obtained from a variety of techniques including observation,[85,135] sound recordings,[442,541,544] video recordings, or simply the parental history.[5,670] The parental history, when compared to a sleep study, may not appear to be compatible according to Croft and colleagues,[135] although whether a one night sleep study should be the final arbiter of what is happening at night is not proven. There are no long-term repeatability studies to see how this problem may fluctuate from night to night.

Polysomnography is accepted by most to be unnecessary in this situation, unless there are doubts about the diagnosis following a simpler study.[85,135,542] However, the problem of how much sleep disturbance is worthy of treatment is, of course, not answered by polysomnography either. Symptoms are still more important when deciding whether a child should be submitted to a tonsillectomy. Clearly one might require more symptoms before operating on a craniofacial abnormality than on simple tonsillar enlargement.

Ideally, systems that are used to assess sleep apnoea in children should be simple, cheap, and useable at home. One clearly wants to avoid an admission to hospital, but home studies need delivery and collection of equipment (perhaps by the parents) as well as requiring the equipment to function unattended. Potsic[442,541] designed a system based on audio recordings that looked for respiratory irregularity and snoring (Fig. 10.7). He felt this would identify those requiring attention. Our system of home oximetry and video recordings certainly identifies sleep disturbance, snoring, and hypoxaemia, but until custom-made equipment is available, it is difficult for the parents to set up. Unless the analysis of snoring and movement is automated the processing of the information is very tedious and time-consuming. As mentioned earlier, oximetry alone is not adequate, because of the marked sleep disruption that can occur due to snoring and upper

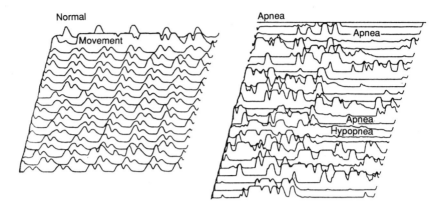

Fig. 10.7 Graphical displays of a sound monitoring system for sleep apnoea in children. (a) A normal child showing the regular inspiratory and expiratory noise. (b) A child with sleep apnoea: note the irregularity and pauses. With permission from Potsic (1987).[541]

airway obstruction in the absence of hypoxaemia.[84,267,544,670] Other systems that could be used are the static charge sensitive bed[395,537,701] and the MESAM IV.[650] Both these systems give indirect information on increased respiratory effort and sleep disturbance, but their use in children has not been fully established.

If the increasing trend to perform tonsillectomy for sleep apnoea rather than for recurrent tonsillitis continues,[582] then it may be necessary to perform more sleep studies on children as part of their assessment. Before this approach is shown to be better than just a good history at deciding who should have an operation, we will need simple and cheap ways to monitor the children, probably for several nights and to look more closely at the outcomes of either operating or not operating.

10.5 Treatment

It will be clear from the earlier sections that the usual treatment for obstructive sleep apnoea is tonsillectomy or adenotonsillectomy. Even when there are other contributory factors such as a craniofacial abnormality, a deposition disorder, Down's syndrome, or obesity, it is still worth trying tonsillectomy first if there is any removable tissue. It has also been observed that the removal of even quite small tonsils can improve matters considerably.[5,135,317,395]

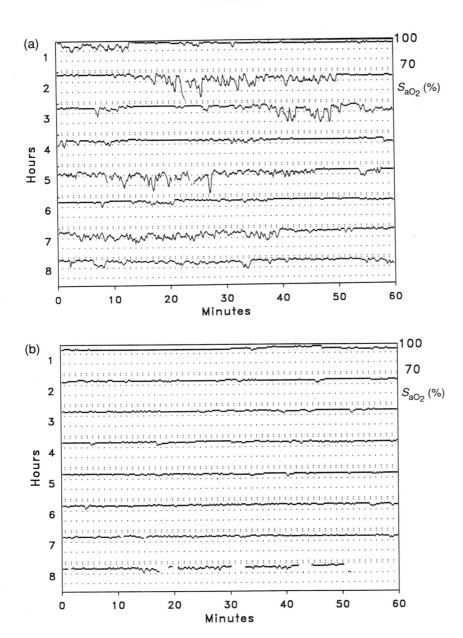

Fig. 10.8 Two all-night oxygen saturation tracings in the same child, (a) pre- and (b) post-adenotonsillectomy for sleep apnoea.

The response to tonsillectomy is usually dramatic (Fig. 10.8) with quieter and more peaceful breathing even in the recovery room.[135,544,670] Operative deaths which have occurred in this situation were probably in severe cases where the secondary consequences on left and right ventricular function had not been recognized.

The effect on daytime symptoms is usually also dramatic and if it is not, then failure to have cured the OSA is likely. This is usually the case when other contributory factors are present. Even so there may have been enough of an improvement to allow postponement of, for example, advancement of the face in a child with a craniosynostosis (for example, Apert's or Creuzon's syndromes).

In Down's syndrome tonsillectomy alone is sometimes not enough but may be.[437,642] It is felt that in these already handicapped children even slight sleep disturbance will further handicap them. Thus, various surgical approaches at treatment have been tried, such as tongue reduction[161,642] or shaving of the lingual tonsils,[524] with some success.

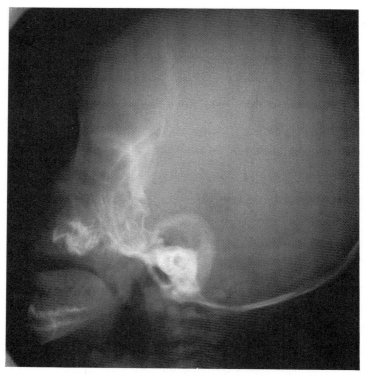

Fig. 10.9 Lateral skull view of a child with Apert's syndrome. Note the hypoplastic and retropositioned maxilla with no retropalatal space.

If surgery is not possible or has failed, then nasal CPAP is an option.[590] Perhaps contrary to expectations, children seem to take to this treatment well. Small nasal masks are available for most of the commercial systems. Using CPAP may allow a craniofacial operation to be delayed until a more appropriate time or indeed to simply improve the child's condition for such an operation. However, our limited experience of nasal CPAP in Apert's and Creuzon's syndromes has not been good, probably because of the poor nasal flow due to posterior displacement of the hard palate against the posterior wall of the nasopharynx (Fig. 10.9).

Children with craniosynostosis and sleep apnoea are difficult to manage, with little data available to help make the clinical decisions. The situation has been made even more complicated recently by the observation that intracranial pressure (ICP) rises dramatically when sleep apnoea occurs in children with craniosynostosis.[233] They are prone to raised ICP because of their smaller and deformed skulls so that such additional rises may push the brainstem into the foramen magnum. The interference to brainstem function may even further affect control of respiration and the upper airway.

Surgery is sometimes possible to relieve OSA in patients with Hunter's or Hurler's syndromes. Again adenotonsillectomy may be adequate, but further surgery can be tried.[586]

10.6 Conclusions

There are many unsolved problems relating to sleep apnoea in children. In many ways less is known about its epidemiology and consequences than in adult sleep apnoea. However, the almost universal response to tonsillectomy, when there is no other specific underlying disorder, is extremely gratifying and makes identifying such children well worth while.

11 Central (non-obstructive) sleep apnoea and hypoventilation

The terms central sleep apnoea or hypopnoea are used to describe reductions in ventilation during sleep where the cause appears to result not from upper airway obstruction, but from failure of ventilatory drive from the respiratory centre. There is no single cause for this phenomenon and the finding of apparent central sleep apnoea should lead to an elucidation of the cause. This is necessary because treatment depends on the cause. Table 11.1 is one attempt at a breakdown of the various causes of apparent central apnoea: other authors have allocated differently.[272] The word 'apparent' is used deliberately here because not all that appears to be central is always so. Each of the types is further discussed below.

11.1 Absent ventilatory drive

11.1.1 Brainstem abnormalities

The two neurological pathways allowing movement of the respiratory pump, involuntary (automatic, chemical) and voluntary, were discussed in Chapter 2 (p. 13). Their neurological pathways are distinct and can be damaged separately, thus producing patients who can breathe voluntarily, but not in response to chemical stimuli.[532] Conversely patients with automatic breathing but no voluntary control have been described.[284,487] This loss of chemical or automatic control may only be very obvious during non-REM sleep when voluntary control is absent. Classically a patient with this problem may seem normal whilst awake, but hypoventilates or is frankly apnoeic, as soon as sleep occurs. This failure of automatic control (so called Ondine's curse) can be congenital[459] or acquired as the result of a stroke,[410] infection,[738] surgical damage,[367] multiple sclerosis,[65] or compression of the respiratory centre by tumour or a syrinx.[59] The congenital problem is very rare and may not be apparent during the first few days or weeks after birth. This delay is thought to be because of the high proportion

Table 11.1 Suggested breakdown of causes of central apnoea

Type of central apnoea	Examples	Daytime arterial CO_2 level
Absent or reduced ventilatory drive (Ondine's curse)	Brainstem damage or congenital abnormality Acquired blunting, e.g. secondary to lung disease.	Raised
Unstable respiratory drive	Sleep onset, hypoxaemia, altitude, heart failure	Normal or low
REM-related oscillations	Normal in REM sleep Due to neuromuscular disorders and respiratory muscle weakness	Normal or raised
Reflex central apnoea	Pharyngeal collapse inhibits inspiration	Normal
Apparent central apnoea (wrongly diagnosed)	Respiratory muscle weakness or gross obesity cause chest wall movement transducers to fail to demonstrate any ventilatory effort during *obstructive* apnoeas	Normal or raised

of REM sleep and low proportion of non-REM sleep during this early period. During REM sleep ventilation may just be adequate because of some 'voluntary' or cortical respiratory signals.[138]

Loss of central control in most of the conditions mentioned above usually occurs fairly suddenly and is obviously part of some catastrophic event. Sometimes the onset is more insidious, for example, as can occur in some forms of CNS degeneration producing autonomic dysfunction (Shy−Drager syndrome). Initially there may be no overt daytime symptoms to suggest an abnormality of ventilation, although a sleep study may reveal problems.[456] Later, there is more sleep disruption leading to daytime hypersomnolence.[104] Originally it was thought that the sleep-related respiratory problems in the Shy−Drager syndrome were entirely central, but it is now clear that many of the previously reported abnormalities were in fact obstructive sleep apnoea due to laryngeal closure. There is a specific denervation atrophy of the laryngeal abductors.[34] However, it does seem as if a wide variety of respiratory abnormalities can develop in this condition.[116]

The factors that will lead one to suspect sleep-related failure of respiratory drive will be signs and symptoms to suggest nocturnal hypoventilation and sleep disruption: morning confusion and headache, restless sleep, hyper-somnolence, and witnessed apnoeas or cyanosis. At presentation the respiratory failure may already be carrying over into the daytime with resting blood gases showing an elevated P_{aCO_2} and perhaps fluid retention with ankle oedema. In the case the of Shy–Drager syndrome there may also be a history of snoring which is usually recognized by relatives as different to real snoring, that is, the inspiratory stridor during sleep due to poor laryngeal abduction.

11.1.2 Acquired secondary loss of ventilatory drive

There are a variety of conditions where respiratory drive may become gradually blunted as a secondary phenomenon. For example, in some of the primary neuromuscular disorders that produce ventilatory failure from respiratory muscle weakness, arterial P_{aCO_2} gradually rises. The ventilatory response to CO_2 will be reduced, mainly due to the muscle weakness, but also because of adaptation (perhaps through changes in brain levels of bicarbonate and other buffers). Thus, at sleep onset the loss of wakefulness drive will produce particularly marked deterioration in blood gases. A secondary factor accentuating the difference between waking and sleeping ventilation will be the loss of adaptation mechanisms (that is, recruitment of accessory muscles of respiration and other non-respiratory muscles) which seem to be much less effective during sleep.

This mechanism may also be operating in the acquired respiratory failure of chronic lung disease (see the section on chronic airways obstruction later in this chapter, p. 207). In some patients with chronic lung disease there is some deterioration in blood gases with the onset of non-REM sleep, but to what extent this is more than occurs with normal subjects is not entirely clear.[105]

There is debate as to whether these non-REM sleep-related deteriorations in ventilation merely reflect the deteriorating respiratory system or whether they might actually contribute to the rate of decline by encouraging a resetting of central control mechanisms.

11.2 Unstable respiratory drive

The control of respiration is made up of several homeostatic loops combined with other drives that are not under feedback control. The complex inter-actions of these drives makes it difficult to predict or understand when the control will become unstable, with consequent periodic breathing or re-current central apnoeas during sleep. Physiologists have been fascinated by phenomena such as Cheyne–Stokes respiration but have not found them easy to explain. The use of computer modelling has improved our under-standing, in particular a useful paper by Khoo *et al.*[355] which, although complex, is well worth the effort required to understand it.

During wakefulness, deliberate hyperventilation to reduce the P_{aCO_2} is followed by ventilation only slightly below resting levels while the P_{aCO_2} slowly climbs back to normal. Post-hyperventilation apnoea is rarely seen during wakefulness except in diffuse brain disorders.[531] However, if a subject is artificially hyperventilated whilst in SWS and this hyper-ventilation is then withdrawn, there *is* apnoea until the P_{aCO_2} rises to a threshold value.[142,158,634] Even quite small reductions in P_{aCO_2} during non-REM sleep (3 mmHg or so) will render a subject temporarily apnoeic. Thus, there *is* an apnoea point when hypocapnic during sleep, which is masked during wakefulness by a fixed wakefulness drive effectively preventing a reduction in ventilation much below the normal resting value.

An important fact about all feedback control systems is that if the slope of the stimulus—response curve (loop gain) is high, then they are intrinsically unstable because of over- and undershoot.[111,223] For example, in the respir-atory system with a high CO_2 gain there will be an exuberant response to a small rise in P_{aCO_2}. This leads to ventilatory overcompensation with an excessive fall in P_{aCO_2}: this leads to a big fall in ventilation that will allow P_{aCO_2} to rise again a little too far, thus perpetuating the cycling. This mechanism is rather like the ventilatory oscillation due to a delayed blood circulation time. A delayed lung to carotid body and brain circulation time means that the results of changes in ventilation are perceived too late by the chemoreceptors such that they are always hunting the correct set point with over- and undershoots of respiratory drive. Given that increased ventilatory drive tends to generate instability of feedback control, it is at first curious that periodic breathing (or Cheyne—Stokes respiration) is much more prevalent during sleep when drives are slightly lower than awake. This section tries to explain the mechanism and circumstances under which the transition from wakefulness to sleep can set up self-sustaining oscillations of respiration.

11.2.1 *Periodic breathing at sleep onset*

Figure 11.1 is a graph of minute ventilation against arterial P_{aCO_2}. The gentle curve (almost horizontal, K to L) describes the effect of ventilation on P_{aCO_2}, that is, the more one deliberately overbreathes, the lower the P_{aCO_2} will go and vice versa. This is called the metabolic production line and its position on the graph will depend on the amount of metabolic CO_2 being produced (and any CO_2 being inhaled): this will fall a little during sleep, but for simplicity this effect has not been shown and we have assumed a fixed line. The diagonal straight lines rising left to right all represent

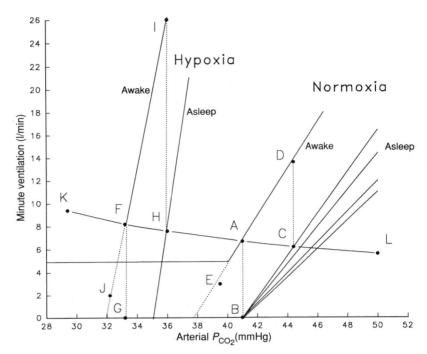

Fig. 11.1 Diagrammatic representation of the changes in ventilatory drive with sleep and altitude. Refer to the text for details.

various ventilatory responses to raised P_{aCO_2}. The diagonal line (D to A) ending in a horizontal line at 5 l/min represents the normal awake response to P_{aCO_2}, including the 'dog's leg' due to the wakefulness drive referred to above. The diagonal lines to the right (labelled 'Asleep') represent an approximate average change in ventilatory response to CO_2 due to the onset of sleep (increasing displacement going from stage 1 through to stage 4).[91,169,355] Point A on the graph represents the ventilation during wakefulness, at rest and is the intersection of the relevant metabolic line and drive line.

As sleep begins the wakefulness drive disappears and the CO_2 drive line moves to the right. This means that the awake P_{aCO_2} of 41 mmHg is too low to drive ventilation and, *without a wakefulness drive*, apnoea or marked hypoventilation *can* occur (point B, Fig. 11.1).

The speed of entry into sleep will determine how quickly these changes in drive occur. If sleep is entered quickly then the subject will go from A to B (with apnoea) and then as CO_2 accumulates and P_{aCO_2} rises, he will progressively breathe more, moving up the CO_2 drive line to C. If sleep comes on very slowly and gently then he will go gradually from A straight to C without going via B and apnoea.

If the subject is now woken from point C (by an outside stimulus or just because sleep onset is hesitant) then the new higher sleep P_{aCO_2} will be inappropriately high for the awake drive line and will cause transient hyperpnoea (point D). The subject will then drive his P_{aCO_2} back down to A to await the onset of sleep again (or overshoot via E if sleep supervenes quickly). As mentioned above, if the slopes of the lines describing the ventilatory response to CO_2 ($\dot{V}/CO_2$) are steep enough, then there will be the potential for under- and overshoot. Whilst awake the presence of the fixed awake drive will prevent undershoot and heavily damp any tendency to oscillations—remove this dampening effect and oscillations can begin. In addition, if there is a big change in the awake to asleep position (A to C) either due to a high basal wakefulness level or a bigger distance between the awake and asleep $\dot{V}/CO_2$ response lines, then there will be bigger swings in ventilation and P_{aCO_2} between awake and asleep. A bigger change in P_{aCO_2} with sleep onset has a subtle effect on the overall gain of the system. In the presence of a higher P_{aCO_2} a certain *change* in ventilation will *alter* P_{aCO_2} more, a rise in so called 'plant gain' which thus increases overall gain. This will increase the potential for instability in just the same way as increasing the $\dot{V}/CO_2$ slope. Khoo *et al.*[355] showed that if the $\dot{V}/CO_2$ response was in the order of 4 l/mmHg/min (very high), with average changes in the wake to asleep (A to C) positions, periodic breathing would occur within non-REM sleep without arousals—simply because of over- and undershoot being self-sustaining. However, this level of CO_2 drive during non-REM sleep, without any additional drives such as hypoxia, would be most unusual.

Another important factor in the generation and maintenance of instability during sleep, not fully explored in Khoo's model, was the effect of fluctuating tidal volumes near and below the anatomical deadspace (about 150 ml). When ventilatory drive is waxing and waning around a low level then a high proportion of the lower tidal volumes will be wasted on deadspace ventilation. As tidal volume increases from below deadspace tidal volumes to above, there will be a sudden increase in alveolar ventilation which means that the effective overall gain of the system is suddenly rising. Thus, similar fluctuations in ventilation at low levels (which, of course, includes periodic breathing with apnoeas) is inherently less stable (and, thus, potentially self-sustaining) than similar fluctuations at high levels of ventilation with tidal volumes well above the anatomical deadspace. This means that if a subject's ventilation can be increased, either by moving him up the CO_2 drive line or by displacing the drive line to the left without necessarily changing the slope, then this will help reduce the instability of their ventilation during sleep. This may be how acetazolamide works in some cases of central sleep apnoea.[741]

What was particularly interesting about Khoo's model was what happened when arousal was triggered *because* of the hyperpnoeic phase. Gleeson *et al.*[224,225] have shown that in normal subjects arousal could be provoked at stimulated ventilations of about 17 l/min. The initial model showed that at $\dot{V}/CO_2$ values of <4 l/mmHg/min, falling asleep without subsequent arousals would only initiate transient oscillations that without arousal simply dampened out, but often the first hyperpnoeic phase in response to the climbing P_{aCO_2} could easily be >17 l/min and thus in theory provoke arousal. This would, of course, move the subject onto the wake CO_2 response line and thus amplify the hyperpnoea and provoke a bigger undershoot of the P_{aCO_2} for the next cycle. Thus, the provocation of an arousal is a destabilizing and amplifying factor that can sustain periodic breathing that otherwise would have dampened out: in fact in Khoo's model $\dot{V}/CO_2$ drives of only 2 l/mmHg/min were associated with continuing oscillation. This was particularly so if the subject fell asleep quickly each time (over approximately 20 s), thus provoking bigger falls in $\dot{V}$ and P_{aO_2} with apnoeas and hence more ventilatory overshoot when P_{aCO_2} levels rise again. Other computer simulations of hypoxia-induced periodic breathing have also demonstrated the importance of arousal in maintaining the periodicity.[602]

Thus, a subject with high $\dot{V}/CO_2$ drives, low threshold to arousal in response to hyperpnoea, a fast wake-to-sleep time, and a big difference between the positions of the awake and asleep $\dot{V}/CO_2$ response lines, will be prone to continuing periodic breathing. He will experience recurrent arousals which are both the result and major cause of this cycling. The prediction from this is that sedative drugs to suppress arousal might prevent this sort of periodic breathing and indeed evidence from Bonnet *et al.*[62] suggests that triazolam is effective in some patients with central sleep apnoea and allows breakthrough into stable stage 4 with improved daytime functioning.

Many groups have shown that the majority of normal subjects experience periodic breathing in light sleep until non-REM sleep consolidates to stages 3 and 4.[508] We all experience the destabilizing effect of sleep onset on ventilation[91] and the extent to which it occurs before dampening out depends on all the factors discussed above: CO_2 drive, the difference between awake and asleep drives, speed of sleep onset, external arousing stimuli, and the arousal threshold to hyperpnoea. The last three will vary to some extent day to day depending on how sleepy one is, thus, the degree of sleep onset periodic breathing is likely to vary from night to night.

Khoo also introduced some upper airway obstruction into his model. Various studies have suggested that at low levels of ventilatory drive the upper airway may collapse when there is still continuing diaphragmatic excursion.[11,318,499] Normal subjects can be made to have a few obstructive apnoeas by provoking marked periodic breathing (with hypoxic gas mixtures) in the presence of an inspiratory resistance (to encourage collapse of the pharynx).[499] The result of introducing this upper airway obstruction at low ventilatory drives made it even easier of course to develop periodic breathing by delaying the effects of rising ventilatory drive. However, a very large hysteresis was required such that occlusion occurred at a ventilatory drive below 1.1 l/min and reopening occurred at a drive of 16.8 l/min. This is unlike real OSA where obstruction appears related to sleep state rather than particular levels of respiratory drive, although this is a ventilatory drive level that might have led to arousal.

As mentioned earlier, many studies have shown that periodic breathing rarely occurs in stages 3 and 4 of sleep.[508] One would expect these stages to be a bit more stable because of the slightly shallower $\dot{V}/CO_2$ response lines. However, this would be a small effect and it is much more likely that because periodic breathing usually needs arousal to perpetuate it, subjects are not able to descend into stages 3 and 4: if arousals stop then they can get down into stages 3 and 4 and breathe regularly. Thus, periodic breathing dictates the sleep state rather than vice versa. There is some evidence that breathing fluctuates with measures of EEG arousal, but deciding whether one leads to the other or whether they both result from something else is difficult.[149,506]

11.2.2 Periodic breathing due to hypoxia (or altitude)

Hypoxia and altitude are well known stimuli for periodic breathing during sleep.[45,283,384,558,736] There is a periodicity even during wakefulness,[716] but sleep increases this periodicity enormously. It appears that this problem of altitude becomes increasingly common over 3500 m or an equivalent sea level inspired oxygen percentage of approximately 12.3 per cent (barometric pressure approximately 490 mmHg, inspired O_2 pressure approximately 94 mmHg). The likely explanations for this are really an extension of the physiology discussed in the previous section.

Hypoxia below a certain level stimulates ventilation, with an ever-increasing steepness of the slope as the P_{aO_2} falls further. If CO_2 responses are measured at different values of P_{aO_2}, then increasing hypoxia steepens the CO_2 response slope. In Fig. 11.1, point F represents a subject newly arrived at altitude who has increased his ventilation in response to hypoxia with a consequent hypocapnia; the P_{aO_2} will be about 50 mmHg (given an S_{aO_2} of approximately 85 per cent). If a CO_2 response measurement were done at this point, the slope would be steeper than at sea level (as well as left-shifted) because of the hypoxaemia. The exact position of the sleep

$\dot{V}/CO_2$ response line during this hypoxia is somewhat speculative, but will certainly move to the right (since P_{aO_2} is known to fall and P_{aCO_2} rise, with sleep onset at altitude) and should be even steeper because of the even greater hypoxaemia. Thus, on falling asleep this subject will move to point H. As described in the previous section, particularly if he falls asleep quickly or if the sleep—wake drive difference is bigger than normal, there will be a marked hypopnoea or apnoea (point G) and then as P_{aCO_2} rises, an overshoot (because of high gain). It will now be even easier to reach transiently the minute ventilation that provokes arousal (approximately 17 l/min) and then there will be particularly brisk hyperventilation to point I. As one might expect, subjects with high hypoxic gains have greater degrees of sleep apnoea and periodicity on arrival at altitude.[384]

At marked levels of hypoxaemia it may be that arousal is being provoked *directly*, and not via the actual ventilatory response to the hypoxaemia. For example, subjects with primary loss of respiratory drive who stop breathing with sleep onset (p. 188) wake up when their blood gases deteriorate, without there being a return of ventilation until they have woken up (oxygen prolongs this period of apnoea). Thus, there must be a direct effect of the carotid body on arousing mechanisms that do *not* need the intermediary of hyperventilation. Removal of the carotid bodies in dogs prevents them from arousing at all in response to hypoxaemia and they die if not resuscitated.[69]

Thus, at altitude, the fall in P_{aO_2} at sleep onset may provoke arousal and a return of ventilation or the return of ventilation may provoke arousal. Either way, arousal is again playing a pivotal role in causing and maintaining periodicity. There is some debate as to whether periodicity can develop due to hypoxaemia or altitude without arousal (due to the higher gains alone). Most studies using EEG recordings have found recurrent transient arousals (sometimes only a few seconds) in association with the periodic breathing[506,558] and all have found worsening of sleep, although micro-arousals may not have been documented.[194,488,736] In addition, there is some evidence that sedatives improve the periodic breathing at altitude.[488] Natives at altitude appear to have normal sleep architecture.[130]

Given this analysis, can any treatments for altitude sleep apnoea be proposed? Clearly added oxygen will reverse the situation, as will return to sea level. The possible benefits of sedation were mentioned above. Two interesting approaches are (1) added inspired CO_2 and (2) the carbonic anhydrase inhibitor acetazolamide. In addition, we need to be able to explain how acclimatization improves altitude sleep apnoea.

Added CO_2 will increase ventilation and so raise the P_{aO_2}. This will decrease the slope of the CO_2 response and this alone should reduce the tendency to oscillate. If hypoxaemia itself is an arousing influence, then the higher P_{aO_2} should help here as well. However Berssenbrugge *et al.*[45]

apparently found that added CO_2 stopped the apnoeas and partially stabilized hypoxia-induced periodic breathing during sleep when S_{aO_2} was *kept constant*, and P_{aCO_2} only rose by approximately 1.5 mmHg. Presumably the extra drive from the added CO_2 is rendering the fluctuations in drive with state changes proportionally less perturbing to the control system. Stability is probably also being improved by moving the overall tidal ventilation further away from the anatomical deadspace ventilation: a beneficial effect described earlier in this chapter (p. 193). In Berssenbrugge's experiments, the mean minute ventilation during periodic breathing (with apnoeas) provoked by hypoxia (S_{aO_2} approximately 67 per cent) was approximately 7.1 l/min. The addition of some added inspired CO_2 raised P_{aCO_2} from 36.7 (approximately) to 38.1 mmHg (approximately) yet minute ventilation went up by over 4 l/min to 11.2 l/min: thus CO_2 drive was approximately 3 l/min/mmHg, the approximate CO_2 response one could expect at an S_{aO_2} of 67 per cent. The general raising of ventilation took the oscillations in V_T away from apnoea and the anatomic deadspace, thus considerably dampening (but not removing) them. Figure 11.2 is from Berssenbrugge's paper showing the effect of adding CO_2 during hypoxia in one subject. This group also claimed that sleep state did not fluctuate during these oscillations but they staged sleep conventionally in 30 s epochs and would have missed any transient movements of the EEG towards wakefulness.

Acetazolamide, by reducing the conversion of CO_2 to H^+ ions in the distal tubule, prevents the reabsorption of HCO_3^- ions thus provoking a metabolic acidosis. This will have the effect of moving the CO_2 response line further to the left and, thus, provoke a higher ventilation (point K). As with added CO_2, this will improve the hypoxaemia and reduce the *slope* of the CO_2 response line, thus reducing instability. As described above, the higher resting drive may also lessen the perturbing effects of state changes and deadspace ventilation. In addition, acetazolamide may have another beneficial effect; an actual *inhibition* of hypoxic drive at the level of the carotid body.[37] This will yet further decrease the effect of hypoxaemia on the CO_2 response slope and promote the return of respiratory stability. This reduction in hypoxic drive is only safe at altitude because of the ventilatory stimulation from the left-shifted CO_2 response line.

The effect of acetazolamide is like natural acclimatization itself. During the days following arrival at altitude, ventilation goes on increasing further, probably as the ventilatory response to CO_2 is left-shifted by a metabolic reduction in the alkalosis produced by the hypocapnia. In a sense this initial respiratory alkalosis temporarily prevents the full and necessary hyperventilation that is needed to correct the hypoxaemia; acetazolamide 'pre-acclimatizes' by rapidly providing a metabolic acidosis that would otherwise take several days for the body to achieve unaided.

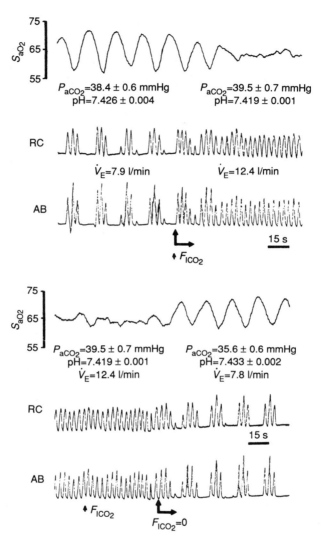

Fig. 11.2 These two panels represent one continual trace demonstrating the effect of raising the P_{aCO_2} during hypoxia-induced periodic respiration. At the start (top left) the subject has marked periodic respiration. At the arrow extra inspired CO_2 is given but the inspired O_2 level is lowered to keep the S_{aO_2} roughly constant. The added CO_2 raised P_{aCO_2} from 38.4 to 39.5 mmHg and ventilation from 7.9 to 12.4 l/min. This is enough to reduce (but not abolish) the periodic respiration and prevent the apnoeas. Removing the added CO_2 at the second arrow allows the apnoeas to return. With permission from Berssenbrugge et al. (1983).[45]

11.2.3 *Periodic breathing due to heart failure*

Periodic breathing as an accompaniment of left ventricular failure was recognized in the last century.[115] It was regarded largely as a medical curiosity[240] until quite recently when it was recognized as a possible cause of symptoms[170,171,274,557] and even contributing to the low cardiac output.[693]

The periodic breathing of heart failure can wax and wane sufficient to produce frank apnoeas, when it is usually called Cheyne–Stokes respiration (CSR). These apnoeas are accompanied by arousal during the resumption of respiration so that if Cheyne–Stokes breathing persists all night, then the patient will experience hundreds of arousals, just as occurs in obstructive sleep apnoea (Fig. 11.3). This suggests that some of the symptoms traditionally ascribed to the poor cardiac output *per se*, may be better explained by the sleep disruption, such as lethargy, sleepiness, and cognitive blunting.

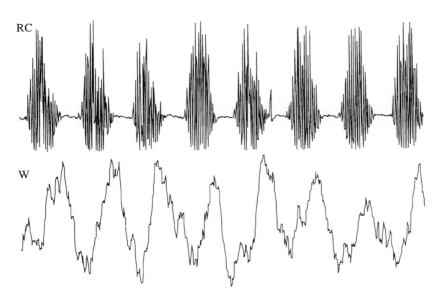

Fig. 11.3 Periodic respiration (monitored from rib-cage movement, RC) and the associated fluctuation in depth of sleep (W) measured second to second from the EEG with a neural network based system. Note how in this particular case the rise in the W trace (meaning increased arousal) seems to follow the return of ventilation or, conversely, sleep deepens during the apnoea. Courtesy of Dr S. Roberts, University of Oxford.

The explanation for the periodic breathing of heart failure is far from clear. Any explanation of its aetiology needs to take account of several facts: it improves with successful treatment of the heart failure[141] but apparently 'dry' patients can still have severe CSR; improvement is seen in response to added oxygen, theophyllines, acetazolamide, and usually to added inspired CO_2.

One of the almost universal findings in heart failure with CSR is a low resting P_{aCO_2} of about 30–36 mmHg. This implies that some additional ventilatory drive is displacing the CO_2 ventilatory response line to the left, but there is no evidence available that this response line is also steeper.[22] In some cases of heart failure there is significant hypoxaemia, which may contribute both to a steeper and left-shifted CO_2 response curve.

This 'heart failure' drive is likely to be due to stimulation of lung receptors by the raised left atrial (and pulmonary venous) pressure. Even small rises in pulmonary venous pressure can stimulate ventilation, probably through activation of both fast and slowly adapting receptors as well as bronchial C-fibres.[342]

How this extra ventilatory drive behaves during sleep is not known. If it also falls with sleep onset, so that there is a bigger change in overall drive than normal, then this (in conjunction with arousals) is probably explanation enough for the CSR. The only evidence related to this point comes from some work on the ventilatory pattern during sleep in patients with interstitial lung disease.[455] The awake tachypnoea in these patients (presumed to be at least in part due to lung receptor stimulation) does reduce with sleep. In the past the delay in lung to brain circulation time found in heart failure has been proposed as the mechanism producing the CSR, but in animal models[269] and with computer modelling, this prolongation has to be considerable (over 2 min). This is longer than is usually seen in practice, however, it could contribute along with the other mechanisms described above.

If the above explanations are true then it is easy to see why added oxygen may help some patients in whom the ventilatory response to CO_2 is left-shifted and steeper due to hypoxia. It is difficult to see how acetazolamide or added inspired CO_2 work unless they provide a further increase in ventilatory drive that is less sensitive to sleep–wake changes (or makes these changes proportionately less important) and, hence, stabilize respiration in that way. As described earlier, moving tidal volumes away from the deadspace volume will help to stabilize ventilation too.

Another facet of this problem has been the finding that nasal continuous positive airway pressure (CPAP), as used in OSA, may improve the CSR and the cardiac function.[693] In the original uncontrolled study on five patients with heart failure and symptoms of sleep apnoea, the CSR certainly did improve with CPAP, as did the left ventricular ejection fraction. This first study was criticized for its lack of controls and the fact that some of the patients may well have had a degree of ordinary OSA. Certainly in patients with OSA, effective treatment is likely to improve heart failure.[433] No other unit has been able to reproduce this work[90,148] although a later paper from the original group has confirmed their earlier findings.[71] It may be that nasal CPAP is simply loading the ventilatory system, increasing functional residual capacity (FRC) and, thus, improving gas exchange and the P_{aO_2}; changes that all effectively flatten the slope of the ventilatory response to CO_2.

If there is any improvement in cardiac function then it may be due to similar mechanisms to those proposed for ordinary positive end expiratory pressure, a treatment used when ventilating patients with pulmonary oedema, which raises intra-alveolar pressure encouraging fluid resorption.

When the CSR of left heart failure is treated successfully there is a definite improvement in symptoms.[273] Clarifying the mechanism of CSR should allow better treatments since simply increasing the antifailure therapy often does not work. This unfortunately is the usual response to a patient with heart failure who complains of episodes of nocturnal breathlessness: presumably based on the assumption that this must be paroxysmal nocturnal dyspnoea (PND) due to pulmonary oedema. However, careful questioning will differentiate PND from CSR: PND goes on for much longer after arousal than the brief disturbance associated with each CSR cycle (only a very small proportion of which will be remembered next morning).

At present there is no satisfactory guidance on the management of CSR with unpleasant symptoms when the heart failure has been adequately treated. The best advice one can give is sequentially to try (or in combination if desperate), added oxygen, acetazolamide, or theophyllines. Added CO_2 will work, but providing it long-term in the home is not easy.

The above explanations for periodic breathing at sleep onset, during hypoxia, and with heart failure are complex and multifactorial. Although computer modelling has helped our understanding considerably, there is still speculation involved in much of the explanations. More experimental data are needed on the sleep–wake changes in the ventilatory drive of hypoxia, hypercapnia, and increased pulmonary venous pressure drives together with better ways of assessing sleep–wake fluctuations during periodic breathing. This information can then be used in yet more sophisticated computer models to aid understanding.

11.3 REM-related respiratory oscillations

The peculiarities of respiratory control during REM sleep (see the section on REM sleep in Chapter 2, p. 16) provide the opportunity for two types of central apnoeas to occur. Apnoeas during this period can be entirely normal or be an indication of problems with the respiratory muscle pump.

11.3.1 Normal REM sleep apnoeas

During REM sleep, ventilation is much less regular than in non-REM sleep due to the 'addition' of fluctuating ventilatory drive that has nothing to do with chemical control, but seems to relate to the phasic events in the brain that also produce the rapid eye movements and muscular twitches.[237,473,485] Gould et al.[237] showed that the diminutions in ventilation were associated with the actual phasic eye movements in normal subjects (Fig. 11.4). It appears that sometimes the phasic activity is sufficiently intense to provoke apnoea. It is likely that these periods of phasic activity are random and do not reflect dream content just as the eye movements are not thought to be 'purposeful' scanning of the dream imagery.[304] The mechanism of the reduction in ventilation appears to be a transient increase in the normal REM sleep paralysis mechanism; hyperpolarization of the lower motorneurones via inhibitory reticulospinal pathways originating in Jouvet's area in the pons (Chapter 2, p. 13).

The extent to which there is suppression of respiratory excursions with the phasic events of REM sleep seems to vary from individual to individual,[485] but is consistent for one subject during a night's study.

11.3.2 Abnormal respiratory pump

In a normal subject the reduction in activity of the non-diaphragm respiratory muscles during REM sleep is of no great consequence, producing only the occasional apnoeas and hypoventilation episodes described above. However, in subjects with compromised respiratory muscle function (particularly of the diaphragm), who rely on accessory muscles of respiration to pump an adequate tidal volume, REM sleep can lead to severely compromised respiration.

There are many diseases where respiratory muscle function is compromised. This can either be primary, that is, a specific abnormality of the muscles or their innervation or secondary, that is, due to problems with the lungs or chest wall which make muscle action less effective. A very complete review of these conditions appears in Shneerson's[625] book on disorders of ventilation.

11.3.2.1 Neuromuscular causes

Many neuromuscular diseases lead to respiratory failure, this often being the primary cause of death. The respiratory system has enormous reserves and the vital capacity (volume exhaled from full inspiration to full

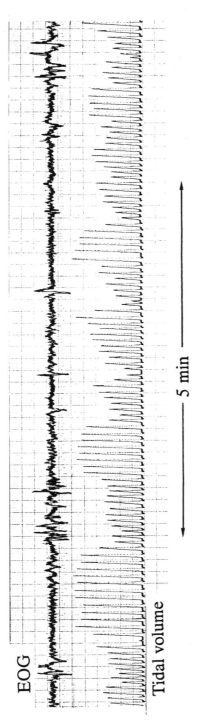

Fig. 11.4 Ventilation (from a face mask) and the effect of bursts of eye movements (EOG) during REM sleep. Note the 'denting' of tidal volume when there are eye movements on the EOG tracing, with recovery in between.

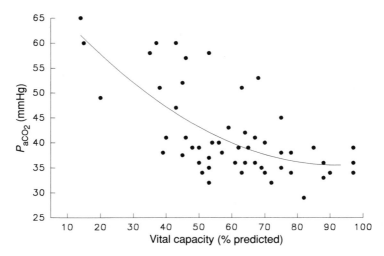

Fig. 11.5 Effect of a reduced vital capacity, due to various myopathies, on arterial CO_2 tension (P_{aCO_2}). Redrawn with permission from Braun *et al.* (1983).[76]

expiration) has to drop considerably before ventilatory failure occurs. There is a correlation between vital capacity and the degree of ventilatory failure[76] as measured by the rise in P_{aCO_2}, but there is a considerable spread (Fig. 11.5). Resting ventilatory failure does not correlate any better with actual muscle strength (using maximal inspiratory and expiratory mouth pressures). There is some evidence that the extent to which the diaphragm is predominantly involved may determine whether or not a patient with a neuromuscular disease develops ventilatory failure early in his disease or not.[486] The best (but rare) example of this is the milder form of acid maltase deficiency.[412] This abnormality of muscle (a glycogen storage disorder) often affects the diaphragm very early on, sometimes before there is much evidence of weakness elsewhere.[583] The presentation is of a middle-aged patient with symptoms of morning headache, orthopnoea, morning confusion and cyanosis, and possibly ankle oedema. Sleep disturbance and hypersomnolence are often present so that night sedation may be prescribed which usually precipitates severe ventilatory failure and hospital admission. The cause of the ventilatory failure may be difficult to ascertain while the patient is lying supine on a ventilator. Attempts at weaning often fail as they are usually attempted with the patient supine, when the weak diaphragm is at its greatest disadvantage due to the abdominal contents pushing up against it. Once spontaneously breathing, the abdominal paradox during inspiration (particularly on sniffing), should be recognized. The simplest test for severe diaphragm weakness is a measurement of vital capacity (VC) done lying and standing. In normal subjects there should be a < 10 per cent fall in VC on lying, but there will be progressively bigger falls with increasing diaphragm weakness.[468] In total diaphragm paralysis, there may be a 50 per cent or more fall in the VC on lying down, again due to the weight of the abdominal contents pushing on the diaphragm. On standing the abdominal contents drop down, thus allowing better lung expansion. The curious point about these patients with acid maltase deficiency is their ability to breathe quite well sitting or standing, yet they can be in severe ventilatory failure.

As mentioned before, during REM sleep the diaphragm may be the only or main muscle left breathing. In the absence of a functioning diaphragm, REM sleep hypoventilation can be profound with long apnoeas.[633,637,672] In a dog model, reversible bilateral diaphragm paralysis was associated with hypoventilation only during REM sleep and, although resting ventilation was not impaired in wakefulness or non-REM sleep, there was a marked inability to cope with any extra ventilatory load,[666] even when awake. Figure 11.6 is an example of REM sleep hypoxaemia in a patient with bilateral diaphragm paralysis.

It appears that repeated arousals are necessary to restore ventilation and blood gases. Whether this REM sleep hypoventilation or apnoea actually accelerates the development of chronic ventilatory failure is not clear; it may be merely a marker of the existence of such a problem. There is some evidence that by suppressing REM sleep with protriptyline[632] there may be a temporary improvement, but in our experience this is not usually sustained. Usually overnight ventilation is required which consistently restores blood gases to normal, day and night. The possible mechanisms of action of this treatment are discussed later (p. 218).

Pure diaphragm paralysis is rare in other neuromuscular disorders, but has been reported, for example, in motor neurone disease,[7] spino-cerebellar degeneration,[467] and bilateral neuralgic amyotrophy.[239] Trauma can avulse both phrenic nerves[392] and, occasionally, they can both be involved in a syndrome similar to Bell's palsy of the facial nerve where a virus infection of unknown type may be responsible.[95,643] This may be the same condition as neuralgic amyotrophy, but without any pain. Although usually unilateral, bilateral damage to the phrenic nerves can occur during cardiac surgery due to the use of crushed ice to preserve the heart. This can produce 'frost bite' of the phrenic nerves which usually recover some months later as the phrenic axons regrow.[362]

In other neuromuscular disorders ventilatory muscle failure usually develops alongside a general muscle failure, but sometimes there is still a profound nocturnal worsening of the blood gases, particularly during REM sleep, which produces symptoms of sleep disturbance and responds to over-night ventilation. Perhaps the best example of this is post-poliomyelitis

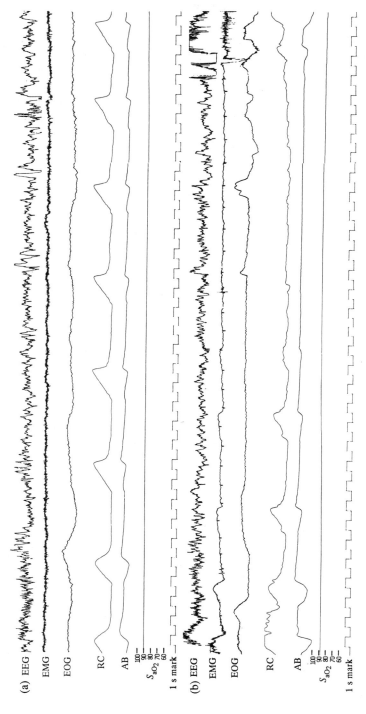

Fig. 11.6 Two separate tracings from a patient with bilateral diaphragm paralysis. (a) Patient in SWS demonstrating the paradoxical abdominal movement. (b) Attempted REM sleep. The tracing starts towards the end of an arousal and as REM sleep starts (falling EMG tone and appearance of eye movements) respiratory activity fades out: S_{aO_2} falls to approximately 80 per cent and another arousal occurs with resumption of ventilation.

syndrome.[160,312,389] Some 30 years or so after the original infection, there can be a return of weakness in the muscles originally affected.[96,140] The mechanism is not clear, but it may just possibly be a reactivation of the poliomyelitis virus.[522,618] It is more likely to be premature ageing of the remaining anterior horn cells that 'took over' more muscle fibres during recovery from the initial illness. If the original disease affected the respiratory muscles or if associated with subsequent scoliosis, then respiratory failure is much more likely to occur as part of the post-polio syndrome.[160] The vital capacity may sometimes be relatively well preserved (> 1.5 l), but dominant involvement of the diaphragm is not particularly obvious. During sleep there is profound hypoxaemia, mainly during REM sleep, usually central, but occasionally with an upper airway obstructive component.[296]

11.3.2.2 Chest wall abnormalities

The respiratory muscles can be put at a severe mechanical disadvantage by conditions that distort the chest wall. The best examples of this are scoliosis and previous thoracoplasty. Thoracoplasty was a chest operation performed until the 1950s, that collapsed a number of the ribs on one side of the chest to squash the underlying lung as a treatment for tuberculosis.

Both these conditions can lead to eventual respiratory failure, even when it appears that there has been no deterioration in respiratory mechanics for some while. The mechanism of the respiratory failure is not understood but a low vital capacity (< 1 l) is usually present. In addition to a stiff rib-cage, there may also be some increase in lung stiffness due to long-term inadequate expansion. Sleep studies in these patients reveal REM sleep hypoxia only, in the early stages, which progresses to all night hypoxaemia once daytime respiratory failure occurs (Fig. 11.7). Respiratory failure due to both scoliosis and thoracoplasty can be treated by overnight ventilation (see later, p. 217).

11.3.2.3 Chronic airways obstruction

Sleep hypoxaemia in chronic airways obstruction (CAWO) excited much attention in the late 1970s and early 1980s. At one stage the presence or absence of sleep hypoxaemia was thought to perhaps underlie the spread of presentations of CAWO, that is, the so-called 'pink puffer' and 'blue bloater' differentiation.[56,196] The CAWO patient with respiratory failure (raised P_{aCO_2} and low P_{aO_2}) and cor pulmonale (ankle oedema from fluid retention) is very different from the patient with preserved blood gases yet who is often breathless. These two different patients might have equally severe airways obstruction, yet one will slip into respiratory failure early and the other only much later (usually as a pre-terminal event). No satisfactory explanation has appeared to account for these two extreme

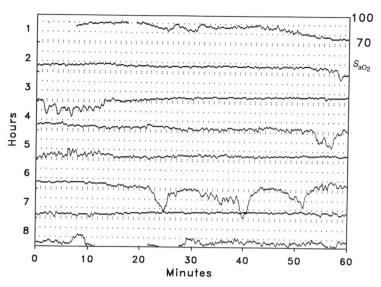

Fig. 11.7 Overnight S_{aO_2} tracing from a patient with scoliosis in mild daytime respiratory failure (P_{aCO_2}, 6.8 kPa). Note the fall in S_{aO_2} to approximately 78 per cent for much of the night (non-REM sleep) and further falls as low as 40 per cent during REM sleep.

presentations of CAWO, although subtle differences in their pathophysiology may be to blame (for example, pre-morbid hypoxic or hypercapnic sensitivity,[27] the exact nature of the ventilation perfusion mismatch,[717] and the degree of respiratory muscle mechanical disadvantage[241]). Thus, the idea that some sleep-related event, provoking extra hypoxia and CO_2 retention, might accelerate the onset of respiratory failure was clearly attractive.

Early work with intermittent sampling of arterial blood showed that there was a deterioration in P_{aO_2} and P_{aCO_2} during sleep in patients with CAWO,[363] but it was only with the arrival of non-invasive oximeters that the full extent of the hypoxaemia could be quantified.[707] When oximetry was combined with sleep staging it was clear that the most severe hypoxaemia was associated with REM sleep.[166,761] Although the hypoxaemia measured on an oximeter (S_{aO_2}) appeared dramatically worse in patients with daytime respiratory failure (Fig. 11.8), this was essentially because of the shape of the haemoglobin dissociation curve.[667] Most CAWO patients will drop their P_{aO_2} levels transiently during REM sleep by approximately 20–30 mmHg, but if they start at an S_{aO_2} of 96 per cent then a fall of 25 mmHg P_{aO_2} will only give an S_{aO_2} of approximately 89 per cent, a fall

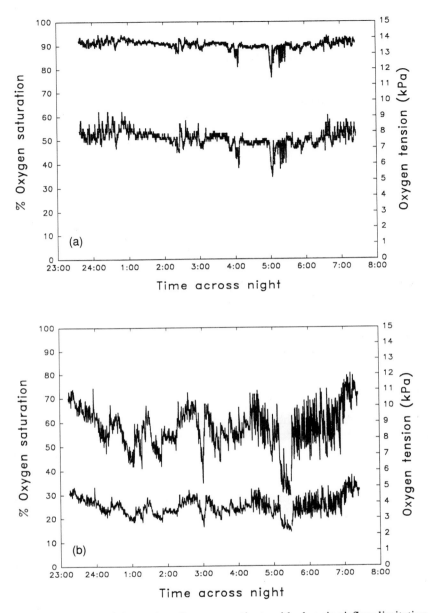

Fig. 11.8 Two overnight tracings from two patients with chronic airflow limitation. The top line in each box is the S_{aO_2} from an oximeter, the lower line in each box is a theoretical conversion to the equivalent P_{aO_2}, assuming a standard haemoglobin/oxygen dissociation curve. (a) This patient is a 'pink puffer' with near normal daytime blood gases and (b) this patient is a 'blue bloater' with daytime hypoxaemia and hypercapnia. Note that although the S_{aO_2} traces look dramatically different, the P_{aO_2} traces are very similar.

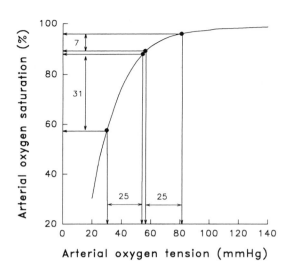

Fig. 11.9 Haemoglobin/oxygen dissociation curve. A 25 mmHg fall in P_{aO_2} produces a much bigger S_{aO_2} fall when the starting P_{aO_2} is already lower. Refer to the text for details.

of only 7 per cent S_{aO_2}. However, if the starting S_{aO_2} is 88 per cent then the same fall in P_{aO_2} will give an S_{aO_2} of 57 per cent, a fall of 31 per cent S_{aO_2} (Fig. 11.9). In one paper, analysing hypoxaemia during sleep in CAWO, the tracings of the 'mildest' and 'severest' desaturations chosen for publication show identical calculated falls in P_{aO_2} (approximately 20 mmHg) during REM sleep, although the first impression is of a dramatic difference.[201] In addition, if the sleep-related change is really a fixed change in pH sensitivity at the brainstem (engendered by the P_{aCO_2} change), then a slightly bigger rise in P_{aCO_2} (and hence fall in P_{aO_2}) would be expected in the initially more hypercapnic patient. This is derived from the fact that pH change is proportional to P_{aCO_2}/HCO_3^-, so that in compensated respiratory acidosis it takes a bigger P_{CO_2} change to produce the same pH change compared to normal. Whether ventilation is more closely related to pH, H^+, or P_{CO_2} in these circumstances is not known.[27]

Overall there is a fairly good relationship between the daytime level of hypoxaemia and the degree of nocturnal hypoxaemia (both mean nocturnal levels and lowest nocturnal values).[105,127,667] However, there is variation about this relationship and some patients experience more than average extra hypoxaemia while others experience less. One of the causes of more than average hypoxaemia is if there is also a degree of obstructive sleep apnoea. This was the case in an early series where patients with primarily sleep apnoea and concomitant lung disease were studied.[250]

Having established that the apparently dramatic falls in S_{aO_2} in the initially hypoxic patients with CAWO are really only a consequence of the shape of the O_2 dissociation curve, do they matter? On the one hand, it has been argued that they are merely a marker of severe hypoxaemia.[667] On the other, that they are an important accelerator of secondary complications of hypoxaemia such as cor pulmonale and polycythaemia.[70,156]

There is conflicting evidence on this point. Early work showed that variations in the red cell mass response to hypoxaemia could be explained entirely by the daytime P_{aO_2} levels and that no extra predictive value is derived from knowing the nighttime P_{aO_2} levels.[667]

In a joint centre study the survival of 97 patients with CAWO was shown not to be significantly related to whether the patients experienced more or less nocturnal hypoxaemia than predicted from their daytime values.[127] Again it was the daytime value of P_{aO_2} that was more predictive of future survival. Two recent studies have looked specifically at CAWO patients with daytime P_{aO_2} levels above 60 mmHg to try and answer this point.[200,409] The first study showed that the patients in whom nocturnal hypoxaemia occurred did have higher pulmonary artery pressures.[409] However, the awake resting S_{aO_2} was significantly lower in this group (91 per cent versus 93.4 per cent, an estimated P_{aO_2} difference of 16 mmHg), suggesting that the one-off arterial blood gas estimation used to select the patients had unfortunately been higher than usual in some cases and therefore unrepresentative. This emphasizes the importance of proper resting measures of arterial oxygenation, perhaps better done with a few minutes of oximetry than a single arterial blood sample. The second parallel study looked at the effects of added nocturnal oxygen versus placebo in a total of 36 patients with CAWO, daytime P_{aO_2} values above 60 mmHg, but evidence of desaturation on overnight oximetry.[200] Although at 3 years there was a small difference in pulmonary artery pressure (7.6 mmHg in favour of O_2 treatment) there was no effect on mortality, red cell mass or lung function. These two groups of 'desaturators' were also compared to a group of 'non-desaturators' who had a much lower mortality rate over three years. However, this 'non-desaturating' group had a resting P_{aO_2} 10 mmHg higher than both the 'desaturating' groups which makes valid comparison impossible.

Whether the nocturnal hypoxaemia is an important extra and variable 'hypoxic insult' reducing survival in CAWO is not just an academic question. If it were important, then the assessment for long-term oxygen therapy *might* be refined by including measures of nocturnal oxygenation. In addition, the flow rate of oxygen used would have to be shown to be adequate to improve the nocturnal as well as the daytime figures. At present there is no evidence to suggest that measures of nocturnal hypoxaemia should be taken into account when assessing suitability for long-term oxygen therapy: the original studies showing benefit in a certain well-defined group did not have nocturnal oxygenation data.[494,677] Until further work is done on this subject there is no justification to do sleep studies routinely on all CAWO patients.

Although it is reasonable to be nihilistic about taking account of nocturnal hypoxaemia in CAWO when prescribing long-term oxygen to improve survival, it may be reasonable to consider it for improvement in sleep quality, which is poor in these patients.[94,195] Again there is conflicting evidence,[94,195,232,454] but raising P_{aO_2} may well reduce the number of arousals during sleep in some patients with hypoxic CAWO. It clearly does not help all such patients, but in our experience some patients sleep much better with consequent improvement in daytime alertness. When looking for such benefits in the clinical setting, the placebo effect of overnight oxygen must not be overlooked.

The exact mechanism of the REM sleep hypoxaemia in CAWO is not fully clear. The ventilation during this period is far from stable and attempts at measuring ventilation/perfusion $(\dot{V}/\dot{Q})$ matching are very inaccurate. Suffice to say that the measured falls in ventilation that occur[314,667] can explain the hypoxaemia (Fig. 11.10). Changes in cardiac output, $\dot{V}O_2$, or $\dot{V}/\dot{Q}$ matching (due to a fall in functional residual capacity) do not need to be invoked, although they may also occur. The hypoventilation is probably explained on the basis of the REM sleep inhibition of the non-diaphragm muscles of respiration upon which these patients are particularly dependent. Johnson and Remmers[336] showed very nicely that during REM sleep in patients with CAWO the loss of activity of muscles, such as the scalenes, resulted in a marked reduction (and even paradoxical movement) in the excursion of the rib-cage with a consequent fall in tidal volume (Fig. 11.11). This loss of intercostal and accessory muscle activity in REM sleep with diminished excursion of the rib-cage, is of course seen in normals[658,692] and is particularly associated with the periods of actual eye movements,[219,237,473] (see the section on REM sleep in Chapter 2, p. 16). Reduction of REM sleep with protriptyline will reduce the degree of sleep hypoxaemia, but side-effects have prevented the long-term evaluation of this approach to treatment.[99]

There is also debate as to how much upper airway obstruction may contribute to the extra hypoxaemia during sleep in patients with CAWO. Most studies have not found an excess of patients with OSA in a group of patients selected primarily for their CAWO[105,219,667] although some have.[201] However, Sullivan's[109] group have suggested recently that during sleep there may be increases in upper airway resistance with snoring, short of actual apnoea, that constitute an extra inspiratory load, thus exacerbating hypoventilation and perhaps long-term ventilatory failure. This work awaits confirmation.

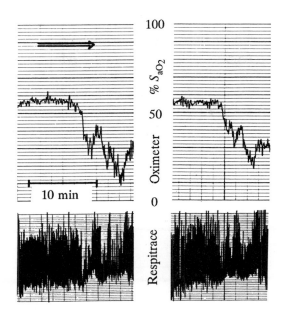

Fig. 11.10 Two short periods of S_{aO_2} and ventilation (from a calibrated respiratory inductance plethysmograph) during REM sleep in a patient with chronic airflow limitation. Note the way S_{aO_2} closely follows the fluctuations in ventilation.

Because many patients with CAWO are large middle-aged men, it would not be surprising if there were patients with additional obstructive sleep apnoea or hypopnoea. The combination of the two probably accelerates the development of cor pulmonale and ventilatory failure.[203,373,731] The clinical consequence of this is that in a patient with CO_2 retention, but a relatively well preserved FEV_1 (perhaps above 1 l), the possibility of associated OSA should be entertained and the right questions about snoring, sleepiness, and witnessed apnoeas asked. Treatment of OSA in the presence of hypercapnic CAWO will improve the P_{aCO_2} and P_{aO_2}.[203] Finally, it has been shown that supplemental oxygen is more likely to provoke CO_2 retention in patients with CAWO if they also have OSA.[232]

11.4 Reflex central apnoea

Central respiratory output can be influenced by a variety of reflexes originating from receptors in the upper airway and lungs. The best known from the lung is the Hering Breuer inflation reflex. The better known

(a)

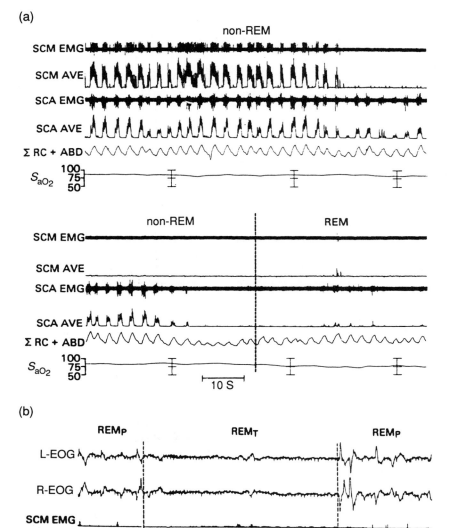

(b)

reflexes from the upper airway are those involved in defending the airway from foreign bodies, such as gagging, coughing, and sneezing. Sleep however can change the efferent limb of such reflexes. For example, laryngeal stimulation provokes coughing whilst awake, but during sleep (in dogs) may provoke complete central apnoea.[683] Most work on laryngeal reflexes has been done under anaesthesia where laryngeal closure and inhibition of inspiration are usually seen in response to stimulation.[451]

In addition to laryngeal reflexes, there are powerful pharyngeal reflexes. Following the recognition of obstructive sleep apnoea, much attention has been paid to the pharynx's ability to defend itself from collapse. There is no doubt that subatmospheric pressures in the pharynx stimulate reflex pharyngeal dilator activity (see p. 24 and Figs 3.7 and 3.8, pp. 30 and 31). Apart from this extra pharyngeal dilation there is also inhibition of inspiration.[450] This presumably reduces inspiratory airflow and reduces the subatmospheric 'sucking effect' on the pharyngeal walls.

This pharyngeal reflex is thought to be the possible explanation for some central apnoeas seen in patients who snore and present clinically as obvious cases of OSA. Sullivan's group[328] first described eight patients with both obstructive and central apnoeas. These patients all had histories of snoring and sleep disruption with daytime sleepiness strongly suggestive of OSA. The central apnoeas in these patients occurred when they were supine, were abolished by nasal CPAP, and in three subjects were converted to ordinary obstructive apnoeas by topical anaesthesia of the pharyngeal mucosa. This suggested to the authors that a pharyngeal reflex, due to collapse of the pharynx and apposition of the mucosal surfaces, was inhibiting inspiration. Also of interest was that in these cases the apnoea was still terminated by arousal suggesting the deterioration in blood gases *per se* was the stimulus to awake, rather than the actual respiratory effort which is now believed to be the usual arousing influence in OSA.[224,225] In our experience these patients can also be recognized on sound and video recordings by the upper

---

Fig. 11.11 Respiratory EMG studies in a patient with chronic airflow limitation. (a) Two continuous tracings taken from a transition period from non-REM to REM sleep. Initially, the scalene and sternocleidomastoid muscles (SCA and SCM, raw and averaged, AVE) are active. As REM sleep appears, first the scalene, and then sternocleidomastoid drop out. Ventilation (the sum of the rib-cage and abdominal movement, RC + ABD) and S_{aO_2} fall simultaneously. (b) A period of REM sleep, initially phasic (REM$_P$), then tonic (REM$_T$), and returning to phasic. The eye movements (R and L EOG) are used to define these phases. During phasic REM there is no activity in the scalene muscle (SCA) and there is rib-cage (RC) paradox. During the tonic phase the activity of the scalene returns and the rib-cage paradox disappears. During this period of normal chest wall movement the S_{aO_2} rises. With permission from Johnson and Remmers (1984).[336]

airway opening noise that can be heard at the end of each apnoea, again suggesting the pharynx was closed. This variant of obstructive sleep apnoea is not common and tends to occur in the less severe patients. In Issa and Sullivan's[328] paper it seemed to be associated with previous brain damage or degeneration, such as a stroke or following brain surgery. They suggested that there might be a release of a more primitive reflex by this brain damage, as is thought to be the explanation for the grasp reflex in this situation.

The Toronto group have also described this OSA variant.[73] They studied 13 normocapnic and obese subjects with central sleep apnoeas who were expected to have obstructive apnoeas on account of their histories of hypersomnolence, snoring, and choking sensations at night. These patients were not hypercapnic during the day, which contrasted with five hypercapnic patients who had central sleep apnoea due to reduced respiratory drive. No connection with possible brain damage was found in this study.

From a clinical point of view it is important not to be put off trying nasal CPAP in such patients where the clinical suspicion of OSA is high, but the sleep study shows dominant central apnoeas.

11.5 Apparent central apnoea

The diagnosis of central sleep apnoeas depends on failing to detect any respiratory effort during the period of absent airflow at the nose and mouth. In a sense the apnoeas found during REM sleep in neuromuscular diseases, particularly with bilateral diaphragm paralysis, are not really central because it is failure of any respiratory muscles to be able to respond to central output that has caused the apnoea. However, these were classified under REM-related sleep oscillations since they occur as a consequence of the peculiar physiology of REM sleep.

Failure to detect evidence of central respiratory output from peripheral indicators (surface movement) may also occur when the respiratory muscles are simply too weak to produce significant expansion of the chest wall when there is upper airway collapse.[636] Examples of this phenomenon are the obstructive apnoeas during sleep seen in Duchenne muscular dystrophy. Figure 11.12 shows the virtual disappearance of surface evidence of respiratory effort (as well as airflow apnoea) but the rib-cage and abdominal signals do continue and the submental EMG shows a respiratory signal[636] indicating that central drive really is continuing.

Work from Khan and Heckmatt[354] has shown that boys with Duchenne dystrophy do indeed get predominantly obstructive apnoeas during REM sleep, often with very minimal rib-cage and abdominal movements to indicate they are obstructive.

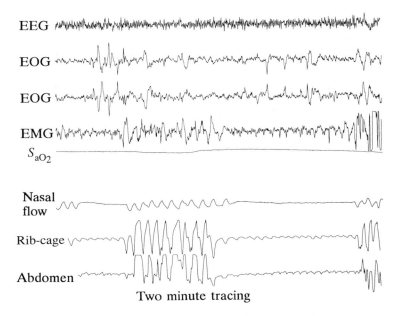

EEG

EOG

EOG

EMG

S_{aO_2}

Nasal flow

Rib-cage

Abdomen

Two minute tracing

Fig. 11.12 Obstructive apnoeas in a boy with Duchenne muscular dystrophy during REM sleep. During the apnoea (no nasal flow) there are tiny rib-cage and abdominal movements that might have been mistaken for cardiac artefact except they are too slow.

Surface movements of the chest and abdomen may also fail to indicate any respiratory effort during obstructive apnoeas in markedly obese subjects. Staats et al.[645] used inductive plethysmography and oesophageal pressure monitoring in 54 patients with different degrees of OSA severity. In three, despite inspiratory efforts of -10 cm H_2O or more, there was no motion measured by the inductance plethysmograph. Thus, surface measurements alone would have led to misclassification of these apnoeas. Again, the clinical message is that in someone in whom OSA is suspected, but respiratory monitoring suggested mainly central apnoeas, it may still be worth trying nasal CPAP.

11.6 Overnight ventilation for central sleep apnoea or hypoventilation

The conditions described in this chapter all have reduced ventilation during sleep and are variously called sleep hypoventilation syndromes, central sleep apnoea, nocturnal hypoventilation syndromes, non-obstructive sleep apnoea, and, in the less severe cases, Cheyne–Stokes breathing or periodic breathing. In each of the individual sections specific treatments, where available, were mentioned, for example, acetazolamide in high altitude periodic breathing or added oxygen in the Cheyne–Stokes breathing of heart failure. In many of these conditions no specific treatment is possible other than to support ventilation during sleep.

The mechanism by which overnight ventilation alone can reverse the diurnal respiratory failure of, for example, a patient with scoliosis is not clear. There are essentially three explanations and it is likely that in any one individual all three play a part. Supporting ventilation overnight will undoubtedly rest the respiratory muscles.[352] This may mean that for the remaining 16 h they can work more effectively. Attempts to measure improved muscle strength have not consistently supported this explanation, but in reality it is muscle *endurance* that is more important and this is much harder to assess.

Alternatively there may be a resetting of the respiratory control mechanisms. By increasing ventilation during sleep there will be a respiratory alkalosis, this will lead to a relative metabolic acidosis in the blood, brain, and CSF, which may keep respiratory stimulation higher during the day. Improvements in the CO_2 response can be demonstrated, but if muscle strength is changing then this cannot be taken as evidence for an increased central response.

Finally, because the tidal volumes generated by the assisted ventilation may be higher than the voluntary vital capacity, an increase in lung and chest wall compliance may occur: simply viewed as an easing of stiffened joints and reversal of atelectatic areas of lung. There is some evidence for this in that the vital capacities of a group of patients with restrictive problems rose approximately 28 per cent after two weeks nocturnal assisted ventilation.[630] Interestingly, even though a patient will have reduced his P_{aCO_2} by breathing more (following a period on overnight ventilation) he will usually be less breathless, rather than more so.

Assisted ventilation during sleep has a long history and grew mainly out of the technology designed to support poliomyelitis victims. An excellent account of the history of negative and positive pressure ventilation is provided by John Shneerson[625] in his book on *Disorders of ventilation*, Chapters 17–19, with splendid photographs of some of the early equipment.

11.6.1 Negative pressure ventilation

The chest wall normally increases in size and pulls the lung out thus drawing air into the alveoli. This action is recreated exactly by surrounding the chest in a rigid container and evacuating the air between the chest wall and the container. The most efficient device is a tank ventilator which encloses the whole body with just the head protruding. There has to be a seal at the neck of course, but otherwise it is quite comfortable to lie in and be ventilated. Although these devices are now a relative rarity, they are still used in many units to ensure a good period of ventilation when patients come in with worsening of their ventilatory failure. There are smaller domiciliary versions available, but the incentive to construct lightweight small domiciliary versions has been reduced by the availability of off the shelf nasal positive airway pressure systems (see p. 220).

Less efficient negative pressure systems are available which do not require a big rigid tank. The jacket system consists of a cage over the chest and abdomen which is further enclosed in an airtight 'anorak' type jacket. The cage provides a space around the chest wall that can be evacuated, although the compliance of the jacket and persistent leaks make the system less efficient than a tank ventilator. Least efficient of all are the cuirass systems that fit around the chest and are specially constructed to fit each individual. They have to be very carefully made to ensure even pressure along the edges with no leaks and no excess pressure areas that will produce pain and discomfort. Few centres have the expertise or facilities to tailor make high quality cuirass shells[88] and again the incentive to gain this expertise has been reduced by the increasing use of nasal positive pressure systems.

The pumps for all these negative pressure systems tend to be bulky and noisy because of the considerable volumes of air that have to be shifted in and out of the space around the chest wall. Smaller versions are available, but are still noisy. Chapter 17 in Shneerson's[625] book describes the various systems available along with their advantages and disadvantages.

There is no doubt that these devices can all be highly effective in reversing the ventilatory failure of a vast range of conditions. Because of their limited efficiency they are less useful when the chest wall is very stiff or when there is a high airways resistance. For example, they will not ventilate very well patients in ventilatory failure due to chronic airways obstruction[106,533] although there was brief enthusiasm for this a few years ago.[131,438,439]

There is a wealth of literature documenting long-term reversal of ventilatory failure, sometimes for decades, in patients who would otherwise have died. For example, Garay et al.[213] demonstrated sustained falls in P_{aCO_2} and improvement in P_{aO_2} in a range of hypoventilation syndromes, as did Loh et al.[416] in patients with bilateral diaphragm paralysis. There is also good evidence for its benefit in patients with chest wall problems such as scoliosis[747] and thoracoplasty.[604]

This kind of therapy has tended to be used only by very specialist centres, partly because of cost, but mainly because of the considerable expertise and time required to successfully establish patients on negative pressure ventilation at home. In addition to the relatively simple problems of careful fitting and leaks, there is also the problem of upper airway obstruction. Normally, spontaneous respiration is accompanied by activation of upper airway dilator muscles to resist the collapsing force of negative intrapharyngeal pressures. During negative pressure ventilation, respiratory drive may be lessened or abolished as the P_{aCO_2} is driven below the apnoea point. This allows inspiratory collapse to occur[231,318] of either (or both) the larynx and pharynx. This may be reversed to some extent by protriptyline[231,631] which increases upper airway muscle activity and reduces REM sleep, when this problem seems most likely to occur. One centre has added nasal CPAP to the negative pressure ventilation[231] with resolution of the obstructive apnoeas, but nasal ventilation alone seems a better solution over all.

11.6.2 The rocking bed

The rocking bed is an extraordinary device which literally rocks, end to end ($\pm 15-25°$), 15 times per minute driving the abdominal contents alternatively up into the lower chest and down again. The result of this is to move the diaphragm passively, thus generating a tidal volume, although the efficiency appears less than that of a jacket ventilator.[230] The advantage of this system over cuirass or jacket ventilators was that no help is required by the patient to use the system each night and he is unencumbered by equipment. The device is effective, if upper airway obstruction does not develop (see previous section) and rather surprisingly is acceptable to patients. The patients with muscle weakness and diaphragm paralysis (but no lung disease) seem to respond best to the rocking bed.[77,319,760]

11.6.3 Positive pressure ventilation

Positive pressure ventilation for long-term use lagged behind the use of negative pressure ventilation until the early 1950s when the poliomyelitis epidemics left many patients requiring mechanical ventilation. The use of a tracheostomy and cuffed tube gave secure control of the airway and allowed much simpler mechanical ventilators to be used. However, for the long-term patient the presence of a tracheostomy and its regular care could be a significant problem. The problems of long-term ventilation via a tracheostomy are well covered by Shneerson,[625] (Chapter 19). Because of these problems a variety of face mask and mouthpiece systems were tried with limited success. The polio patients showed enormous ingenuity in designing assisted ventilation systems, some of which travelled with them on their wheelchairs. The use of mouthpieces during nocturnal ventilation does work in some units, but in others has been difficult due to discomfort and poor sealing.[32,179]

It was the arrival of nasal masks, developed for the treatment of obstructive sleep apnoea, that produced a very rapid boom in the use of chronic intermittent positive pressure ventilation. By using the nasal route, humidification was rarely required. This approach was initially used for short periods[31,154] but was then used continuously overnight.[98,179] The use of 'off the shelf' equipment meant that long delays fabricating cuirass shells for oddly shaped chests could be bypassed. This relative ease of use, along with much increased efficiency, has ensured the almost universal replacement of negative pressure systems by nasal intermittent positive airway pressure ventilation (NIPPV).

For NIPPV to be successful still requires careful attention to detail and there are some pitfalls. In our experience almost any ventilator *can* be used although certain features are desirable. Although the ventilator takes over breathing once asleep, when awake it is often triggered. Thus, a ventilator with a trigger makes it easier for the patient to get used to any particular machine.

Our practice is to spend time with a patient during the day practising breathing with the ventilator: getting used to the sensation of being 'blown up' takes time. The approximate settings for inspiratory time, expiratory time, and pressure (or volume) are worked out during these trials. The correct size nasal mask (Fig. 7.3, p. 123) is chosen and a chin support and mouth cover prepared in case it is needed. Alternatively, the intranasal cushion system (Adams' circuit, see Fig. 7.4, p. 124) may be more appropriate. In patients with neuromuscular diseases alone the inflation pressures need only be about 10–20 cm H_2O depending on the particular ventilator. In patients with chest wall restriction or a degree of airway obstruction, higher pressures will be necessary. Beyond about 25 cm H_2O requires very careful fitting of the mask to avoid uncomfortable pressure effects at the rim of contact between mask and skin (see Plate 5).

Prior to the patient's usual sleep time the patient is set up on the ventilator, again in the triggered mode. The success of the system is continuously monitored with finger oximetry: this being compared to a previous night's tracing with no ventilatory support. Because the patient is usually sleep-deprived there is often little problem getting to sleep initially. Whether ventilation then remains adequate with only a triggered machine is unpredictable. Sometimes breathing simply stops with sleep onset and a default, back-up, rate for the ventilator has to be chosen that is not far short of the awake rate. On other occasions, in our experience much less commonly, the ventilator will go on being paced by the patient with adequate S_{aO_2} levels.

It is not advisable to try and return S_{aO_2} to normal on the first night, but to aim for abolition of the big REM sleep-related dips and a modest improvement in the S_{aO_2} at other times. If S_{aO_2} is returned too closely towards normal, then hypocapnia and alkalosis will inevitably also occur. Apart from sometimes making the patient uncomfortable, alkalosis may also explain why the larynx can close and prevent NIPPV working.[155] This problem appears quite suddenly when all seems to be going well; the chest and abdomen will stop moving, the ventilator continues blowing, inflation pressures may rise with greater outward distention of the neck or leakage around the mask or at the nose. The explanation for this is thought to be laryngeal closure,[155] and sometimes asynchronous respiratory movements of the chest and abdomen return before the patient wakes and the ventilator appears to be assisting breathing again. Although the full explanation for this phenomenon has not been found, it appears to be avoidable if one does not try to improve the oxygenation too quickly, presumably allowing acid/base adjustments to the falling P_{aCO_2}.

The second, more prevalent problem is leakage of air at the mouth following onset of sleep when muscle tone falls. In patients with OSA, who often have big soft palates, there is good sealing of the nasopharynx. The rise in air pressure blows the soft palate onto the back of the tongue with no leakage into the buccal cavity and out the mouth. In many patients having overnight ventilatory support, this sealing mechanism does not seem to work. Their soft palates are often smaller and they may have orofacial muscle weakness as well. This leads to the jaw falling open with considerable air leakage that prevents adequate ventilation. Even if a chin support is used to keep the jaw up, there can still be leakage through the lips. There are two approaches to this. Firstly, the pressure or tidal volume of the ventilator can be increased to 'beat' the leak or a mouth cover can be used. Trying to 'beat' the leak produces very uncomfortable buccal drying, variable performance depending on the exact degree of leakage and a variation in the system's efficiency depending on the lung and chest wall compliance. For example, if there is an increase in effective lung compliance due to infection or bronchospasm, then more air will escape through the mouth, with less ventilating the lungs. A mouth cover will provide support to the lips and, along with a chin support, prevent most leaks. However, such an arrangement is considerably more claustrophobic and may be intolerable.

In our experience, mouth leaks are the biggest problem setting up overnight ventilation. Various other approaches have been tried, such as oral prostheses to keep the jaw closed and lips supported, but to our knowledge these are not a significant improvement over chin supports and mouth covers.

Nasal blockage can be a problem, often exacerbated by the NIPPV. This usually responds to intranasal steroids and anticholinergics (ipratropium). Occasionally the anterior nares collapse and a mechanical dilator such as the Nozovent can be useful. The Adams' nasal cushions system will bypass this problem (see Fig. 7.4, p. 124).

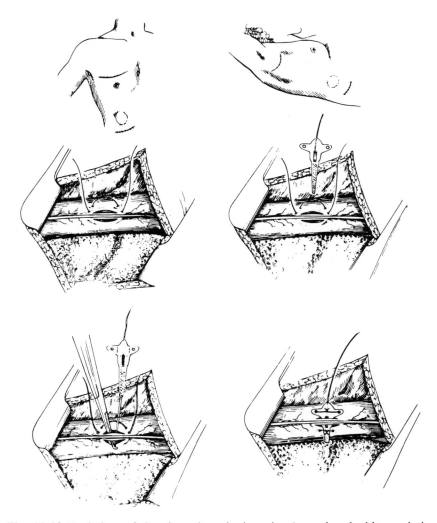

Fig. 11.13 Technique of phrenic pacing wire insertion (reproduced with permission from Glenn and Sairenji (1985)).[226]

If instituted successfully, there is no doubt that remarkable improvements can be obtained. The chronic respiratory failure can be reversed with normalization of P_{aO_2} and P_{aCO_2} levels.[98,216,295,720] Hypersomnolence can disappear along with greatly improved energy levels.[216,295,352] Clear benefit has been shown in a variety of neuromuscular disorders[179,216,285,295,563] and chest wall deformities.[98,180] There is also early evidence that this approach may be beneficial in some cases of chronic airways obstruction with CO_2 retention.[98,216,573]

11.6.4 Diaphragm pacing

When respiratory failure is due to inadequate central drive, particularly during sleep and the phrenic nerves and diaphragm are intact, then electrical pacing becomes a possibility. Attempts to stimulate the phrenic nerve to support ventilation have a long history. In the late 19th century Duchenne showed that stimulation of the phrenic nerve in the neck produced diaphragmatic contraction. In the 1920s adequate ventilation in neonates was shown to be possible with this approach.[625] Successful long-term use of implantable phrenic electrodes was first shown by Judson and Glenn[338] in 1966.

The main phrenic nerves can be exposed in the neck (distal to the point where all the nerve roots have joined) and bipolar or quadripolar electrodes sewn to the nerve bundles. Because of proximity to the brachial plexus and the risk of stimulating other nerves, as well as being able to ensure that the C_5 contribution is proximal to the attachment, it is now usual to place the phrenic electrode via a thoracic approach and, if at all possible, on two separate occasions (Fig. 11.13). The pacing wires connect to pick up coils placed under the skin, usually on the anterior chest wall.[226,625] Two weeks after implantation, the subcutaneous coils are pulsed with an external coil that generates a current in the implanted coil via induction. The mode of pulsing is critical to the long-term viability of the implanted electrodes. If establishing bilateral pacing, the nerves can be stimulated simultaneously or alternatively (some hours each side or alternate breaths each side). With lower frequency pacing it is possible to pace continuously which provides a better physiological result. An initially weak and atrophied diaphragm can recover over time.[748]

Few centres outside Glenn's unit at Yale have wide experience of this technique. When ventilatory assistance is only required at night, the extra cost and invasiveness of diaphragmatic pacing means that nasal IPPV is the first choice.

12 Differential diagnosis of sleepiness in adults

Any clinician primarily looking after patients with disorders of sleep and breathing will inevitably come across other causes of excessive daytime sleepiness. The recognition of the sleep apnoea syndromes has pushed these conditions off centre stage and certainly a general sleep disorders clinic will now see mainly sleep apnoea as a cause of hypersomnia.[87,461,484,764]

Table 12.1 is a list of the 'commoner' disorders and situations that can provoke hypersomnia. It is not an exhaustive list, but contains those likely to be met in everyday practice.

12.1 Intrinsic causes

This group of disorders appear to be due to abnormalities of the brain whereas the conditions in subsequent sections are due to external effects.

12.1.1 Narcolepsy

Narcolepsy appears to be a disorder of the control of REM sleep and its associated atonia (see Chapter 2). Normally REM sleep is tightly linked to sleep as a whole: REM sleep normally occurring in approximately equally spaced batches, the first appearing after approximately 90 min of non-REM sleep. In narcolepsy this is no longer the case: REM sleep and/or the associated atonia come on at any time during the day or night. The cardinal symptoms of narcolepsy relate closely to this problem and at present the diagnosis is made more on the history than any tests.

Cataplexy is the term for the sudden onset of general muscle weakness coming on whilst awake, almost exclusively in response to some exciting event or strong emotion. It can vary between complete collapsing on the floor to a mild drooping of the head, the period of weakness lasting for a few seconds up to several minutes. A typical story would be that during a good laugh the knees give way with collapse onto the floor; indeed this is thought to be the origin of the expression 'going weak at the knees with

Table 12.1 Differential diagnosis of sleepiness in adults

Intrinsic causes	Extrinsic causes	Circadian rhythm problems	Other conditions
Narcolepsy	Poor 'sleep hygiene'	Jet lag	Depression
Recurrent hypersomnia (Kleine–Levin syndrome)	Environmental causes	Shift work	Alcoholism
Idiopathic hypersomnia	Insufficient sleep	Irregular sleep–wake cycle	Parkinsons
Post-traumatic hypersomnia	Hypnotic/sedative abuse	Delayed sleep phase	
Periodic movements of the legs/restless sleep	Alcohol abuse		
The sleep apnoea syndromes			

After Thorpy,[704] *International classification of sleep disorders. Diagnostic and coding manual, 1990.* American Sleep Disorders Assocation, Rochester, Minnesota.

laughter'. To an onlooker, the sufferer may appear to have passed out as he is too weak to respond to questions and his eyes may be closed. However, on recovery, usually some seconds to a few minutes later, the patient will remember what was said whilst he was 'unconscious'. These 'drop attacks' can occur in response to a variety of emotional events such as laughter, sexual intercourse, anger, and intense pleasure. One of our patients lost his arm in a piece of machinery, having fallen into it after being told a joke.

This REM atonia may persist upon awakening. The patient is aware that he is paralysed. The period of paralysis can be as long as 5 min but may only last a few seconds. The patient feels that if only he could move a small part of his body he could break the whole paralysis. Although breathing continues, there is often a feeling of suffocation and impending doom. Because there may also be some frightening dreams and imagery with it, the whole experience can be intensely frightening and disturbing such that patients do not want to talk about it. Occasionally a few grunts may be possible during the sleep paralysis which will alert a bed partner to what is going on. A gentle push or noise, appears sometimes to be able to break the paralysis. Sleep paralysis occurs as an isolated unrelated event in some people and, although one of the cardinal symptoms of narcolepsy, does not allow a diagnosis of narcolepsy to be made unless other features are present.

Again because of the disordered REM sleep control, early onset dreaming with above average dream recall is common in narcolepsy. Average dream recall is perhaps zero to two per week but sometimes patients with narcolepsy can remember several per night. Particularly during daytime naps, the patient will be aware that he can wake after only a few minutes of sleep, having already had a dream. Sometimes the dreaming will come on almost in advance of sleep and is also referred to as hypnagogic hallucinations. These dreams, or hallucinations, are often particularly strange and frightening.

The usual presenting symptom and, hence, the possibility for confusion with sleep apnoea, is daytime sleepiness. The mechanism of this daytime sleepiness is not entirely clear. The sleepiness is often overwhelming and varies throughout the day. In contrast to sleep apnoea, the short daytime naps can be very refreshing and are used prophylactically to ward off sleepiness. Some of the sleepiness is probably due to very restless nighttime sleep. Polysomnography reveals more disturbed sleep,[766] possibly because of the rather random arrival of REM sleep interfering with the restorative potential of the non-REM sleep. This is unlikely to be the whole explanation, however.

Although severe cases of narcolepsy will have all these features, there are all grades of severity. Indeed minor examples may not be diagnosed when mild daytime sleepiness and occasional sleep onset dreaming are the only symptoms.

Narcolepsy has the highest human leukocyte antigen (HLA) association of any disorder so far looked at.[391] If definite cataplexy is required for the diagnosis then there is a virtual 100 per cent association with HLA DR2 and HLA DQW1. This particular HLA type being present in approximately 20–30 per cent of the population. The negroid population does not show such a high association with HLA DR2/DQW1. The association with an HLA type does not imply that narcolepsy is an immunological disorder, there being very little evidence to support this hypothesis. Presumably between DR2 and DQW1 there is a gene coding for a protein, probably a receptor, involved in the control of REM atonia. Initially a cholinergic receptor was thought to be the candidate,[356] but more recently an alpha adrenergic receptor subtype has been thought to be more likely.[492,493]

Narcolepsy certainly appears to be dominantly inherited and family histories are often positive.[35] As mentioned above, the diagnosis of narcolepsy may not have been made in a particular relative, but questioning will reveal that this is, or was, the likely diagnosis.

Most authors maintain that a diagnosis of classical narcolepsy requires cataplexy and at least one of the other three symptoms; sleepiness, sleep paralysis, and sleep onset dreaming (or hypnagogic hallucinations). If laboratory confirmation is required then the multiple sleep latency test can be performed (see the section on measuring daytime sleepiness in Chapter 4, p. 68). If two or more of four sleeps during a day have REM sleep onset then this is considered diagnostic. This may also be seen of course during a conventional polysomnographic sleep study. However, some of the sleep apnoea syndromes, particularly those that are much worse during REM sleep, can produce sufficient pressure for REM sleep to cause REM sleep onset. This phenomenon may explain some of the apparent association between sleep apnoea and narcolepsy. HLA typing can be done; the finding of the HLA DR2/DQW1 suggesting the possibility of narcolepsy and their absence virtually ruling it out, except in the negroid population.

Narcolepsy is much less common than sleep apnoea, the lifetime prevalence being approximately 0.06 per cent depending on the population studied. The prevalence in any population depends on the frequency of the HLA DR2 gene in that population. In Israeli Jews, for example, the gene frequency is only 11 per cent (compared to 25 per cent in the general North American population) and narcolepsy much rarer.[403] The converse is true in Japan where the DR2 gene frequency is nearer 35 per cent.[303] General sleep clinics now see perhaps ten times as many OSA patients as narcoleptics.[461,484,764] The peak age of onset is adolescence and young adulthood, with a range between five and 55 years. Males are very slightly more affected than females. Once present, the symptoms rarely regress and usually worsen slowly as the years progress.

Treatment of narcolepsy essentially falls into three categories: appropriate prophylactic behaviour, tricyclic antidepressants, and CNS stimulating drugs.

Regular sleeping schedules are important with fixed bed times and wake up times. The reverse to this is that any kind of shift work exacerbates the symptoms of narcolepsy. Regular prophylactic naps of 10–20 min can be very useful, limited by alarm clock if necessary. Some patients may benefit from reducing carbohydrate intake. If possible, active work should be sought rather than sedentary and boring jobs. Long-term support is often necessary for these patients, the patient associations and self-help groups being particularly helpful here.

If the above is inadequate in controlling the daytime sleepiness then a tricyclic antidepressant can be used, initially just at night. Through its REM suppressing action sleep seems to be improved and, particularly if a sedating version is used (for example, imipramine), more consolidated. Daytime sleepiness is often better on quite small doses. The tricyclic antidepressants are also used if cataplexy is a problem. Here again the suppressant action on REM sleep seems to extend to the awake REM atonia.

Finally, if these approaches fail, then simple CNS stimulants may be required. Caffeine can be adequate in some, but stronger agents are usually needed. Although amphetamines can still be prescribed for this purpose (for example, dextroamphetamine), other agents are preferred. Methylphenindate is a more CNS-specific sympathomimetic agent than the amphetamines, but unfortunately still has a high addictive potential. Weaker alternatives, with lower addictive potential, are mazindol (introduced as an appetite suppressant) and pemoline. These can be used on an 'as required' basis, before any activity where particular vigilance is required. They should not be used on a regular basis if at all possible.

This is only a brief description of narcolepsy and fuller, interesting, accounts are available from Broughton[82] and Parkes.[511]

12.1.2 Recurrent hypersomnia

This is a rare condition that is also known as the Kleine–Levin syndrome.[133] It is characterized by recurrent episodes of hypersomnia lasting several days to several weeks, occurring on average about twice a year. The patient is usually a male adolescent (but not always) and the episodes of prolonged sleeping are associated with bouts of binge eating and indiscrete hypersexuality. In about half the cases a flu-like illness or head injury precedes the onset of symptoms.[50] The condition usually gradually improves and the ultimate prognosis is said to be good. However, during the period of maximum activity there can be severe psychosocial and developmental problems. The main differential would be a psychiatric cause.

There is no known cause and there are no specific features on classical polysomnography. The value of sleep studies and brain imaging is to exclude other diagnoses that might present with weight gain, sleepiness, and behaviour changes such as hypothalamic tumours.

12.1.3 Idiopathic hypersomnia

This condition presents in a similar way to narcolepsy with daytime sleepiness and sleep episodes, particularly during periods of low activity. The periods of sleep during the day tend to be longer than in narcolepsy (often hours). There are *no* features of REM sleep abnormalities such as cataplexy, sleep paralysis, or sleep onset dreaming. Sometimes there are other non-specific symptoms such as headache, fainting episodes, and Raynaud-like coldness of the hands and feet.

The condition is usually progressive and lifelong, appearing mainly during adolescence or early adulthood. The prevalence is not known but accounts for perhaps 10 per cent of the patients at a general sleep clinic. The cause is unknown but there appears to be a familial version with possible dominant inheritance.

There are no useful investigations other than those excluding alternative causes of sleepiness. The main differential will be psychiatric problems and it is important to recognize these before embarking on stimulant therapy. The use of CNS stimulants such as methylphenindate and pemoline is less successful than in narcolepsy, partly because of an increase in side-effects such as palpitations and irritability.

Essentially this diagnosis is a diagnosis of exclusion in a patient with genuine sleepiness but no other apparent cause.

12.1.4 Post-traumatic hypersomnia

Following traumatic injury to the brain, a period of excessive sleepiness and tiredness is quite common. This trauma may be due to a blow to the head, a stroke, or surgical. Sleepiness may be more likely to follow such trauma when certain parts of the brain (posterior hypothalamus, IIIrd ventricle, and posterior fossa) are involved but the evidence for this is limited.

This excessive daytime sleepiness may persist for the rest of the patient's life and greatly exacerbate any other neurological problems that resulted from the injury. The diagnosis is again very much one of exclusion in association with a relevant injury. It may be difficult to exclude psychiatric problems, particularly if there are compensation issues relating to the original accident.

12.1.5 *Periodic movements of the limbs during sleep, restless legs*

Ekbom[178] described the restless legs syndrome which is characterized by unpleasant creeping or aching sensations in the legs producing an irresistible urge to move them. This can occur predominantly prior to sleep, producing insomnia. There is usually no obvious cause but the syndrome can be associated with pregnancy, uraemia, heart failure, tricyclic antidepressants, monoamine oxidase inhibitors, and sedative withdrawal. The severity of the condition varies enormously with perhaps 10 per cent of the population experiencing similar symptoms from time to time. A severer form, probably dominantly inherited, can be very troublesome.

This problem of restless legs seems to blend with the condition of periodic movements of the limbs during sleep (PMLS), also sometimes called nocturnal myoclonus.[126,424] The definition of this is periodic episodes of repetitive and highly stereotyped limb movements that occur during non-REM sleep.

These movements, usually of the legs but also sometimes the arms, consist of extension of the foot and flexion of the ankle, knee, and sometimes the hip. One or both legs may be involved and the frequency is about one per 20–50 s. Each movement lasts between 0.5 and 5 s. There is much night to night variability and different degrees of sleep disruption. Each limb movement is followed by an arousal, both cortical and autonomic. It is debatable whether their presence always leads to daytime symptoms. The prevalence of these movements increases with age, figures of up to 30 per cent being quoted in those over 60 years.

Because periodic limb movements are seen in other sleep disorders, for example, sleep apnoea and following its treatment with CPAP, it can be difficult to decide if the leg movements are causing the arousal or vice versa. A particular problem is when there are recurrent arousals in association with leg movements on a polysomnographic study, but no apparent cause. It is tempting to label this periodic movement of the limbs (PMLS), but the real cause of the arousals may have been missed. It is difficult to prove, but it is possible, that some cases of snoring-induced arousals have been labelled as PMLS because the part played by increasing upper airway resistance in the arousal was not recognized on polysomnography.[264,549] Thus, the prevalence of symptomatic PMLS is far from clear.

If judged worthy of treatment, then the options are limited. Either the underlying cause can be treated or the associated arousal suppressed with hypnotics. Clonazepam has been used in this condition, but whether it is any better than other hypnotics is not clear. If the leg movements are in fact caused by the arousals from recurrent upper airway narrowing or snoring, then clonazepam may make this problem worse.

12.2 Extrinsic causes

Modern life has led to a variety of behaviour patterns that can interfere with sleep to the point where daytime symptoms of sleepiness become a problem. The abandonment of a siesta in cooler climates may have contributed. In North America the behaviour leading to poor sleep and daytime symptoms is put under the heading of poor 'sleep hygiene' conjuring up, as it does, the image of dirty sleep habits.

Most of the behaviour patterns interfering with sleep are known from common sense and are listed in Table 12.2. Sleeping during the day reduces the nocturnal sleep requirement and tends to perpetuate the continuing requirement for daytime naps. This may then be interpreted as daytime sleepiness. Sleep needs to be reconsolidated back into one period of nocturnal sleep by enforced wakefulness during the day. Varying the wake-up and bed-times can disrupt the quality and amount of refreshing sleep in some individuals, particularly as one gets older. Weekend lie-ins on a Sunday morning make it harder to get up on the Monday morning! This is because the circadian clock is quick to lengthen but finds it hard to be shortened. Caffeine and nicotine are CNS stimulants and prevent or fragment sleep. Even subjects who deny poor sleep after caffeine can be shown to have more fragmented sleep after three cups of coffee.[344] Nicotine has a short half-life, but that of caffeine is approximately 5 h. Roasted and ground coffee has about 85 mg of caffeine per 5 oz cup, 500 mg (6 cups) being equivalent in cortical arousal to approximately 5 mg of dextroamphetamine.[512]

If too much coffee is drunk in the evening then there will be increased wakefulness, sometimes later on in the night when the sleep pressure has reduced, which will produce some daytime sleepiness the following day. This may then be combated with increasing coffee consumption which perpetuates the problem.

Alcohol is a CNS sedative and, in common with other sedatives, produces a rebound in alertness or arousal when blood levels fall.[431,757] This means that although a few drinks will aid sleep onset, by 3 or 4 a.m. there is actually an alerting effect which reduces the overall amount of sleep. If caffeine has been taken as well, then the problem is compounded with two separate reasons for poorer sleep later on in the night (Fig. 12.1).

Although exercise in the early evening may improve sleep later that night, if the exercise is too near bedtime the opposite occurs.

It is not always obvious why someone's sleep quality is poor and the individuals themselves may not realize that they are being disturbed by external noises or influences. The pressures of modern life may also require an individual to persistently reduce his sleeping hours. Although this is

Table 12.2 Factors predisposing to poor sleep and its daytime consequences (poor 'sleep hygiene')

Daytime naps
Variable wake-up and bed-times
Weekend lie-ins
Recreational drug abuse (alcohol, caffeine, and nicotine)
Vigorous exercise immediately prior to bed
Excessive mental stimulation immediately prior to bed
Use of bed for reading, eating, television, etc.
Poor sleep environment
Ruminating on the day's problems in bed

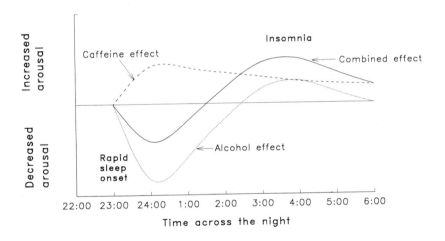

Fig. 12.1 Diagrammatic representation of the effects of combining pre-sleep alcohol and caffeine on level of brain arousal. Initially, alcohol's sedative properties may overcome caffeine's alerting properties. Once the alcohol has metabolized (much faster than caffeine) then the combination of the post-alcohol rebound alerting effect, plus the remaining caffeine effect, is a potent provoker of insomnia.

possible without detriment for a few days, it is usually unsustainable with recuperation required at weekends and consequently the additional problems of shifting wake-up times referred to above. It is extraordinary, but sometimes patients complain of sleepiness, are referred to a sleep clinic, and these simple and obvious points have not been considered before.

Chronic abuse of sedatives and alcohol produce considerable long-term problems of sleep quality and daytime sleepiness. The problem of poor sleep in alcoholics can persist for some years after abstinence.[408]

12.3 Circadian rhythm problems

The normal spontaneous human circadian rhythm is approximately 25 h and is entrained back to 24 h by the time cues provided by the environment. Within this 24 h cycle there are two periods of greatly increased sleep propensity, maximal at about 2 or 3 p.m. and from 11 p.m. to 5 a.m.[398] These periods have been described as 'sleep gates' when sleep is possible and at other times it may be almost impossible ('forbidden zones'), even when sleepy (Fig. 12.2). These gates vary between individuals both in their exact timing and their strength. The consequence of these gates is that sleep is not usually possible at *all* times during the 24 h cycle. Hence, the effects of jet lag and shift work.

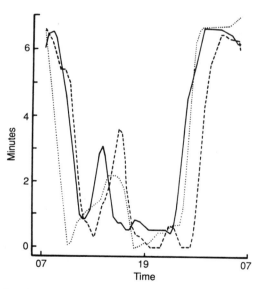

Fig. 12.2 Example of the two peaks of sleep propensity in one subject tested three times. The vertical axis is the number of minutes slept (out of a maximum of 7 min allowed) measured every 20 min throughout the 24 h cycle. Most subjects show this bimodal pattern with an afternoon increase in sleep propensity as well as the night time one. With permission from Lavie (1991).[399]

Flying west across time zones lengthens the 24 h cycle. A flight across the Atlantic to the USA usually means arrival in the middle of one's own 'night'. Sleep is usually able to commence within one's own 'night', albeit rather late. The body also finds it easier to elongate the 24 h cycle so that this westward flight, with about a 6 h time elongation is not difficult to cope with. The extra 6 h is rapidly lost in two or three slightly longer circadian cycles. The return journey is different. The flights are usually overnight and only a short sleep period is possible, often before reaching the usual nocturnal sleep gate. The body finds it almost impossible to shorten the 24 h cycle, this eastward flight would need two cycles of 21 h or perhaps three of 22 h. The alternative is to try and have one long day of 42 h or several less long days. This eastward flight produces much more disruption of the circadian rhythm (as measured by the body temperature change and melatonin release) which can take up to 10 days or longer to resynchronize with the local day/night timing.[359] There is considerable effort by pharmaceutical companies going into producing drugs which will rapidly reset the circadian cycle to local time and thus minimize the effects on performance and well being of jet lag (and shift work). This approach may also be useful in the field of hypnotics. Melatonin, a naturally occurring hormone, is released from the pineal gland during the night and suppressed by bright light. This excretion pattern is under circadian control and not affected by whether sleep occurs or not. The amount released at night does however depend on the previous day's level of light intensity. More light causes less melatonin to be released subsequently. There is some preliminary evidence that by manipulating melatonin levels, with oral melatonin or exposure to bright lights, it is possible to reset circadian rhythms quicker than would occur naturally.[174,581]

The function of melatonin is not known but it may be important as a link between the environment and the neurohumoural system, giving photo period information and seasonal time clues: the latter clearly important for some species.

Of far greater importance than jet lag is the disrupting effect on people's lives of shift working.[6] Constantly changing shifts can be very destructive to a sense of well being and alertness. There is a selection process in shift working industries, only those who can cope with the time changes stay in the industry. Certain shift work patterns are worse than others. For example, a three, 8 h, shift system rotating onwards by 8 h each week is much less destructive than rotating backwards, that is, a week of mornings (8.00 until 16.00) should be followed by a week of evenings (16.00 until 24.00) and then by a week of nights (24.00 until 8.00). This means that each week the time change is equivalent to a westward flight from the UK to the east coast of the USA. The alternative of mornings followed by nights followed by evenings etc., is like the eastward flight every week. There is evidence that the former shift system is attended by less absenteeism and staff turnover than the latter.[139] Despite this some companies refuse to change their shift patterning. Personnel directors of companies with shift workers would be well advised to read some of the work of Akerstedt.[6]

As a shift worker gets older he may find it harder and harder to cope with the increasing problems of daytime sleepiness and lethargy. These symptoms may be used to negotiate retirement on health grounds which will complicate assessment. Clearly any other cause of sleep disruption (sleep apnoea, heavy snoring, alcohol, narcolepsy, etc.) will have a bigger impact in a shift worker, already struggling to cope, than in someone with a regular sleep/wake schedule.

Nurses often have fairly chaotic oscillations between shifts, having days off after night duty, but not before. They rarely sleep the day before going onto night duty and by the end of their first night they effectively have had one night's sleep deprivation. Figure 4.2 (p. 70) shows the reaction times of 20 nurses at 8.00 a.m. coming fresh onto the ward for an early shift, compared to their performance at 8.00 a.m. after their first night on night duty.

Delayed sleep phase syndrome is a situation that many people may get into from time to time. If bed time is delayed (rather akin to a westward flight) then the circadian rhythm will elongate a little quite readily. After a few nights of later bed times, but the same wake-up time, sleepiness will appear. This may lead to an attempt to re-establish the earlier bed time. This may be very difficult because the 'sleep gate' may not be that early any more and sleep will only occur later on. Trying to drag back the sleep onset time to its previous point can be very difficult, because of the reluctance of the body to accept a shorter circadian rhythm than normal. Thus, a situation is established of inability to sleep at night until 2.00 or 3.00 a.m., difficulty getting up in the morning, and daytime sleepiness.

In some sleep centres treatment may consist of allowing the subject to go to sleep 2 h later each day so that the sleep time moves right around the clock to 10 p.m. a process that takes approximately 10 days. The alternative (and simpler) approach is to prevent sleep entirely for one or two days and nights so that the subject is so sleep-deprived that he will be able to fall asleep earlier at 10 p.m. and, thus, reset the sleep gates.

12.4 Other conditions

Sleepiness may be the dominant symptom in certain other conditions where it may be severe enough to provoke referral to a sleep clinic. Depression may provoke the complaint of sleepiness. This may be genuine sleepiness or be really tiredness and lethargy which lead to inactivity and sleep by default.

The problem of alcohol has been discussed earlier. Current and ex-alcoholics are likely to have irregular sleep—wake schedules; the sleep disrupting effects of alcohol and possibly some permanent brain damage from the alcohol, producing fragmented and poorly refreshing sleep.[408] Because alcohol decreases upper airway tone,[63,576] increased degrees of sleep apnoea may compound the problem,[324] an effect that seems to persist through unknown mechanisms even whilst subsequently abstaining from alcohol.[694,713]

Appendix

Osler Chest Unit Sleep Questionnaire

NAME .... DATE ....

HOSP NO .... DOB .... AGE ....

ADDRESS ....

....

Presentation and main complaints ....

....

....

....

....

....

Epworth Sleepiness Score .... Shiftwork? ....

Occupation ....

Past Medical History ....

....

....

....

Drug history ....

....

....

Social History ....

....

Weight and Collar size history

Age .... Weight .... Collar size ....

Age .... Weight .... Collar size ....

Age .... Weight .... Collar size ....

(1) Do you have difficulty getting to sleep?

    1 = never 2 = rarely 3 = sometimes 4 = often

(2) Do you fall asleep reading or watching television?

    1 = never 2 = rarely 3 = sometimes 4 = often

(3) Do you fall asleep during the day, particularly when not busy?

    1 = never 2 = rarely 3 = sometimes 4 = often

(4) Do you fall asleep during the day against your will?

    1 = never 2 = rarely 3 = sometimes 4 = often

(5) Do you have to pull off the road whilst driving due to sleepiness?

    1 = never 2 = rarely 3 = sometimes 4 = often

(6) Have you almost had an accident whilst driving due to sleepiness?

   1 = never   2 = once   3 = 2 to 4   4 = more than 4 . . .

(7) Do you think you might have ever had a car accident through sleepiness?

   1 = never   2 = once   3 = 2 to 4   4 = more than 4 . . .

(8) How long do you estimate you sleep altogether per 24 hours?

   1 = 4/5 hrs 2 = 6/7 hrs 3 = 8/9 hrs   4 = more than 10 . . .

(9) Do you have sudden attacks of muscle weakness or falling?

   1 = never   2 = rarely   3 = sometimes   4 = often

(10) As you fall asleep, do you have strange or frightening dreams?

   1 = never   2 = rarely   3 = sometimes   4 = often

(11) As you fall asleep or wake up, do you ever feel paralysed for a few moments?

   1 = never   2 = rarely   3 = sometimes   4 = often

(12) Are you a restless sleeper, or have you been told that you move your arms and legs around a lot during sleep?

   1 = never   2 = rarely   3 = sometimes   4 = often

(13) Do you get choking or shortness of breath sensations at night?

   1 = never   2 = rarely   3 = sometimes   4 = often

(14) Do you snore or have you been told that you do?

   1 = never   2 = rarely   3 = sometimes   4 = often

(15) When did your snoring start?

   1 = <1 yr   2 = 1–3 yrs   3 = 4–9 yrs   4 >10 yrs

(16) Do you snore . . .

    1 = On back only   2 = In all positions

(17) Is your snoring worse after alcohol?

    1 = No different   2 = A little worse   3 = Much worse

(18) Is your snoring worse if your nose is blocked with colds or hayfever?

    1 = No different   2 = A little worse   3 = Much worse

(19) Has your partner ever told you that you stop breathing while asleep?

    1 = no   2 = yes

(20) Do you get morning fatigue, fogginess or wake up feeling unrefreshed?

    1 = never 2 = rarely 3 = sometimes 4 = often

(21) How many times do you have to get up at night to pass urine?

    1 = never   2 = once   3 = twice   4 = more than twice

(22) Do you ever wake up with headaches?

    1 = never 2 = rarely 3 = sometimes 4 = often

(23) Roughly how much alcohol do you drink a day?
(Units = half pint of beer or a single short)

    1 = <1 2 = 1 to 3 3 = 4 to 7   4 = >7

(24) Do you smoke cigarettes?

    1 = none   2 = 1–5/day   3 = 6–15/day   4 = >15/day

(25) Do you get a stuffy or blocked nose? (eg hayfever)

    1 = never 2 = rarely 3 = sometimes 4 = often

(26) Have you ever damaged your nose or had surgery to it?

     1 = no   2 = damaged   3 = surgery   4 = both

Specify ....

....

(27) Have you ever had your tonsils taken out?

     1 = yes   2 = no

(29) Do you take any tranquillisers or sleeping tablets?

     1 = never 2 = rarely 3 = sometimes 4 = often

MEASUREMENTS

Height ....

Weight ....

Collar size ....

EXAMINATION

Pharyngeal appearance

Nasal Patency ....

Nasal PIFR ....

Jaw ....

Teeth ....

Blood Pressure ....

INVESTIGATIONS (tick if ordered)

FBC .... Hb .... WBC .... PLTS ....

U&E .... Normal .... Abnormal .... HCO_3^- ....

THYROID FUNCTION   TSH .... T3 .... T4 ....

BLOOD GASES PaO_2 ...... $PaCO_2$ ...... pH ...... Base excess ......

LATERAL NECK X-RAY ....

....

....

FEV1/FVC ..../..........   Predicted FEV1/FVC ..../..........

FEV1/FVC ratio .... %   %Pred FEV1 ....   %Pred FVC ......

References

1. Minutes from the Clinical Society of London. *Br Med J* 1889; 1: 358.
2. Abbey NC, Cooper KR, Kwentus JA. Benefit of nasal CPAP in obstructive sleep apnea is due to positive pharyngeal pressure. *Sleep* 1989; 12: 420–2.
3. Aber WR, Block AJ, Hellard DW, Webb WB. Consistency of respiratory measurements from night to night during the sleep of elderly men. *Chest* 1989; 96: 747–51.
4. Abroug F, Dougui M, Knani J, Hmouda H, Belghith M, Khouaja F, *et al.* [Sleep apnea syndromes and Arnold–Chiari malformation]. *Rev Mal Respir* 1990; 7: 159–61.
5. Ahlqvist-Rastad J, Hultcrantz E, Svanholm H. Children with tonsillar obstruction: indications for and efficacy of tonsillectomy. *Acta Paediatr Scand* 1988; 77: 831–5.
6. Akerstedt T. Sleepiness at work: effects of irregular work hours. In: Monk TH. ed. *Sleep, sleepiness and performance*. Chichester, UK: John Wiley & Sons, 1991: 129–52.
7. Al-Shaikh B, Kinnear W, Higenbottam TW, Smith HS, Shneerson JM, Wilkinson I. Motor neurone disease presenting as respiratory failure. *Br Med J* 1986; 292: 1325–6.
8. Aldrich M, Eiser A, Lee M, Shipley JE. Effects of continuous positive airway pressure on phasic events of REM sleep in patients with obstructive sleep apnea. *Sleep* 1989; 12: 413–19.
9. Aldrich MS. Automobile accidents in patients with sleep disorders. *Sleep* 1989; 12: 487–94.
10. Aldrich MS, Chauncey JB. Are morning headaches part of obstructive sleep apnea? *Arch Intern Med* 1990; 150: 1265–7.
11. Alex CG, Onal E, Lopata M. Upper airway occlusion during sleep in patients with Cheyne–Stokes respiration. *Am Rev Respir Dis* 1986; 133: 42–5.
12. Ali NJ, Davies RJ, Fleetham JA, Stradling JR. Periodic movements of the legs during sleep associated with rises in systemic blood pressure. *Sleep* 1991; 14: 163–5.
13. Ali NJ, Davies RJO, Fleetham JA, Stradling JR. The acute effects of continuous positive airway pressure and oxygen administration on blood pressure during obstructive sleep apnea. *Chest* 1992; 101: 1526–32.
14. Ali NJ, Pitson D, Stradling JR. Daytime behaviour in 4–5 year old children with mild to moderate sleep disordered breathing. *Thorax* 1992; 47: 220 (Abstract).
15. Ali NJ, Pitson DJ, Stradling JR. Snoring, sleep disturbance and behaviour in 4–5 year olds. *Arch Dis Child* 1993; 68: 360–6.

16. Ancoli-Israel S, Klauber MR, Butters N, Parker L, Kripke DF. Dementia in institutionalized elderly: relation to sleep apnea. *J Am Geriatr Soc* 1991; 39: 258–63.

17. Ancoli-Israel S, Kripke DF. Epidemiology of sleep apnea in three populations of elderly. In: Horne J. ed. *Sleep '88*. Stuttgart: G.F.Verlag, 1989: 258–9.

18. Ancoli-Israel S, Kripke DF, Mason W, Messin S. Sleep apnea and nocturnal myoclonus in a senior population. *Sleep* 1981; 4: 349–58.

19. Anderson HT. Physiological adaptations in diving vertebrates. *J Appl Physiol* 1964; 19: 417–22.

20. Andersson L, Brattstrom V. Cephalometric analysis of permanently snoring patients with and without obstructive sleep apnea syndrome. *Int J Oral Maxillofac Surg* 1991; 20: 159–62.

21. Andreas S, Hajak G, v.Breska B, Ruther E, Kreuzer H. Changes in heart rate during obstructive sleep apnoea. *Eur Respir J* 1992; 5: 853–7.

22. Andreas S, v.Breska B, Kopp E, Siegener MS, Figulla HR, Kreuzer H. Sleep and periodic breathing in patients with dilated cardiomyopathy. *J Sleep Res* 1992; 1(suppl 1): 10 (Abstract).

23. Andrews JM, Guilleminault C, Holdway RA. Retaining devices and mandibular positioning appliances. *Bull Eur Physiopathol Respir* 1983; 19: 611.

24. Angell-James JE, DeBurgh-Daly M. Cardiovascular responses in apnoeic asphyxia: role of arterial chemoreceptors and the modification of their effects by a pulmonary inflation reflex. *J Physiol Lond* 1969; 201: 87–104.

25. Anonymous. Obstructive sleep apnoea and lower airways obstruction. *Lancet* 1987; 2: 774–6.

26. Anonymous. Pulse oximeters. *Health Devices* 1989; 18: 185–230.

27. Anthonisen NR, Cherniack RM. Ventilatory control in lung disease. In: Hornbein TF. ed. *Regulation of breathing* (part 2). *Lung biology in health and disease*. New York: Marcel Dekker, 1981: 965–87.

28. Aserinsky E, Kleitman N. Regularly occurring periods of eye motility and concomitant phenomena during sleep. *Science* 1953; 118: 273–4.

29. Asher T, Leiberman A, Margulis G, Sofer S. Ventricular dysfunction in children with obstructive sleep apnea. *Pediatr Pulmonol* 1988; 4: 139–43.

30. Aubert-Tulkens G, Culee G, Harmant-Van Rijckevorsel K, Rodenstein DO. Ambulatory evaluation of sleep disturbance and therapeutic effects in sleep apnea syndrome by wrist activity monitoring. *Am Rev Respir Dis* 1987; 136: 851–6.

31. Bach JR, Alba A, Mosher R, Delaubier A. Intermittent positive pressure ventilation via nasal access in the management of respiratory insufficiency. *Chest* 1987; 92: 168–70.

32. Bach JR, Alba AS, Bohatiuk G, Saporito L, Lee M. Mouth intermittent positive pressure ventilation in the management of post-polio respiratory insufficiency. *Chest* 1987; 91: 859–64.

33. Balter MS, Chapman KR, Maleki-Yazdi MR, Leenen FH, Rebuck AS. Effects of oxygen withdrawal on catecholamine release in patients on home oxygen therapy. *Clin Sci* 1990; 79: 155–9.

34. Bannister R, Gibson W, Michaels L, Oppenheimer DR. Laryngeal abductor paralysis in multiple system atrophy. *Brain* 1981; 104: 351–68.

35. Baraitser M, Parkes JD. Genetic study of narcoleptic syndrome. *J Med Genet* 1987; 15: 254—9.

36. Baruzzi A, Cappelli M, Cirignotta F, Riva R, Zucconi M, Lugaresi E. Atrial natriuretic peptide (ANP) in obstructive sleep apnea syndrome (OSAS). *Sleep Res* 1989; 18: 195 (Abstract).

37. Bashir Y, Kann M, Stradling JR. The effect of acetazolamide on hypercapnic and eucapnic/poikilocapnic hypoxic ventilatory responses in normal subjects. *Pulmonary Pharmacology* 1990; 3: 151—4.

38. Bass C. *Somatization*. Oxford: Blackwell Scientific, 1990.

39. Bate TWP, Price DA, Holme CA, McGucken RB. Short stature caused by obstructive sleep apnoea during sleep. *Arch Dis Child* 1984; 59: 78—80.

40. Bear SE, Priest JH. Sleep apnea syndrome: correction with surgical advancement of the mandible. *J Oral Surg* 1980; 38: 543—9.

41. Berkenbosch A, DeGroede J, Olievier CN, Schuitmaker JJ. A pseudo rebreathing technique for assessing the ventilatory response to carbon dioxide in cats. *J Physiol Lond* 1986; 381: 483—95.

42. Berrettini WH. Paranoid psychosis and sleep apnea syndrome. *Am J Psych* 1980; 137: 493—4.

43. Berry DT, Webb WB, Block AJ, Switzer DA. Sleep-disordered breathing and its concomitants in a subclinical population. *Sleep* 1986; 9: 478—83.

44. Berry RB, Desa MM, Branum JP, Light RW. Effect of theophylline on sleep and sleep-disordered breathing in patients with chronic obstructive pulmonary disease. *Am Rev Respir Dis* 1991; 143: 245—50.

45. Berssenbrugge A, Dempsey J, Iber C, Skatrud J, Wilson P. Mechanisms of hypoxia-induced periodic breathing during sleep in humans. *J Physiol Lond* 1983; 343: 507—26.

46. Berthon-Jones M, Sullivan CE. Ventilatory and arousal responses to hypoxia in sleeping humans. *Am Rev Respir Dis* 1982; 125: 632—9.

47. Berthon-Jones M, Sullivan CE. Ventilation and arousal responses to hypercapnia in normal sleeping adults. *J Appl Physiol* 1984; 57: 59—67.

48. Berthon-Jones M, Sullivan CE. Time course of change in ventilatory response to CO_2 with long-term CPAP therapy for obstructive sleep apnea. *Am Rev Respir Dis* 1987; 135: 144—7.

49. Biernacki H, Douglas NJ. Evaluation of a computerised polysomnography system. *Thorax* 1992; 47: 234p (Abstract).

50. Billiard M. The Kleine—Levin syndrome. In: Kryger MH, Roth T, Dement WC. eds. *Principles and practices of sleep medicine*. Philadelphia: W.B. Saunders, 1989: 377—8.

51. Black N. Geographical variation in use of surgery for glue ear. *J R Soc Med* 1985; 78: 631—7.

52. Blair D, Habicht JP, Sims EAH, Sylvester D, Abraham S. Evidence for an increased risk for hypertension with centrally located body fat and the effect of race and sex on this risk. *Am J Epidermol* 1984; 119: 526—40.

53. Bliwise D, Carskadon M, Carey E, Dement WC. Longitudinal development of sleep-related respiratory disturbance in adult humans. *J Gerontol* 1984; 39: 290—3.

54. Bliwise DL, Nekich JC, Partinen M, Dement WC. Neuropsychological test performance and sleep apnea in the elderly. *Sleep Res* 1991; 20: 209 (Abstract).

55. Block AJ, Berry D, Webb W. Nocturnal hypoxemia and neuropsychological deficits in men who snore. *Eur J Respir Dis Suppl* 1986; 146: 405–8.

56. Block AJ, Boysen PG, Wynne JW. The origins of cor pulmonale a hypothesis. *Chest* 1979; 75: 109–10.

57. Bloom JW, Kaltenborn WT, Quan SF. Risk factors in a general population for snoring. Importance of cigarette smoking and obesity. *Chest* 1988; 93: 678–83.

58. Bogle RL, Skatrud JB. Effect of lung volume on expiratory muscle recruitment during wakefulness and NREM sleep. *Am Rev Respir Dis* 1989; 139(No. 4, pt 2): A82 (Abstract).

59. Bokinsky GE, Hudson LD, Weil JV. Impaired peripheral chemosensitivity and acute respiratory failure in Arnold–Chiari malformation and syringomyelia. *N Engl J Med* 1973; 288: 947–8.

60. Bonnet M, Carley D, Carskadon M, Easton P, Guilleminault C, Harper R, *et al*. EEG arousals: scoring rules and examples. A preliminary report from the Sleep Disorders Atlas Task Force of the American Sleep Disorders Association. *Sleep* 1992; 15(2): 173–84.

61. Bonnet MH. Sleep restoration as a function of periodic awakening, movement, or electroencephalographic change. *Sleep* 1987; 10: 364–73.

62. Bonnet MH, Dexter JR, Arand DL. The effect of triazolam on arousal and respiration in central sleep apnea patients. *Sleep* 1990; 13: 31–41.

63. Bonora M, Shields GI, Knuth SL, Barlett D Jr, St John WM. Selective depression by ethanol of upper airway respiratory motor activity in cats. *Am Rev Respir Dis* 1984; 130: 156–61.

64. Bonora M, St John WM, Bledsoe TA. Differential elevation by protriptyline and depression by diazepam of upper airway respiratory motor activity. *Am Rev Respir Dis* 1985; 131: 41–5.

65. Boor JW, Johnson RJ, Canales L, Dunn DP. Reversible paralysis of automatic respiration in multiple sclerosis. *Arch Neurol* 1977; 34: 686–9.

66. Born J, Muth S, Fehm HL. The significance of sleep onset and slow wave sleep for nocturnal release of growth hormone (GH) and cortisol. *Psychoneuroendocrinology* 1988; 13: 233–43.

67. Bornstein SK. Respiratory monitoring during sleep: polysomnography. In: Guilleminault C. ed. *Sleeping and waking disorders*. California: Addison-Wesley, 1982: 183–212.

68. Boudoulas H, Schmidt H, Gelens P, Clark RW, Lewis RP. Case reports on deterioration of sleep apnea during therapy with propranolol—preliminary studies. *Res Commun Chem Pathol Pharmacol* 1983; 39: 3–10.

69. Bowes G, Townsend ER, Kozar LF, Bromley SM, Phillipson EA. Effect of carotid body denervation on arousal response to hypoxia in sleeping dogs. *J Appl Physiol* 1981; 51: 40–5.

70. Boysen PG, Block AJ, Wynne JW, Hunt LA, Flick MR. Nocturnal pulmonary hypertension in patients with chronic pulmonary disease. *Chest* 1979; 76: 536–42.

71. Bradley TD, Holloway RM, McLaughlin PR, Ross BL, Walters J, Liu PP. Cardiac output response to continuous positive airway pressure in congestive heart failure. *Am Rev Respir Dis* 1992; 145: 377—82.

72. Bradley TD, Martinez D, Rutherford R, Lue F, Grossman RF, Moldofsky H, *et al.* Physiological determinants of nocturnal arterial oxygenation in patients with obstructive sleep apnea. *J Appl Physiol* 1985; 59: 1364—8.

73. Bradley TD, McNicholas WT, Rutherford R, Popkin J, Zamel N, Phillipson EA. Clinical and physiologic heterogeneity of the central sleep apnea syndrome. *Am Rev Respir Dis* 1986; 134: 217—21.

74. Bradley TD, Rutherford R, Grossman RF, Lue F, Zamel N, Moldofsky H, *et al.* Role of daytime hypoxemia in the pathogenesis of right heart failure in the obstructive sleep apnea syndrome. *Am Rev Respir Dis* 1985; 131: 835—9.

75. Bradley TD, Rutherford R, Lue F, Moldofsky H, Grossman RF, Zamel N, *et al.* Role of diffuse airway obstruction in the hypercapnia of obstructive sleep apnea. *Am Rev Respir Dis* 1986; 134: 920—4.

76. Braun NMT, Arora NS, Rochester DF. Respiratory muscle and pulmonary function in polymyositis and other proximal myopathies. *Thorax* 1983; 38: 616—23.

77. Braun NMT, Faulkner J, Hughes RL, Roussos C, Sahgal V. When should respiratory muscles be exercised? *Chest* 1983; 84: 76—84.

78. Broadbent WH. Cheyne—Skokes respiration in cerebral haemorrhage. *Lancet* 1877; 1: 307—9.

79. Brodsky L, Adler E, Stanievich JF. Naso- and oropharyngeal dimensions in children with obstructive sleep apnea. *Int J Pediatr Otorhinolaryngol* 1989; 17: 1—11.

80. Brodsky L, Moore L, Stanievich JF. A comparison of tonsillar size and oro- pharyngeal dimensions in children with obstructive adenotonsillar hypertrophy. *Int J Pediatr Otorhinolaryngol* 1987; 13: 149—56.

81. Broughton RJ. Sleep attacks, naps, and sleepiness in medical sleep disorders. In: Dinges DF, Broughton RJ. eds. *Sleep and alertness: chronobiological, behavioral, and medical aspects of napping.* New York: Raven Press, 1989: 267—98.

82. Broughton RJ. Narcolepsy. In: Thorpy MJ. ed. *Handbook of sleep disorders.* New York: Marcel Dekker, 1990: 197—216.

83. Brouillette RT, Thach BT. Control of genioglossus muscle inspiratory activity. *J Appl Physiol* 1980; 49: 801—8.

84. Brouillette RT, Fernbach SK, Hunt CE. Obstructive sleep apnea in infants and children. *J Pediatr* 1982; 100: 31—9.

85. Brouillette RT, Hanson D, David R, Klemka L, Szatkowski A, Fernbach SF, *et al.* A diagnostic approach to suspected obstructive sleep apnea in children. *J Pediatr* 1984; 105: 10—14.

86. Brouillette RT, Thach BT. A neuromuscular mechanism maintaining extra- thoracic airway patency. *J Appl Physiol* 1979; 46: 722—79.

87. Browman CP, Unruh MM, Winslow DH. Differential diagnosis of the hyper- somnolent patient. *Sleep Res* 1989; 18: 207 (Abstract).

88. Brown L, Kinnear W, Sergeant K-A, Shneerson J. Artificial ventilation by external negative pressure—a method for manufacturing cuirass shells. *Physiotherapy* 1985; 71: 181–3.

89. Brownell LG, West P, Sweatman P, Acres JC, Kryger MH. Protriptyline in obstructive sleep apnea: a double-blind trial. *N Engl J Med* 1982; 307: 1037–42.

90. Buckle P, Kerr P, Millar T, Steljes D, Kryger M. The effect of acute nasal CPAP on sleep and respiration in congestive heart failure. *Am Rev Respir Dis* 1991; 143: 592 (Abstract).

91. Bulow K. Respiration and wakefulness in man. *Acta Physiol Scand* 1963; 59 (suppl 209): 1–110.

92. Burwell CS, Robin ED, Whaley RD, Bickelmann AG. Extreme obesity associated with alveolar hypoventilation—a Pickwickian syndrome. *Am J Med* 1956; 21: 811–24.

93. Caldarelli DD, Cartwright R, Lillie JK. Severity of sleep apnea as a predictor of successful treatment by palatopharyngoplasty. *Laryngoscope* 1986; 96: 945–7.

94. Calverley PMA, Brezinova V, Douglas NJ, Catterall JR, Flenley DC. The effect of oxygenation on sleep quality in chronic bronchitis and emphysema. *Am Rev Respir Dis* 1982; 126: 206–10.

95. Camfferman F, Bogaard JM, Van Der Meche FGA, Hilvering C. Idiopathic bilateral diaphragmatic paralysis. *Eur J Respir Dis* 1985; 66: 65–71.

96. Campbell AMG, Williams ER, Pearce J. Late motor neuron degeneration following poliomyelitis. *Neurology* 1969; 19: 1101–6.

97. Carrol J, Loughlin GM. Diagnostic criteria for obstructive sleep apnea syndrome in children. *Pediatr Pulmonol* 1992; 14: 71–4.

98. Carroll N, Branthwaite MA. Control of nocturnal hypoventilation by nasal intermittent positive pressure ventilation. *Thorax* 1988; 43: 349–53.

99. Carroll N, Parker RA, Branthwaite M. The use of protriptyline for respiratory failure in patients with chronic airflow limitation. *Eur Respir J* 1990; 3: 746–51.

100. Carskadon MA. Ontogeny of human sleepiness as measured by sleep latency. In: Dinges DF, Broughton RJ. eds. *Sleep and alertness: chronobiological, behavioral, and medical aspects of napping.* New York: Raven Press, 1989: 53–69.

101. Carskadon MA, Dement WC, Mitler MM, Roth T, Westbrook PR, Keenan S. Guidelines for the multiple sleep latency test (MSLT): a standard measure of sleepiness. *Sleep* 1986; 9: 519–24.

102. Carskadon MA, Rechtschaffen A. Monitoring and staging human sleep. In: Kryger MH, Roth T, Dement WC. eds. *Principles and practice of sleep medicine.* Philadelphia: W.B. Saunders, 1989: 665–83.

103. Cartwright R, Ristanovic R, Diaz F, Caldarelli D, Alder G. A comparative study of treatments for positional sleep apnea. *Sleep* 1991; 14: 546–52.

104. Castaigne P, Laplane D, Autret A, Bousser MG, Gray F, Baron JC. Syndrome de Shy et Drager avec troubles du rhythme respiratoire et de la vigilance. *Revue Neurologique* 1977; 133: 455–66.

105. Catterall JR, Douglas NJ, Calverley PMA, Shapiro CM, Brezinova V, Brash HM, *et al*. Transient hypoxaemia during sleep in chronic obstructive pulmonary disease is not a sleep apnea syndrome. *Am Rev Respir Dis* 1983; 128: 24–9.

106. Celli B, Lee H, Criner G, Bermudez M, Rassulo J, Gilmartin M, *et al*. Controlled trial of external negative pressure ventilation in patients with severe chronic airflow obstruction. *Am Rev Respir Dis* 1989; 140: 1251–6.

107. Chadwick GA, Crowley P, Fitzgerald MX, O'Regan RG, McNicholas WT. Obstructive sleep apnea following topical oropharyngeal anesthesia in loud snorers. *Am Rev Respir Dis* 1991; 143: 810–13.

108. Chalmers DC, Stewart I, Silva P, Mulvena A. *Otitis media with effusion in children—the Dunedin study* (Clinics in Developmental Medicine, volume 108). London: MacKeith Press, 1989.

109. Chan CS, Bye PTP, Woolcock AJ, Sullivan CE. Eucapnia and hypercapnia in patients with chronic airflow limitation. *Am Rev Respir Dis* 1990; 141: 861–5.

110. Chan CS, Grunstein RR, Bye PT, Woolcock AJ, Sullivan CE. Obstructive sleep apnea with severe chronic airflow limitation. Comparison of hypercapnic and eucapnic patients. *Am Rev Respir Dis* 1989; 140: 1274–8.

111. Chapman KR, Bruce EN, Gothe B, Cherniack NS. Possible mechanisms of periodic breathing during sleep. *J Appl Physiol* 1988; 64: 1000–8.

112. Chase MH, Chandler SH, Nakamura Y. Intracellular determination of membrane potential of trigeminal motorneurons during sleep and wakefulness. *J Neurophysiol* 1980; 44: 349–58.

113. Check WA. Does drop in T and A's pose new issue of adenotonsillar hypertrophy? *JAMA* 1982; 247: 1229–30.

114. Cheshire K, Engleman H, Deary I, Shapiro C, Douglas NJ. Factors impairing daytime performance in patients with the sleep apnoea/hypopnoea syndrome. *Arch Intern Med* 1992; 152: 538–41.

115. Cheyne JA. A case of apoplexy in which the fleshy part of the heart was converted into fat. *Dublin Hospital Rep* 1818; 2: 216–22.

116. Chokroverty S. Sleep and breathing in neurological disorders. In: Edelman NH, Santiago TV. eds. *Breathing disorders of sleep*. New York: Churchill Livingston, 1986: 225–64.

117. Christensen G, Bugge JF, Ostensen J, Kiil F. Atrial natriuretic factor and renal sodium excretion during ventilation with PEEP in hypervolemic dogs. *J Appl Physiol* 1992; 72: 993–7.

118. Cirignotta F, D'Alessandro R, Partinen M, Zucconi M, Cristina E, Gerardi R, *et al*. Prevalence of every night snoring and obstructive sleep apneas among 30–69-year-old-men in Bologna, Italy. *Acta Psychiatr Scand* 1989; 79: 366–72.

119. Clark LA, Denby L, Pregibon D, Harshfield GA, Pickering TG, Blank S, *et al*. A quantitative analysis of the effects of activity and time of day on the diurnal variations of blood pressure. *J Chron Dis* 1987; 40: 671–81.

120. Clark RW, Boudoulas H, Schael SF, Schmidt HS. Adrenergic hyperactivity and cardiac abnormality in primary disorder of sleep. *Neurology* 1980; 30: 113–19.

121. Clarke RW, Schmidt HS, Sweatman P. Sleep apnea: treatment with pro-triptyline. *Neurology* 1979; 29: 1287−92.

122. Coccagna G, Mantovani M, Brignani F, Manzini A, Lugaresi E. Arterial pressure changes during spontaneous sleep in man. *Electroencephalog Clin Neurophysiol* 1971; 31: 277−81.

123. Coccagna G, Mantovani M, Brignani F, Parchi C, Lugaresi E. Continuous recording of the pulmonary and systemic arterial pressure during sleep in syndromes of hypersomnia with periodic breathing. *Bull Eur Physiopathol Respir* 1972; 8: 1159−72.

124. Cohn M. Surgical treatment in sleep apnea syndrome. In: Fletcher EC. ed. *Abnormalities of respiration during sleep*. Orlando: Grune & Stratton, 1986: 117−39.

125. Cole RJ, Kripke DF. Progress in automatic sleep/wake scoring by wrist actigraph. *Sleep* 1988; 17: 331 (Abstract).

126. Coleman RM, Pollak CP, Weitzman ED. Periodic movements in sleep (nocturnal myoclonus): relation to sleep disorders. *Ann Neurol* 1980; 8: 416−21.

127. Connaughton JJ, Catterall JR, Elton RA, Stradling JR, Douglas NJ. Do sleep studies contribute to the management of patients with severe chronic obstructive pulmonary disease? *Am Rev Respir Dis* 1988; 138: 341−4.

128. Conners CK. A teacher rating scale for use in drug studies with children. *Am J Psych* 1969; 126: 884−8.

129. Conway W, Fujita S, Zorick F, Roehrs T, Wittig R, Roth T. Uvulopalato-pharyngoplasty: 1 year follow-up. *Chest* 1985; 88: 385−7.

130. Coote JH, Stone BM, Tsang G. Sleep of Andean high altitude natives. *Eur J Appl Physiol* 1992; 64: 178−81.

131. Copp T, DiMarco AF, Altose MD. Effects of intermittent assisted ventilation in patients with severe COPD. *Am Rev Respir Dis* 1984; 129(suppl): A34 (Abstract).

132. Corbo GM, Fuciarelli F, Foresi A, De-Benedetto F. Snoring in children: association with respiratory symptoms and passive smoking [published erratum appears in *BMJ* 1990 Jan 27; 300(6719): 226]. *Br Med J* 1989; 299: 1491−4.

133. Critchley M, Hoffman HL. The syndrome of periodic somnolence and morbid hunger (Kleine−Levin syndrome). *Br Med J* 1942; 1: 137−9.

134. Crocker BD, Olson LG, Saunders NA, Hensley MJ, McKeon JL, Allen KM, *et al*. Estimation of the probability of disturbed breathing during sleep before a sleep study. *Am Rev Respir Dis* 1990; 142: 14−18.

135. Croft CB, Brockbank MJ, Wright A, Swanston AR. Obstructive sleep apnoea in children undergoing routine tonsillectomy and adenoidectomy. *Clin Otolaryngol* 1990; 15: 307−14.

136. Croft CB, Golding-Wood DG. Uses and complications of uvulopalato-pharyngoplasty. *J Laryngol Otol* 1990; 104: 871−5.

137. Crumley RL, Stein M, Gamsu G, Golden J, Dermon S. Determination of obstructive site in obstructive sleep apnea. *Laryngoscope* 1987; 97: 301−8.

138. Curzi-Dascalova L, Checoury A, Plouin P, Vasseur O. Respiration of artificially ventilated infants: degree of dependance on the ventilator and sleep states. *Rev EEG Neurophysiol* 1982; 12: 227−32.

139. Czeisler CA, Moore-Ede MC, Coleman RM. Rotating shift work schedules that disrupt sleep are improved by applying circadian principles. *Science* 1982; 217: 460–3.

140. Dalakas MC, Elder G, Hallet M, Ravits J, Baker M, Papadopoulos N, *et al.* A long-term follow-up of patients with post-poliomyelitis neuromuscular symptoms. *N Engl J Med* 1986; 314: 959–63.

141. Dark DS, Pingleton SK, Kerby GR, Crabb JE, Gollub SB, Glatter TR, *et al.* Breathing pattern abnormalities and arterial oxygen desaturation during sleep in the congestive heart failure syndrome. *Chest* 1987; 91: 833–6.

142. Datta AK, Shea SA, Horner RL, Guz A. The influence of induced hypocapnia and sleep on the endogenous respiratory rhythm in humans. *J Physiol Lond* 1991; 440: 17–33.

143. Davies RJ, Stradling JR. The relationship between neck circumference, radiographic pharyngeal anatomy, and the obstructive sleep apnoea syndrome. *Eur Respir J* 1990; 3: 509–14.

144. Davies RJO, Ali NJ, Fleetham J, Stradling JR. Observations on the mechanisms of blood pressure swings during central sleep apnoea and periodic movement of the legs. *Am Rev Respir Dis* 1991; 143(No. 4, pt 2): 383 (Abstract).

145. Davies RJO, Ali NJ, Stradling JR. Neck circumference and other clinical features in the diagnosis of the obstructive sleep apnoea syndrome. *Thorax* 1992; 47: 101–5.

146. Davies RJO, Belt PJ, Robert SJ, Ali NJ, Stradling JR. Arterial blood pressure responses to graded transient arousal from sleep in normal man. *J Appl Physiol* 1993; 74: 1123–30.

147. Davies RJO, Vardi-Visy K, Clarke M, Stradling JR. Nighttime blood pressure in obstructive sleep apnoea, snoring, and normal sleep. *J Sleep Res* 1992; 1 (Suppl): 52 (Abstract).

148. Davies RJO, Harrington KJ, Ormerod OJM, Stradling JR. Nasal continuous positive airway pressure in chronic heart failure with sleep disordered breathing. *Am Rev Respir Dis* 1993; 147: 630–4.

149. Davies RJO, Roberts SJ, Channon KJ, Stradling JR. Cyclical EEG and blood pressure changes during Cheyne–Stokes respiration. *Thorax* 1993; 48: 413 (Abstract).

150. Davies RJO, Turner R, Stradling JR. Fasting blood lipid and insulin levels in OSA patients, snorers, and matched controls. *Thorax* 1993; 48: 447 (Abstract).

151. Davies RJO, Vardi-Visy K, Clarke M, Stradling JR. Night time blood pressure in obstructive sleep apnoea, snoring, and normal sleep. *Thorax* 1992; 47: 216–17p (Abstract).

152. Dayall VS, Phillipson EA. Nasal surgery in the management of sleep apnea. *Ann Otol Rhinol Laryngol* 1985; 94: 550–4.

153. de Berry-Borowiecki B, Kukwa AA, Blanks RHI. Indications for palato-pharyngoplasty. *Arch Otolaryngol Head Neck Surg* 1985; 111: 659–63.

154. Delaubier A. (ed.) Traitement de l'insuffisance respiratoire chronique dans les dystrophies musculaires. In: *Memoires de certificat d'etudes superieuresde reeducation et readaptation fonctionelles*. Paris: Universite R Descartes, 1984: 1–124.

155. Delguste P, Aubert-Tulkens G, Rodenstein DO. Upper airway obstruction during nasal intermittent positive-pressure hyperventilation in sleep. *Lancet* 1991; 338: 1295–7.

156. DeMarco FJJ, Wynne JW, Block AJ, Boysen PG, Taasan VC. Oxygen desaturation during sleep as a determinant of the "blue and bloated" syndrome. *Chest* 1981; 79: 621–5.

157. Dement WC, Carskadon MA, Richardson G. Excessive daytime sleepiness in the sleep apnea syndrome. In: Guilleminault C, Dement WC. eds. *Sleep apnea syndromes*. New York: Alan R. Liss, 1978: 23–46.

158. Dempsey JA, Skatrud JB. A sleep-induced apneic threshold and its consequences. *Am Rev Respir Dis* 1986; 133: 1163–70.

159. Derderian SS, Bridenbaugh RH, Rajagopal KR. Neuropsychologic symptoms in obstructive sleep apnea improve after treatment with nasal continuous positive airway pressure. *Chest* 1988; 94: 1023–7.

160. Dolmage TE, Avendano MA, Goldstein RS. Respiratory function during wakefulness and sleep among survivors of respiratory and non-respiratory poliomyelitis. *Eur Respir J* 1992; 5: 864–70.

161. Donaldson JD, Redmond WM. Surgical management of obstructive sleep apnea in children with Down syndrome. *J Otolaryngol* 1988; 17: 398–403.

162. Dorlas JC, Nijboer JA, Butijn WT, van-der-Hoeven GM, Settels JJ, Wesseling KH. Effects of peripheral vasoconstriction on the blood pressure in the finger, measured continuously by a new noninvasive method (the Finapres). *Anesthesiology* 1985; 62: 342–5.

163. Douglas NJ. Control of ventilation during sleep. In: Kryger MH. ed. *Clinics in chest medicine* (Vol. 6, No. 4), *sleep disorders*. Philadelphia: Saunders, 1985: 563–75.

164. Douglas NJ. Funding treatment for sleep apnoea. *Br J Hosp Med* 1992; 47: 323–4.

165. Douglas NJ, Brash HM, Wraith PK, Calverley PMA, Leggett RJE, McElderry L, *et al*. Accuracy, sensitivity to carboxyhaemoglobin, and speed of response of the Hewlett Packard 47201A ear oximeter. *Am Rev Respir Dis* 1979; 119: 311–13.

166. Douglas NJ, Calverley PMA, Leggett RJE, Brash HM, Flenley DC, Brezinova V. Transient hypoxaemia during sleep in chronic bronchitis and emphysema. *Lancet* 1979; 1: 1–4.

167. Douglas NJ, Thomas S, Jan MA. Clinical value of polysomnography. *Lancet* 1992; 339: 347–50.

168. Douglas NJ, White DP, Weil JV, Pickett CK, Martin RJ, Hudgel DW, *et al*. Hypoxic ventilatory response decreases during sleep in normal men. *Am Rev Respir Dis* 1982; 125: 286–9.

169. Douglas NJ, White DP, Weil JV, Pickett CK, Zwillich CW. Hypercapnic ventilatory response in sleeping adults. *Am Rev Respir Dis* 1982; 126: 758–62.

170. Dowdell WT, Javaheri S, McGinnis W. Cheyne–Stokes respiration presenting as sleep apnea syndrome. *Am Rev Respir Dis* 1990; 141: 871–9.

171. Dowell AR, Buckley CE, Cohen R, Whalen RE, Sieker HO, Durham NC. Cheyne—Stokes respiration, a review of clinical manifestations and critique of physiological mechanisms. *Arch Intern Med* 1971; 127: 712—26.

172. Downey R, Bonnet MH. Performance during frequent sleep disruption. *Sleep* 1987; 10: 354—63.

173. Dunleavy D, Brezinova V, Oswald I, MacLean AW, Tinker M. Changes during weeks in effects of tricyclic drugs on the human sleeping brain. *Br J Psychiatry* 1972; 120: 663—72.

174. Eastman CI, Miescke KJ. Entrainment of circadian rhythms with 26-h bright light and sleep-wake schedules. *Am J Physiol* 1990; 259: 1189—97.

175. Eccles R. The central rhythm of the nasal cycle. *Acta Otolaryngol* 1978; 86: 464—8.

176. Edlund MJ, McNamara ME, Millman RP. Sleep apnea and panic attacks. *Compr Psychiatry* 1991; 32: 130—2.

177. Ehlenz K, Peter JH, Schneider H, Elle T, Scheere B, von Wichert P, *et al.* Renin secretion is substantially influenced by obstructive sleep apnea syndrome. In: Horne J. ed. *Sleep '90.* Bochum: Pontenagel Press, 1990: 193—5.

178. Ekbom KA. Restless legs syndrome. *Neurology* 1960; 10: 868—73.

179. Ellis ER, Bye PTB, Bruderer JW, Sullivan CE. Treatment of respiratory failure during sleep in patients with neuromuscular disease. *Am Rev Respir Dis* 1987; 135: 148—52.

180. Ellis ER, Grunstein RR, Chan S, Bye PT, Sullivan CE. Noninvasive ventilatory support during sleep improves respiratory failure in kyphoscoliosis. *Chest* 1988; 94: 811—15.

181. Escourrou P, Jirani A, Nedelcoux H, Duroux P, Gaultier C. Systemic hypertension in sleep apnea syndrome. Relationship with sleep architecture and breathing abnormalities. *Chest* 1990; 98: 1362—5.

182. Evans RA. Gastric stapling and sleep apnea [letter]. *Tex Med* 1988; 84: 7—8.

183. Fairbanks D. Complications of nasal packing. *Otolaryngol Head Neck Surg* 1986; 94: 412—15.

184. Fairbanks DNF, Fujita S, Ikematsu T, Simmons FB. *Snoring and obstructive sleep apnea.* New York: Raven Press, 1987.

185. Farney RJ, Walker LE, Jensen RL, Walker JM. Ear oximetry to detect apnea and differentiate rapid eye movement (REM) and non-REM (NREM) sleep. Screening for the sleep apnea syndrome. *Chest* 1986; 89: 533—9.

186. Fillenz M, Widdicombe JG. Receptors of the lungs and airways. In: Neil E. ed. *Handbook of sensory physiology,* Vol. 3. Berlin: Springer-Verlag, 1971: 81—112.

187. Findley LJ, Bonnie RJ. Sleep apnea and auto crashes. *Chest* 1988; 94: 225—6.

188. Findley LJ, Fabrizio M, Thommi G, Suratt PM. Severity of sleep apnea and automobile crashes [letter]. *N Engl J Med* 1989; 320: 868—9.

189. Findley LJ, Fabrizio MJ, Knight H, Norcross BB, LaForte AJ, Suratt PM. Driving simulator performance in patients with sleep apnea. *Am Rev Respir Dis* 1989; 140: 529—30.

190. Findley LJ, Ries AL, Tisi GM, *et al.* Hypoxemia during apnea in normal subjects: mechanisms and impact of lung volume. *J Appl Physiol* 1983; 55: 1777—83.

191. Findley LJ, Unverzagt ME, Suratt PM. Automobile accidents in patients with obstructive sleep apnea. *Am Rev Respir Dis* 1988; 138: 337–40.

192. Findley LJ, Weiss JW, Jabour ER. Drivers with untreated sleep apnea. A cause of death and serious injury. *Arch Intern Med* 1991; 151: 1451–2.

193. Finkelstein JW, Roffwarg HP, Boyar RM, Kream J, Hellman L. Age-related change in the twenty-four-hour spontaneous secretion of growth hormone. *J Clin Endocrinol Metab* 1972; 35: 665–70.

194. Finnegan TP, Abraham P, Docherty TB. Ambulatory monitoring of the electroencephalogram in high altitude mountaineers. *Electroencephalog Clin Neurophysiol* 1985; 60: 220–4.

195. Fleetham J, West P, Mezon B, Conway W, Roth T. Sleep, arousals, and oxygen desaturation in chronic obstructive pulmonary disease. *Am Rev Respir Dis* 1982; 126: 429–33.

196. Flenley DC. Clinical hypoxia: causes, consequences, and correction. *Lancet* 1978; 542–6.

197. Fletcher EC. *Abnormalities of respiration during sleep*. Orlando, Florida: Grune & Stratton, 1986,

198. Fletcher EC. History, techniques, and definitions in sleep related respiratory disorders. In: Fletcher EC. ed. *Abnormalities of respiration during sleep*. Orlando, Florida: Grune & Stratton, 1986: 1–19.

199. Fletcher EC, DeBehnke RD, Lovoi MS, Gorin AB. Undiagnosed sleep apnea in patients with essential hypertension. *Ann Intern Med* 1985; 103: 190–5.

200. Fletcher EC, Luckett RA, Goodnight-White S, Miller CC, Qian W, Costarangos Galarza C. A double-blind trial of nocturnal supplemental oxygen for sleep desaturation in patients with chronic obstructive pulmonary disease and a daytime P_{aO_2} above 60 mmHg. *Am Rev Respir Dis* 1992; 145: 1070–6.

201. Fletcher EC, Miller J, Divine GW, Fletcher JG, Miller T. Nocturnal oxyhemoglobin desaturation in COPD patients with arterial oxygen tensions above 60 mmHg. *Chest* 1987; 92: 604–8.

202. Fletcher EC, Miller J, Schaaf JW, Fletcher JG. Urinary catecholamines before and after tracheostomy in patients with obstructive sleep apnea and hypertension. *Sleep* 1987; 10: 35–44.

203. Fletcher EC, Schaaf JW, Miller J, Fletcher JG. Long-term cardiopulmonary sequelae in patients with sleep apnea and chronic lung disease. *Am Rev Respir Dis* 1987; 135: 525–33.

204. Franceschi M, Zamproni P, Crippa D, Smirne S. Excessive daytime sleepiness: a 1-year study in an unselected inpatient population. *Sleep* 1982; 5: 239–47.

205. Freidman M, Rosenman R, Carroll V. Changes in the serum cholestrol and blood clotting time in men subjected to cyclic variations of occupational stress. *Circulation* 1958; 17: 852–61.

206. Froehling B, Seidenburg M, Georgemiller R, Romano C. Neuropsychological and affective dysfunction in sleep apnea syndrome: response to nasal continuous positive airway pressure treatment. *Sleep Res* 1991; 20: 244 (Abstract).

207. Fry J. Are all ''T's and A's'' really necessary? *Br Med J* 1957; 1: 124–9.

208. Fujita S. Surgical treatment of obstructive sleep apnea: UPPP and linguoplasty (laser midline glossectomy). In: Guilleminault C, Partinen M. eds. *Obstructive sleep apnea syndrome*. New York: Raven Press, 1990: 129–51.

209. Fujita S, Conway W, Zorick F, Roth T. Surgical correction of anatomic abnormalities in obstructive sleep apnea syndrome: uvulopalatopharyngoplasty. *Otolaryngol Head Neck Surg* 1981; 89: 923–34.

210. Fujita S, Conway WA, Sicklesteel JM, Wittig RM, Zorick FJ, Roehrs TA, *et al*. Evaluation of the effectiveness of uvulopalatopharyngoplasty. *Laryngoscope* 1985; 95: 70–4.

211. Gabrielczyk MR. Acute airway obstruction after uvulopalatopharyngoplasty for obstructive sleep apnea syndrome. *Anesthesiology* 1988; 69: 941–3.

212. Gaddy JR, Doghramji K. Daytime sleepiness after nCPAP treatment. *Sleep Res* 1991; 20: 245 (Abstract).

213. Garay SM, Turino GM, Goldring RM. Sustained reversal of chronic hypercapnia in patients with alveolar hypoventilation syndromes. *Am J Med* 1981; 70: 269–74.

214. Gardner AMN, Fox RH. *The return of blood to the heart*. London: John Libbey, 1989: 70–5.

215. Gastaut H, Tassinari CA, Duron B. Polygraphic study of the episodic diurnal and nocturnal (hypnic and respiratory) manifestations of the Pickwick syndrome. *Brain Res* 1966; 2: 167–86.

216. Gay PC, Patel AM, Viggiano RW, Hubmayr RD. Nocturnal nasal ventilation for treatment of patients with hypercapnic respiratory failure. *Mayo Clin Proc* 1991; 66: 695–703.

217. George C, Nickerson PW, Hanly PJ, Millar TW, Kryger MH. Sleep apnoea patients have more automobile accidents. *Lancet* 1987; 2: 447 (Letter).

218. George CF, Millar TW, Kryger MH. Identification and quantification of apneas by computer-based analysis of oxygen saturation. *Am Rev Respir Dis* 1988; 137: 1238–40.

219. George CF, West P, Kryger MH. Oxygenation and breathing pattern during phasic and tonic REM in patients with chronic obstructive pulmonary disease. *Sleep* 1987; 10: 234–43.

220. Gislason T, Almqvist M, Eriksson G, Taube A, Boman G. Prevalence of sleep apnea syndrome among Swedish men—an epidemiological study. *J Clin Epidemiol* 1988; 41: 571–6.

221. Gislason T, Lindholm CE, Almqvist M, Birring E, Boman G, Eriksson G, *et al*. Uvulopalatopharyngoplasty in the sleep apnea syndrome. Predictors of results. *Arch Otolaryngol Head Neck Surg* 1988; 114: 45–51.

222. Gleadhill I, Patterson C, McCrum E, Evans A, MacMahon J. Prevalence of nocturnal hypoxic dips in men. *Thorax* 1991; 46: 320p (Abstract).

223. Gleeson K, Zwillich CW. Adenosine infusion and periodic breathing during sleep. *J Appl Physiol* 1992; 72: 1004–9.

224. Gleeson K, Zwillich CW. Adenosine stimulation, ventilation, and arousal from sleep. *Am Rev Respir Dis* 1992; 145: 453–7.

225. Gleeson K, Zwillich CW, White DP. The influence of increasing ventilatory effort on arousal from sleep. *Am Rev Respir Dis* 1990; 142: 295–300.

226. Glenn WWL, Sairenji H. Diaphram pacing in the treatment of chronic respiratory insufficiency. In: Roussos C, Macklem PT. eds. *The thorax: lung biology in health and disease.* New York: Marcel Dekker, 1985: 1407–40.

227. Gold AR, Bleeker ER, Smith PL. A shift from central and mixed sleep apnea to obstructive sleep apnea resulting from low-flow oxygen. *Am Rev Respir Dis* 1985; 132: 220–3.

228. Goldman JM, Ireland RM, Berthon-Jones M, Grunstein RR, Sullivan CE, Biggs JC. Erythropoietin concentrations in obstructive sleep apnoea. *Thorax* 1991; 46: 25–7.

229. Goldstein DS. Plasma catecholamines and essential hypertension. *Hypertension* 1983; 5: 86–99.

230. Goldstein RS, Molotiu N, Skrastins R, Long S, Contreras M. Assisting ventilation in respiratory failure by negative pressure ventilation and by rocking bed. *Chest* 1987; 92: 470–4.

231. Goldstein RS, Molotiu N, Skrastins R, Long S, de Rosie J, Contreras M, *et al.* Reversal of sleep-induced hypoventilation and chronic respiratory failure by nocturnal negative pressure ventilation in patients with restrictive ventilatory impairment. *Am Rev Respir Dis* 1987; 135: 1049–55.

232. Goldstein RS, Rancharan V, Bowes G, McNicholas WT, Bradley D, Phillipson EA. Effect of supplemental nocturnal oxygen on gas exchange in patients with severe obstructive lung disease. *N Engl J Med* 1984; 310: 425–9.

233. Gonsalez S, Lane R, Stocks J, Dinwiddie R, Hayward R, Mackersie A. The relationship between upper airway obstruction (UAO) and raised intracranial pressure (ICP) during sleep in children with craniosynostosis. *Eur Respir J Suppl* 1992; 5(suppl 15): 25s (Abstract).

234. Gonzalez-Rothi RJ, Foresman GE, Block AJ. Do patients with sleep apnea die in their sleep? *Chest* 1988; 94: 531–8.

235. Gothe B, Altose MD, Goldman MD, Cherniack NS. Effect of quiet sleep on resting and CO_2-stimulated breathing in humans. *J Appl Physiol* 1981; 50: 724–30.

236. Gothe B, Strohl KP, Levin S, Chernick NS. Nicotine: a different approach to treatment of obstructive sleep apnea. *Chest* 1985; 87: 11–17.

237. Gould GA, Gugger M, Molloy J, Tsara V, Shapiro CM, Douglas NJ. Breathing pattern and eye movement density during REM sleep in humans. *Am Rev Respir Dis* 1988; 138: 874–7.

238. Gould GA, Whyte KF, Rhind GB, Airlie MA, Catterall JR, Shapiro CM, *et al.* The sleep hypopnea syndrome. *Am Rev Respir Dis* 1988; 137: 895–8.

239. Graham AN, Martin PD, Haas LF. Neuralgic amyotrophy with bilateral diaphragmatic palsy. *Thorax* 1985; 40: 635–6.

240. Greene JA. Clinical studies on respiration: IV. Some observations on Cheyne–Stokes respiration. *Ann Intern Med* 1933; 52: 454–63.

241. Gribbin HR, Gardiner IT, Heinz GJ, Gibson GJ, Pride NB. Role of impaired inspiratory muscle function in limiting the ventilatory response to carbon dioxide in chronic airflow obstruction. *Clin Sci* 1983; 64: 487–95.

242. Grunstein RR, Handelsman DJ, Lawrence SJ, Blackwell C, Caterson ID, Sullivan CE. Neuroendocrine dysfunction in sleep apnea: reversal by continuous positive airways pressure therapy. *J Clin Endocrinol Metab* 1989; 68: 352–8.

243. Grunstein RR, Sullivan CE. Sleep apnea and hypothyroidism: mechanisms and management. *Am J Med* 1988; 85: 775–9.

244. Grunstein RR, Yang TS, Wilcox I. Sleep apnea and pattern of obesity. *Am Rev Respir Dis* 1991; 143(No. 4, pt 2): A380 (Abstract).

245. Guilhaume A, Benoit O, Gourmelen M, Richardet JK. Relationship between sleep stage IV deficit and reversible HGH deficiency in psychosocial dwarfism. *Pediatr Res* 1982; 16: 299–303.

246. Guilleminault C. Benzodiazepines, breathing, and sleep. *Am J Med* 1990; 88: 25S–8S.

247. Guilleminault C. Treatments in obstructive sleep apnea. In: Guilleminault C, Partinen M. eds. *Obstructive sleep apnea syndrome*. New York: Raven Press, 1990: 99–118.

248. Guilleminault C, Connolly SJ, Winkle RA. Cardiac arrhythmias and conduction disturbances during sleep in 400 patients with sleep apnea syndrome. *Am J Cardiol* 1983; 52: 490–4.

249. Guilleminault C, Cummiskey J, Dement WC. Sleep apnea syndrome: recent advances. *Adv Int Med* 1980; 26: 347–72.

250. Guilleminault C, Cummiskey J, Motta J. Chronic obstructive airflow disease and sleep studies. *Am Rev Respir Dis* 1980; 122: 397–406.

251. Guilleminault C, Cummiskey J, Motta J, Lynne-Davies P. Respiratory and hemodynamic study during wakefulness and sleep in myotonic dystrophy. *Sleep* 1978; 1: 19–31.

252. Guilleminault C, Dement WC. Sleep apnea syndromes and related sleep disorders. In: Williams RL, Karacan I, Moore CA. eds. *Sleep disorders: diagnosis and treatment*. New York: John Wiley & Sons, 1988: 47–71.

253. Guilleminault C, Hayes B. Naloxone, theophylline, bromocriptine, and obstructive sleep apnea. Negative results. *Bull Eur Physiopathol Respir* 1983; 19: 632–4.

254. Guilleminault C, Hill MW, Simmons FB, Dement WC. Obstructive sleep apnea: electromyographic and fibreoptic studies. *Exp Neurol* 1978; 62: 48–67.

255. Guilleminault C, Korobkin R, Winkle R. A review of 50 children with obstructive sleep apnea syndrome. *Lung* 1981; 159: 275–87.

256. Guilleminault C, Partinen M. *Obstructive sleep apnea syndrome*. New York: Raven Press, 1990: xv.

257. Guilleminault C, Quera-Salva MA. Obstructive sleep apnoea: is prevention ever possible? *Eur Respir J Suppl* 1990; 11: 539s–42s.

258. Guilleminault C, Riley R, Powell N. Obstructive sleep apnea and abnormal cephalometric measurements. Implications for treatment. *Chest* 1984; 86: 793–4.

259. Guilleminault C, Riley RW, Powell NB. Surgical treatment of obstructive sleep apnea. In: Kryger MH, Roth T, Dement WC. eds. *Principles and practice of sleep medicine*. Philadelphia: W.B. Saunders, 1989: 571–83.

260. Guilleminault C, Rosekind M. The arousal threshold: sleep deprivation, sleep fragmentation, and obstructive sleep apnea syndrome. *Bull Eur Physiopathol Respir* 1981; 17: 341–9.

261. Guilleminault C, Shiomi T, Stoohs R, Schnittger I. Echocardiographic studies in adults and children presenting with obstructive sleep apnea or heavy snoring. In: Gaultier C, Escourrou P, Curzi-Dascalova L. eds. *Sleep and cardiorespiratory control*. Montrouge: John Libbey, 1991: 95–103.

262. Guilleminault C, Simmons FB, Motta J, Cummiskey J, Rosekind M, Schroeder JS, *et al*. Obstructive sleep apnea syndrome and tracheostomy. *Arch Intern Med* 1981; 141: 985–8.

263. Guilleminault C, Stoohs R, Clerk A, Labanowski M, Simmons J. Upper airway resistance, increased breathing frequency and sleep. *J Sleep Res* 1992; 1(suppl): 89 (Abstract).

264. Guilleminault C, Stoohs R, Duncan S. Snoring (I). Daytime sleepiness in regular heavy snorers. *Chest* 1991; 99: 40–8.

265. Guilleminault C, Tilkian A, Dement WC. The sleep apnea syndromes. *Ann Rev Med* 1976; 27: 465–84.

266. Guilleminault C, Van den Hoed J, Mitler MM. Sleep apnea syndromes. In: Guilleminault C, Dement WC. eds. *Clinical overview of the sleep apnea syndromes*. New York: Alan R. Liss, 1978.

267. Guilleminault C, Winkle R, Korbkin R, Simmons B. Children and nocturnal snoring: evaluation of the effects of sleep related respiratory resistive load and daytime functioning. *Eur J Pediatr* 1982; 139: 165–71.

268. Guy Grand B, Apfelbaum M, Crepaldi G, Gries A, Lefebvre P, Turner P. International trial of long-term dexfenfluramine in obesity. *Lancet* 1989; 2: 1142–5.

269. Guyton AC, Crowell JH, Moore JW. Basic oscillating mechanism of Cheyne–Stokes breathing. *Am J Physiol* 1956; 187: 385–98.

270. Guyton AC, Lindsey AW, Abernathy B, Richardson T. Venous return at various right atrial pressures, and the normal venous return curve. *Am J Physiol* 1957; 189: 609–15.

271. Gyulay S, Gould D, Sawyer B, Pond D, Mant A, Saunders N. Evaluation of a microprocessor-based portable home monitoring system to measure breathing during sleep. *Sleep* 1987; 10: 130–42.

272. Hanly PJ. Mechanisms and management of central sleep apnea. *Lung* 1992; 170: 1-17.

273. Hanly PJ, Millar TW, Steljes DG, Baert R, Frais MA, Kryger MH. The effect of oxygen on respiration and sleep in patients with congestive heart failure. *Ann Intern Med* 1989; 111: 777–82.

274. Hanly PJ, Millar TW, Steljes DG, Baert R, Frais MA, Kryger MH. Respiration and abnormal sleep in patients with congestive heart failure. *Chest* 1989; 96: 480–8.

275. Haponik EF, Bleeker ER, Allen RP, Smith PL, Kaplan J. Abnormal inspiratory flow–volume curves in patients with sleep-disordered breathing. *Am Rev Respir Dis* 1981; 124: 571–4.

276. Haponik EF, Smith PL, Bohlman ME, Allen RP, Goldman SM, Bleeker ER. Computerised tomography in obstructive sleep apnea: correlation of airway

size with physiology during sleep and wakefulness. *Am Rev Respir Dis* 1983; 127: 221–6.

277. Haraldsson PO, Carenfelt C, Diderichsen F, Nygren A, Tingvall C. Clinical symptoms of sleep apnea syndrome and automobile accidents. *J Otorhinolaryngol Relat Spec* 1990; 52: 57–62.

278. Haraldsson PO, Carenfelt C, Persson HE, Sachs C, Tornros J. Simulated long-term driving performance before and after uvulopalatopharyngoplasty. *J Otorhinolaryngol Relat Spec* 1991; 53: 106–10.

279. Haraldsson PO, Carenfelt C, Tingvall C. Sleep apnea syndrome symptoms and automobile driving in a general population. *J Clin Epidemiol* 1992; 45: 821–5.

280. Harmon JD, Morgan W, Chaudhary B. Sleep apnea: morbidity and mortality of surgical treatment. *South Med J* 1989; 82: 161–4.

281. Haustein W, Pilcher J, Klink J, Schulz H. Automatic analysis overcomes limitations of sleep stage scoring. *Electroencephalog Clin Neurophysiol* 1986; 64: 364–74.

282. He J, Kryger MH, Zorick FJ, Conway W, Roth T. Mortality and apnea index in obstructive sleep apnea. Experience in 385 male patients. *Chest* 1988; 94: 9–14.

283. Heath D, Williams DR. *High altitude medicine and pathology.* London: Butterworths, 1989.

284. Hebertson WM, Talbert OR, Cohen MI. Respiratory apraxia and anosognia. *Trans Am Neurol Assoc* 1959; 84: 176–9.

285. Heckmatt JZ, Loh L, Dubowitz V. Night-time nasal ventilation in neuro-muscular disease. *Lancet* 1990; 335: 579–82.

286. Hedemark LL, Kronenberg RS. Ventilatory and heart rate responses to hypoxia and hypercapnia during sleep in adults. *J Appl Physiol* 1982; 53: 307–12.

287. Hedner J, Ejnell H, Caidahl K. Left ventricular hypertrophy independent of hypertension in patients with obstructive sleep apnoea. *J Hypertens* 1990; 8: 941–6.

288. Hedner J, Ejnell H, Sellgren J, Hedner T, Wallin G. Is high and fluctuating muscle nerve sympathetic activity in the sleep apnoea syndrome of pathogenetic importance for the development of hypertension? *J Hypertens Suppl* 1988; 6: S529–31.

289. Hedner J, Ejnell H, Wallin G, Carlsson J, Caidahl K. Consequences of increased sympathetic activity in sleep apnea. A pathogenetic mechanism for cardiovascular complications? In: Horne J. ed. *Sleep '90.* Bochum: Pontenagel Press, 1990: 435–9.

290. Heimer D, Schaaf SM, Lieberman A, Lavie P. Sleep apnea syndrome treated by repair of deviated nasal septum. *Chest* 1983; 84: 184–5.

291. Hendley JD. Tonsillectomy: justified but not mandated in special patients. *N Engl J Med* 1984; 310: 717–18.

292. Hendricks JC, Morrison AR, Mann GL. Different behaviors during paradoxical sleep without atonia depend on pontine lesion site. *Brain Res* 1982; 239: 81–105.

293. Henke KG, Sullivan CE. Activation of upper airway muscles by high frequency oscillatory pressures. *Am Rev Respir Dis* 1991; 143(No. 4, pt 2): A405 (Abstract).

294. Hernandez SF. Palatopharyngoplasty for the obstructive sleep apnea syndrome: technique and preliminary report of results in ten patients. *Am J Otolaryngol* 1982; 3: 229–34.

295. Hill NS, Eveloff SE, Carlisle CC, Goff SG. Efficacy of nocturnal nasal ventilation in patients with restrictive thoracic disease. *Am Rev Respir Dis* 1992; 145: 365–71.

296. Hill R, Robbins AW, Messing R, Arora NS. Sleep apnea syndrome after poliomyelitis. *Am Rev Respir Dis* 1983; 127: 129–31.

297. Hillerdal G, Hetta J, Lindholm CE, Hultcrantz E, Boman G. Symptoms in heavy snorers with and without obstructive sleep apnea. *Acta Otolaryngol Stockh* 1991; 111: 574–81.

298. Hirshkowitz M, Karacan I, Gurakar A, Williams RL. Hypertension, erectile dysfunction, and occult sleep apnea. *Sleep* 1989; 12: 223–32.

299. Hoddes E, Zarcone V, Smythe H, Phillips R, Dement W. Quantification of sleepiness: a new approach. *Psychophysiology* 1973; 10: 431–6.

300. Hoffstein V, Rubinstein I, Mateika S, Slutsky AS. Determinants of blood pressure in snorers. *Lancet* 1988; 2: 992–4.

301. Hoffstein V, Wright S, Zamel N. Flow–volume curves in snoring patients with and without obstructive sleep apnea. *Am Rev Respir Dis* 1989; 139: 957–60.

302. Holschneider AM, Bliesener JA, Abel M. [Brain stem dysfunction in Arnold–Chiari II syndrome]. *Z Kinderchir* 1990; 45: 67–71.

303. Honda Y, Juji T, Matsuki K, Naohara T, Satake M, Inoko H, *et al*. HLA-DR2 and Dw2 in narcolepsy and in other disorders of excessive somnolence without cataplexy. *Sleep* 1986; 9: 133–42.

304. Hong CC, Gillin C, Callaghan G, Potkin S. Correlation of rapid eye movement density with dream report length and not with movements in the dream: evidence against the scanning hypothesis. *Sleep Res* 1992; 21: 127 (Abstract).

305. Horne J. *Why we sleep*. Oxford: Oxford University Press, 1988.

306. Horne JA. Dimensions to sleepiness. In: Monk TH. ed. *Sleep, sleepiness and performance*. Chichester: John Wiley & Sons, 1991: 169–96.

307. Horner RL, Innes JA, Holden HB, Guz A. Afferent pathway(s) for pharyngeal dilator reflex to negative pressure in man: a study using upper airway anaesthesia. *J Physiol Lond* 1991; 436: 31–44.

308. Horner RL, Innes JA, Murphy K, Guz A. Evidence for reflex upper airway dilator muscle activation by sudden negative airway pressure in man. *J Physiol Lond* 1991; 436: 15–29.

309. Horner RL, Mohiaddin RH, Lowell DG, Shea SA, Burman ED, Longmore DB, *et al*. Sites and sizes of fat deposits around the pharynx in obese patients with obstructive sleep apnoea and weight matched controls. *Eur Respir J* 1989; 2: 613–22.

310. Horner RL, Shea SA, McIvor J, Guz A. Pharyngeal size and shape during wakefulness and sleep in patients with obstructive sleep apnoea. *Q J Med* 1989; 72: 719–35.

311. Howard GF. Laboratory assessment of sleep and related functions. In: Riley TL. ed. *Clinical aspects of sleep and sleep disturbance*. Boston: Butterworth, 1985: 197–228.

312. Howard RS, Wiles CM, Spencer GT. The late sequelae of poliomyelitis. *Q J Med* 1988; 66: 219–32.

313. Hudgel DW, Hendricks C. Palate and hypopharynx—sites of inspiratory narrowing of the upper airway during sleep. *Am Rev Respir Dis* 1988; 138: 1542–7.

314. Hudgel DW, Martin RJ, Capehart M, Johnson B, Hill P. Contribution of hypoventilation to sleep oxygen desaturation in chronic obstructive pulmonary disease. *J Appl Physiol* 1983; 55: 669–77.

315. Huggare J, Kylamarkuza S. Morphology of the first cervical vertebra in children with enlarged adenoids. *Eur J Orthod* 1985; 7: 93–6.

316. Hultcrantz E, Larson M, Hellquist R, Ahlqvist-Rastad J, Svanholm H, Jakobsson OP. The influence of tonsillar obstruction and tonsillectomy on facial growth and dental arch morphology. *Int J Pediatr Otorhinolaryngol* 1991; 22: 125–34.

317. Hultcrantz E, Svanholm H, Ahlqvist-Rastad J. Sleep apnea in children without hypertrophy of the tonsils. *Clin Pediatr Phila* 1988; 27: 350–2.

318. Hyland RH, Hutcheon MA, Perl A, Bowes G, Anthonisen NR, Zamel N, *et al*. Upper airway occlusion induced by diaphragm pacing for primary alveolar hypoventilation: implications for the pathogenesis of obstructive sleep apnea. *Am Rev Respir Dis* 1981; 124: 180–5.

319. Hyland RH, Jones NL, Powles ACP, Lenkie SCM, Vanderlinden RG, Epstein SW. Primary alveolar hypoventilation treated with nocturnal electrophrenic respiration. *Am Rev Respir Dis* 1978; 117: 165–72.

320. Iber C, Berssenbrugge A, Skatrud JB, Dempsey JA. Ventilatory adaptations to resistive loading during wakefulness and non-REM sleep. *J Appl Physiol* 1982; 52: 607–14.

321. Ikematsu T. Study of snoring. 4th report. Therapy (in Japanese). *J Jpn Otol Rhinol Laryngol* 1964; 64: 434–5.

322. Imes NK, Orr WC, Smith RO, Rogers RM. Retrognathia and sleep apnea: a life-threatening condition masquerading as narcolepsy. *JAMA* 1977; 237: 1596–7.

323. Ingrassia TS, Nelson SB, Harris CD, Hubmayr RD. Influence of sleep state on CO_2 responsiveness. A study of the unloaded respiratory pump in humans. *Am Rev Respir Dis* 1991; 144: 1125–9.

324. Issa FG, Sullivan CE. Alcohol, snoring and sleep apnea. *J Neurol Neurosurg Psych* 1982; 45: 353–9.

325. Issa FG, Sullivan CE. Arousal and breathing responses to airway occlusion in healthy sleeping adults. *J Appl Physiol* 1983; 55: 1113–19.

326. Issa FG, Sullivan CE. Upper airway closing pressures in obstructive sleep apnea. *J Appl Physiol* 1984; 57: 520–7.

327. Issa FG, Sullivan CE. Upper airway closing pressures in snorers. *J Appl Physiol* 1984; 57: 528–35.

328. Issa FG, Sullivan CE. Reversal of central sleep apnea using nasal CPAP. *Chest* 1986; 90: 165–71.

329. Jamal K, McMahon G, Edgell G, Fleetham JA. Cough and arousal responses to inhaled citric acid in sleeping humans. *Am Rev Respir Dis* 1983; 127(pt 2): 237 (Abstract).

330. Jamieson A, Guilleminault C, Partinen M, Quera-Salva MA. Obstructive sleep apneic patients have craniomandibular abnormalities. *Sleep* 1986; 9: 469–77.

331. Jennum P. Cortisol and adrenergic activity in patients suffering from obstructive sleep apnea before and after nasal CPAP treatment. In: Horne J. ed. *Sleep '90*. Bochum: Pontenagel Press, 1990: 426–8.

332. Johns MW. A new method for measuring daytime sleepiness: the Epworth sleepiness scale. *Sleep* 1991; 14: 540–5.

333. Johnson D, Drenick ET. Therapeutical fasting in morbid obesity: long-term follow-up. *Arch Intern Med* 1977; 137: 1381–2.

334. Johnson JT, Sanders MH. Breathing during sleep immediately after uvulopalatopharyngoplasty. *Laryngoscope* 1986; 46: 1236–8.

335. Johnson LC, Lubin A. The orienting reflex during waking and sleeping. *Electroencephalog Clin Neurophysiol* 1967; 22: 11–21.

336. Johnson MW, Remmers JE. Accessory muscle activity during sleep in chronic obstructive pulmonary disease. *J Appl Physiol* 1984; 57: 1011–17.

337. Jouvet M, Delorme F. Locus Coeruleus et sommeil paradoxal. *C R Soc Biol (Paris)* 1965; 159: 895–9.

338. Judson JP, Glenn WWL. Radiofrequency electrophrenic respiration. *J Am Med Assoc* 1968; 203: 1033–7.

339. Jurado JL, Luna-Villegas G, Buela-Casal G. Normal human subjects with slow reaction times and larger time estimations after waking have diminished delta sleep. *Electroencephalog Clin Neurophysiol* 1989; 73: 124–8.

340. Kales A, Bixler ED, Cadieux RJ, Schneck DW, Shaw LC, Locke TW, *et al.* Sleep apnoea in a hypertensive population. *Lancet* 1984; 2: 1005–8.

341. Kales A, Tan T-L, Kollar EJ, Naitoh P, Preston TA, Malmstrom EJ. Sleep patterns following 205 hours of sleep deprivation. *Psychosomatic Medicine* 1970; 32: 189–200.

342. Kappagoda CT, Man GC, Teo KK. Behaviour of canine pulmonary vagal afferent receptors during sustained acute pulmonary venous pressure elevation. *J Physiol Lond* 1987; 394: 249–65.

343. Karacan I, Rosenbloom AL, Williams RL, Finley WW, Hursch CJ. Slow wave sleep deprivation in relation to plasma growth hormone concentration. *Behavior Neuropsychiat* 1971; 2: 11–14.

344. Karacan I, Thornby JI, Anch AM, Booth GH, Williams RL, Salis PJ. Dose-related sleep disturbances induced by coffee and caffeine. *Clin Pharmacol Ther* 1976; 20: 682–9.

345. Katsantonis GP, Friedman WH, Krebs FJ, Walsh JK. Nasopharyngeal complication following uvulopalatopharyngoplasty. *Laryngoscope* 1987; 97: 309–14.

346. Katsantonis GP, Schweiter PK, Branham GH, Chambers G, Walsh JK. Management of obstructive sleep apnea: comparison of various treatment modalities. *Laryngoscope* 1988; 98: 304–9.

347. Katsantonis GP, Walsh JK. Somnofluoroscopy: its role in the selection of candidates for uvulopalatopharyngoplasty. *Otolaryngol Head Neck Surg* 1986; 94: 56−60.

348. Katz I, Stradling J, Slutsky AS, Zamel N, Hoffstein V. Do patients with obstructive sleep apnea have thick necks? *Am Rev Respir Dis* 1990; 141: 1228−31.

349. Katz I, Zamel N, Slutsky AS, Rebuck AS, Hoffstein V. An evaluation of flow−volume curves as a screening test for obstructive sleep apnea. *Chest* 1990; 98: 337−40.

350. Kauffmann F, Annesi I, Neukirch F, Oryszczyn MP, Alperovitch A. The relation between snoring and smoking, body mass index, age, alcohol consumption and respiratory symptoms. *Eur Respir J* 1989; 2: 599−603.

351. Keenan SP, Burt H, Ryan CF, Fleetham JA. Chronic nasal CPAP therapy reduces systemic hypertension in patients with obstructive sleep apnea. *Am Rev Respir Dis* 1991; 143(No. 4, pt 2): A608 (Abstract).

352. Kerby GR, Mayer LS, Pingleton SK. Nocturnal positive pressure ventilation via nasal mask. *Am Rev Respir Dis* 1987; 135: 738−40.

353. Kern W, Ripberger R, Schafer J, Born J, Fehm HL. Nocturnal growth hormone and cortisol secretion in patients with sleep apnea syndrome. In: Horne J. ed. *Sleep '90*. Bochum: Pontenagel Press, 1990: 196−9.

354. Khan Y, Heckmatt JZ. Breathing during sleep in Duchenne muscular dystrophy. *Am Rev Respir Dis* 1992; 145: A863 (Abstract).

355. Khoo MCK, Gottschalk A, Pack AI. Sleep-induced periodic breathing and apnea: a theoretical study. *J Appl Physiol* 1991; 70: 2014−24.

356. Kilduff TS, Bowersox SS, Kaitin KI, Baker TL, Ciaranello RD, Dement WC. Muscarinic cholinergic receptors in the canine model of narcolepsy. *Sleep* 1986; 9: 102−6 (Abstract).

357. Kimmelman CP, Levine SB, Shore ET, Millman RP. Uvulopalatopharyngoplasty. A comparison of two techniques. *Laryngoscope* 1985; 95: 1488−90.

358. Kinney HC, Filiano JJ, Harper RM. The neuropathology of the sudden infant death syndrome. A review. *J Neuropathol Exp Neurol* 1992; 51: 115−26.

359. Klein KE, Hermann H, Kuklinski P, Wegmann HM. Circadian performance rhythms. Experimental studies in air operation. In: Mackie JR. ed. *Vigilance, theory, operational performance and physiological correlates*. New York: Plenum Press, 1977: 117−32.

360. Knight H, Millman RP, Gur RC, Saykin AJ, Doherty JU, Pack AI. Clinical significance of sleep apnea in the elderly. *Am Rev Respir Dis* 1987; 136: 845−50.

361. Koenig JE, Thach BT. Effects of mass loading on the upper airway. *J Appl Physiol* 1988; 64: 2294−9.

362. Kohorst WR, Schonfield SA, Altman M. Bilateral diaphragmatic paralysis following topical cardiac hypothermia. *Chest* 1984; 85: 65−8.

363. Koo KW, Sax DS, Snider GL. Arterial blood gases and pH during sleep in chronic obstructive pulmonary disease. *Am J Med* 1975; 58: 663−70.

364. Koopmann CF, Feld RA, Coulthard SW. Sleep apnea syndrome associated with a neck mass. *Otolaryngol Head Neck Surg* 1981; 89: 949−52.

365. Koskenvuo M, Kaprio J, Partinen M, Langinvainio H, Sarna S, Heikkila K. Snoring as a risk factor for hypertension and angina pectoris. *Lancet* 1985; 1: 893–6.

366. Koskenvuo M, Kaprio J, Telakivi T, Partinen M, Heikkila K, Sarna S. Snoring as a risk factor for ischaemic heart disease and stroke in men. *Br Med J* 1987; 294: 16–19.

367. Krieger AJ. Sleep apnea produced by cervical cordotomy and other neurosurgical lesions in man. In: Guilleminault C, Dement WC. eds. *Sleep apnea syndromes*. New York: Alan R. Liss, 1978: 273–94.

368. Krieger J, Follenius M, Sforza E, Brandenberger G, Peter JD. Effects of treatment with nasal continuous positive airway pressure on atrial natriuretic peptide and arginine vasopressin release during sleep in patients with obstructive sleep apnoea. *Clin Sci* 1991; 80: 443–9.

369. Krieger J, Imbs JL, Schmidt M, Kurtz D. Renal function in patients with obstructive sleep apnea. Effects of nasal continuous positive airway pressure. *Arch Intern Med* 1988; 148: 1337–40.

370. Krieger J, Laks L, Wilcox I, Grunstein RR, Costas LJ, McDougall JG, et al. Atrial natriuretic peptide release during sleep in patients with obstructive sleep apnoea before and during treatment with nasal continuous positive airway pressure. *Clin Sci* 1989; 77: 407–11.

371. Krieger J, Mangin P, Kurtz D. Effects of almitrine in the treatment of sleep apnea syndrome. *Bull Eur Physiopathol Respir* 1983; 19: 630.

372. Krieger J, Schmidt M, Sforza E, Lehr L, Imbs JL, Coumaros G, et al. Urinary excretion of guanosine 3′:5′-cyclic monophosphate during sleep in obstructive sleep apnoea patients with and without nasal continuous positive airway pressure treatment. *Clin Sci* 1989; 76: 31–7.

373. Krieger J, Sforza E, Apprill M, Lampert E, Weitzenblum E, Ratomaharo J. Pulmonary hypertension, hypoxemia, and hypercapnia in obstructive sleep apnea patients. *Chest* 1989; 96: 729–37.

374. Kripke DF, Ancoli-Israel S, Mason WJ, Kaplan O. Correlates of sleep apnea and periodic leg movements in sleep among representative elderly. In: Horne J. ed. *Sleep '88*. Stuttgart: G.F.Verlag, 1989: 262–3.

375. Kripke DF, Mason WJ, Bloomquist J, Cobarrubias M, Engler R, Ancoli-Israel S. Relationship of respitrace apnea–hypopnea counts and 4% desaturations. *Sleep Res* 1988; 17: 208 (Abstract).

376. Kripke DF, Mullaney DJ, Messin S, Wyborney VG. Wrist actigraph measures of sleep and rhythms. *Electroencephalog Clin Neurophysiol* 1978; 44: 674–8.

377. Kryger M, Quesney LF, Holder D, Gloor P, MacLeod P. The sleep deprivation syndrome of the obese patient. *Am J Med* 1974; 56: 531–9.

378. Kryger MH. Sleep apnea. From the needles of Dionysius to continuous positive airway pressure. *Arch Intern Med* 1983; 143: 2301–3.

379. Kryger MH, Roth T, Dement WC. *Principles and practice of sleep medicine*. Philadelphia: W.B. Saunders, 1989.

380. Kuhlo W, Doll E, Frank MD. Erfolgreiche behandlung eines Pickwick-syndroms durch eine dauertrachealkanule. *Dtsch Med Wochenschr* 1969; 94: 1286–90.

381. Kuo PC, West RA, Bloomquist DS, McNiel RW. The effect of mandibular osteotomy in three patients with hypersomnia sleep apnea. *Oral Surg* 1979; 48: 385—92.

382. Kurono T, Sakuma T, Shinozaki T, Kouchiyama S, Masuyama S, Kunitomo F, et al. [A case of obstructive sleep apnea syndrome remarkably improved by gastric restriction surgery]. *Nippon Kyobu Shikkan Gakkai Zasshi* 1990; 28: 767—72.

383. Kurtz D, Krieger J, Kowalski J, Hoff E, Mangin P. Nycterohemeral variations in plasma growth hormone (GH) levels and sleep apnea syndromes: their relationship with obesity. *Rev EEG Neurophysiol* 1980; 10: 366—75.

384. Lahiri S, Maret K, Sherpa MG. Dependence of high altitude sleep apnea on ventilatory sensitivity to hypoxia. *Respir Physiol* 1983; 52: 281—301.

385. Lahive KC, Weiss JW, Weinberger SE. Alpha-methyldopa selectively reduces alae nasi activity. *Clin Sci* 1988; 74: 547—51.

386. Lahive KC, Weiss JW, Weinberger SE. Low dose aminophylline selectively increases upper airway motor activity in normals. *Respir Physiol* 1988; 72: 163—70.

387. Lakshminarayan S, Sahn SA, Hudson L, Weil JV. Effect of diazepam on ventilatory responses. *Clin Pharmacol Ther* 1976; 20: 178—83.

388. Lamphere J, Roehrs T, Wittig R, Zorick F, Conway WA, Roth T. Recovery of alertness after CPAP in apnea. *Chest* 1989; 96: 1364—7.

389. Lane DJ, Hazleman B, Nichols PJR. Late onset respiratory failure in patients with previous poliomyelitis. *Q J Med* 1974; 43: 551—68.

390. Langanke P, Podszus T, Penzel T, Peter JH, Bonzel T, von Wichert P. Venous return during upper airway obstruction in obstructive sleep apnea. *Sleep Res* 1991; 20: 275 (Abstract).

391. Langdon N, Welsh KI, van Dam M, Vaughan RW, Parkes D. Genetic markers in narcolepsy. *Lancet* 1985; 2: 1178—80.

392. Laroche CM, Carroll N, Moxham J, Green M. Clinical significance of severe isolated diaphragm weakness. *Am Rev Respir Dis* 1988; 138: 862—6.

393. Larsson B, Svardsudd K, Welin L, Wilhelmsen L, Bjorntorp P, Tibblin G. Abdominal adipose tissue distribution, obesity, and risk of cardiovascular disease and death: 13 year follow up of participants in the study of men born in 1913. *Br Med J* 1984; 288: 1401—4.

394. Larsson SG, Gislason T, Lindholm CE. Computed tomography of the oropharynx in obstructive sleep apnea. *Acta Radiol* 1988; 29: 401—5.

395. Laurikainen E, Erkinjuntti M, Alihanka J, Rikalainen H, Suonpaa . Radiological parameters of the bony nasopharynx and the adenotonsillar size compared with sleep apnea episodes in children. *Int J Pediatr Otorhinolaryngol* 1987; 12: 303—10.

396. Lavie P. Incidence of sleep apnea in a presumably healthy working population. *Sleep* 1983; 6: 312—18.

397. Lavie P. Nothing new under the moon. Historical accounts of the sleep apnea syndrome. *Arch Intern Med* 1984; 144: 2025—8.

398. Lavie P. Ultra short sleep—waking schedule III. "Gates" and forbidden "zones" for sleep. *Electroencephalog Clin Neurophysiol* 1986; 63: 414—25.

399. Lavie P. The 24-hour sleep propensity function (SPF): practical and theoretical implications. In: Monk TH. ed. *Sleep, sleepiness and performance*. Chichester: John Wiley & Sons, 1991: 65−93.

400. Lavie P, Ben-Yosef R, Rubin AE. Prevalence of sleep apnea syndrome among patients with essential hypertension. *Am Heart J* 1984; 108: 373−6.

401. Lavie P, Fischel N, Zomer J, Eliaschar I. The effects of partial and complete mechanical occlusion of the nasal passages on sleep structure and breathing in sleep. *Acta Otolaryngol* 1983; 95: 161−6.

402. Lavie P, Gertner R, Zomer J, Podoshin L. Breathing disorders in sleep associated with ''microarousals'' in patients with allergic rhinitis. *Acta Otolaryngol* 1981; 92: 529−64.

403. Lavie P, Peled R. Narcolepsy is a rare disease in Israel. *Sleep* 1987; 6: 608−9.

404. Lea S, Ali NJ, Goldman M, Loh L, Fleetham J, Stradling JR. Systolic blood pressure swings reflect inspiratory effort during simulated obstructive sleep apnoea. In: Horne J. ed. *Sleep '90*. Bochum: Pontenagel Press, 1990: 178−81.

405. Leiter JC, Knuth SL, Bartlett D. The effect of sleep deprivation on activity of the genioglossus muscle. *Am Rev Respir Dis* 1985; 132: 1242−5.

406. Leiter JC, Knuth SL, Krol RC, Bartlett D. The effect of diazepam on genioglossal muscle activity in normal human subjects. *Am Rev Respir Dis* 1985; 132: 216−19.

407. Lenders H, Schaefer J, Pirsig W. Turbinate hypertrophy in habitual snorers and patients with obstructive sleep apnea: findings of acoustic rhinometry. *Laryngoscope* 1991; 101: 614−18.

408. Lester BK, Rundell OH, Cowden LC, Williams HL. Chronic alcoholism, alcohol and sleep. *Adv Exp Med Biol* 1973; 35: 261−79.

409. Levi-Valensi P, Weitzenblum E, Rida Z, Aubry P, Braghiroli A, Donner C, *et al*. Sleep-related oxygen desaturation and daytime pulmonary haemodynamics in COPD patients. *Eur Respir J* 1992; 5: 301−7.

410. Levin BE, Margolis G. Acute failure of automatic respirations secondary to a unilateral brainstem infarct. *Ann Neurol* 1977; 1: 583−6.

411. Levine OR, Simpser M. Alveolar hypoventilation and cor pulmonale associated with chronic airway obstruction in infants with Downs syndrome. *Clin Paediatr* 1982; 21: 25−9.

412. Lightman NI, Schooley RT. Adult-onset acid maltase deficiency. *Chest* 1977; 72: 250−2.

413. Liistro G, Stanescu DC, Veriter C, Rodenstein DO, Aubert-Tulkens G. Pattern of snoring in obstructive sleep apnea patients and in heavy snorers. *Sleep* 1991; 14: 517−25.

414. Linder-Aronson S. Effects of adenoidectomy on dentition and nasopharynx. *Am J Orthod* 1974; 65: 1−15.

415. Linder-Aronson S, Woodside DG, Lundstrom A. Mandibular growth direction following adenoidectomy. *Am J Orthod* 1986; 89: 273−84.

416. Loh L, Hughes JMB, Newsom Davis J. Gas exchange problems in bilateral diaphragm paralysis. *Bull Eur Physiopathol Respir* 1979; 15(suppl): 137−41.

417. Longobardo GS, Gothe B, Goldman MD, Cherniack NS. Sleep apnea considered as a control system instability. *Respir Physiol* 1982; 50: 311−33.

418. Loomis AL, Harvey EN, Hobart GA. Cerebral states during sleep, as studied by human brain potentials. *J Exp Physiol* 1937; 21: 127–44.

419. Lopes JM, Tabachnik E, Muller NL, Levison H, Bryan AC. Total airway resistance and respiratory muscle activity during sleep. *J Appl Physiol* 1983; 54: 773–7.

420. Lovett Doust JW, Schneider RA. Studies on the physiology of awareness: anoxia and the levels of sleep. *Br Med J* 1952; 1: 449–55.

421. Lowe A, Fleetham J, Ryan F, Mathews B. Effects of a mandibular re-positioning appliance used in the treatment of obstructive sleep apnea on tongue muscle activity. *Prog Clin Biol Res* 1990; 345: 395–404.

422. Lowe AA, Gionhaku N, Takeuchi K, Fleetham JA. Three dimensional CT reconstructions of tongue and airway in adult subjects with obstructive sleep apnea. *Am J Orthod* 1986; 90: 364–74.

423. Luchsinger J, Garshick E, Schaul N, Hackshaw R, Scharf SM. Criteria for defining sleep disordered breathing events are non-uniform. *Sleep Res* 1990; 19: 370 (Abstract).

424. Lugaresi E, Cirignotta F, Coccagna G, Montagna P. Nocturnal myoclonus and restless legs syndrome. *Adv Neurol* 1986; 43: 295–306.

425. Lugaresi E, Cirignotta F, Coccagna G, Piana C. Some epidemiological data on snoring in cardiocirculatory disturbances. *Sleep* 1980; 3: 221–4.

426. Lugaresi E, Cirignotta F, Coccogna G, Montagna P. Clinical significance of snoring. In: Saunders NA, Sullivan CE. eds. *Sleep and breathing*. New York: Marcel Dekker, 1984: 283–98.

427. Lugaresi E, Cirignotta F, Montagna P. Pathogenic aspects of snoring and obstructive apnea syndrome. *Schweiz Med Wochenschr* 1988; 118: 1333–7.

428. Lugaresi E, Cirignotta F, Montagna P. Snoring: pathogenic, clinical and therapeutic aspects. In: Kryger MH, Roth T, Dement WC. eds. *Principles and practice of sleep medicine*. Philadelphia: W.B. Saunders, 1989: 494–500.

429. Lugaresi E, Coccagna G, Mantovani M, Lebrun R. Some periodic phenomena arising during drowsiness and sleep in man. *Electroencephalog Clin Neurophysiol* 1972; 32: 701–5.

430. Lugaresi E, Mondini S, Zucconi M, Montagna P, Cirignotta F. Staging of heavy snorers' disease. A proposal. *Bull Eur Physiopathol Respir* 1983; 19: 590–4.

431. MacLean AW, Cairns J. Dose–response effects of ethanol on the sleep of young men. *J Stud Alcohol* 1982; 43: 434–44.

432. Mahboubi S, Marsh RR, Potsic WP, Pasquariello PS. The lateral neck radiograph in adenotonsillar hyperplasia. *Int J Pediatr Otorhinolaryngol* 1985; 10: 67–73.

433. Malone S, Liu PP, Holloway R, Rutherford R, Xie A, Bradley TD. Obstructive sleep apnoea in patients with dilated cardiomyopathy: effects of continuous positive airway pressure. *Lancet* 1991; 338: 1480–4.

434. Mant A, Saunders NA, Eyland AE, Pond CD, Chancellor AH, Webster IW. Sleep-related respiratory disturbance and dementia in elderly females. *J Gerontol* 1988; 43: M140–4.

435. Mant A, Saunders NA, Eyland EA, Pond CD, Sawyer B, Saltman DC. Sleep habits and sleep related respiratory disturbances in an elderly population. In: Horne J. ed. *Sleep '88*. Stuttgart: G.F.Verlag, 1989: 260–1.

436. Marabini A, Chan-Yeung M, Fleetham JA, Ward H. Smoking and obesity indicators as predictors of snoring and sleep-apnea. Relation with diastolic blood pressure. *Am Rev Respir Dis* 1992; 145: A867 (Abstract).

437. Marcus CL, Keens TG, Bautista DB, von Pechmann WS, Ward SL. Obstructive sleep apnea in children with Down syndrome. *Pediatrics* 1991; 88: 132–9.

438. Marino W. The acute effects of negative pressure mechanical ventilation on patients with chronic respiratory insufficiency. *Am Rev Respir Dis* 1986; 133(suppl): A167 (Abstract).

439. Marino W, Braun N. Reversal of the clinical sequelae of respiratory muscle fatigue by intermittent mechanical ventilation. *Am Rev Respir Dis* 1982; 125(pt 2): A85 (Abstract).

440. Marrone O, Bellia V, Ferrara G, Milone F, Romano L, Salvaggio A, *et al.* Transmural pressure measurements. Importance in the assessment of pulmonary hypertension in obstructive sleep apneas. *Chest* 1989; 95: 338–42.

441. Marrone O, Stallone A, Salvaggio A, Milone F, Bellia V, Bonsignore G. Occurrence of breathing disorders during CPAP administration in obstructive sleep apnoea syndrome. *Eur Respir J* 1991; 4: 660–6.

442. Marsh RR, Potsic WP, Pasquariello C. Recorder for assessment of upper airway disorders. *Otolaryngol Head Neck Surg* 1983; 5: 584–5.

443. Martin RJ, Block AJ, Cohn MA, Conway WA, Hudgel DW, Powles ACP, *et al.* Indications and standards for cardiopulmonary sleep studies. *Sleep* 1985; 8: 371–9.

444. Martin RJ, Sanders MH, Garay BA, Pennock BE. Acute and long-term ventilatory effects and hyperoxia in the adult sleep apnea syndrome. *Am Rev Respir Dis* 1982; 125: 175–80.

445. Mason EE. Vertical banded gastroplasty for obesity. *Arch Surg* 1982; 117: 701–6.

446. Masuyama S, Shinozaki T, Kohchiyama S, Okita S, Kimura H, Honda Y, *et al.* Heart rate depression during sleep apnea depends on hypoxic chemosensitivity. A study at high altitude. *Am Rev Respir Dis* 1990; 141: 39–42.

447. Mateika JH, Mateika S, Slutsky AS, Hoffstein V. The effect of snoring on mean arterial blood pressure during non-REM sleep. *Am Rev Respir Dis* 1992; 145: 141–6.

448. Mathew OP. Upper airway negative-pressure effects on respiratory activity of upper airway muscles. *J Appl Physiol* 1984; 56: 500–5.

449. Mathew OP, Abu-Osba YK, Thach BT. Influence of upper airway pressure changes on genioglossus muscle respiratory activity. *J Appl Physiol* 1982; 52: 438–44.

450. Mathew OP, Farber JP. Effect of upper airway negative pressure on respiratory timing. *Respir Physiol* 1983; 54: 259–68.

451. Mathew OP, Sant'Ambrogio FB. Laryngeal reflexes. In: Mathew OP, Sant'Ambrogio G. eds. *Respiratory function of the upper airway. Lung biology in health and disease*. New York: Marcel Dekker, 1988: 259–302.

452. Maw AR. Tonsillectomy today. *Arch Dis Child* 1986; 61: 421–3.
453. Mayer J, Brandenburg U, Ploch T, Weichler U, Moser R, Peter JH. Blood pressure and sleep apnea. Results after long-term therapy with nCPAP. *European Sleep Research Society (Strasbourg)* 1991; 410 (Abstract).
454. McKeon JL, Murre-Allen K, Saunders NA. Supplemental oxygen and quality of sleep in patients with chronic obstructive lung disease. *Thorax* 1989; 44: 184–8.
455. McNicholas WT, Coffey M, Fitzgerald MX. Ventilation and gas exchange during sleep in patients with interstitial lung disease. *Thorax* 1986; 41: 777–82.
456. McNicholas WT, Rutherford R, Grossman R, Moldofsky H, Zamel N, Phillipson EA. Abnormal respiratory pattern generation during sleep in patients with autonomic dysfunction. *Am Rev Respir Dis* 1983; 128: 429–33.
457. McNicholas WT, Tarlo S, Cole P, Zamel N, Rutherford R, Griffin D, *et al.* Obstructive apneas during sleep in patients with seasonal allergic rhinitis. *Am Rev Respir Dis* 1982; 126: 625–8.
458. Meier-Ewert K, Brosig B. Treatment of sleep apnea by prosthetic mandibular advancement. In: Peter JH, Podszus T, von Wichert P. eds. *Sleep-related disorders and internal disease.* Munich: Springer-Verlag, 1987: 341–6.
459. Mellins RB, Balfour HH, Turino GM, Winters R. Failure of automatic control of ventilation (Ondine's curse). Report of an infant born with this syndrome and review of the literature. *Medicine* 1970; 49: 487–504.
460. Menashe VD, Farrehi C, Miller M. Hypoventilation and cor pulmonale due to chronic airway obstruction. *J Pediatr* 1965; 67: 198–203.
461. Mendelson WB. Clinical sleep disorder patients in Stony Brook: an overview. *Sleep Res* 1991; 20: 291 (Abstract).
462. Mendelson WB, Garnett D, Gillin JC. Flurazepam induced sleep apnea syndrome in a patient with insomnia and mild sleep-related respiratory changes. *J Nerv Ment Dis* 1981; 169: 261–4.
463. Mendelson WB, Gujavarty K, Slintak C, Schwartz J, Maczaj M. Endocrine measures and reported sexual dysfunction in obstructive sleep apnea. In: Horne J. ed. *Sleep '90.* Bochum: Pontenagel Press, 1990: 200–2.
464. Metes A, Hoffstein V, Mateika S, Cole P, Haight JS. Site of airway obstruction in patients with obstructive sleep apnea before and after uvulopalato-pharyngoplasty. *Laryngoscope* 1991; 101: 1102–8.
465. Metes A, Ohki M, Cole P, Haight JS, Hoffstein V. Snoring, apnea and nasal resistance in men and women. *J Otolaryngol* 1991; 20: 57–61.
466. Mezzanotte WS, Tangel DJ, White DP. Waking genioglossus (GG) EMG in sleep apnea patients versus normal controls (a neuromuscular compensatory mechanism). *Am Rev Respir Dis* 1991; 143(No. 4, pt 2): A792 (Abstract).
467. Mier A, Brophy C, Havard CW, Green M. Severe diaphragmatic weakness in spinocerebellar degeneration. *Thorax* 1988; 43: 78–9.
468. Mier A, Brophy C, Moxham J, Green M. Assessment of diaphragm weakness. *Am Rev Respir Dis* 1988; 137: 877–83.
469. Miles L, Austin S, Guilleminault C. Secretion of glucose, growth hormone, and cortisol during sleep in patients with obstructive sleep apnea.

In: Guilleminault C, Dement WC. eds. *Sleep apnea syndromes*. New York: Alan R. Liss, 1978: 323−32.

470. Miles LE, Bushek GD, McClintock DP, Miles SC, Narvios LR, Wang YX. Development and application of two automatic nasal CPAP calibration procedures for use in the unsupervised home environment. *J Sleep Res* 1992; 1(suppl 1): 150 (Abstract).

471. Miller AJ, Vargervik K, Chierici G. Sequential neuromuscular changes in rhesus monkeys during the initial adaptation to oral respiration. *Am J Orthod* 1982; 81: 99−107.

472. Millikan GA. The oximeter, an instrument for measuring continuously the oxygen saturation of arterial blood in man. *Rev Sci Instrum* 1942; 13: 434−44.

473. Millman RP, Knight H, Kline LR, Shore ET, Chung DC, Pack A. Changes in compartmental ventilation in association with eye movements during REM sleep. *J Appl Physiol* 1988; 65: 1196−202.

474. Millman RP, Redline S, Carlisle CC, Assaf AR, Levinson PD. Daytime hypertension in obstructive sleep apnea. Prevalence and contributing risk factors. *Chest* 1991; 99: 861−6.

475. Milner AD, Ruggins N. Sudden infant death syndrome. *Br Med J* 1989; 298: 689−90.

476. Mitler MM. The multiple sleep latency test as an evaluation for excessive somnolence. In: Guilleminault C. ed. *Sleep and waking disorders*. Menlo Park: Addison-Wesley, 1982: 145−53.

477. Molhoek GP, Wesseling KH, Settels JJM, Van Vollenhoven E, Weeda HWH, De Witn B, *et al*. Evaluation of the Penaz servo-plethysmo-manometer for the continuous, non-invasive measurement of finger blood pressure. *Basic Res Cardiol* 1984; 79: 598−609.

478. Morrison AR. A window on the sleeping brain. *Sci Am* 1983; 248: 86−94.

479. Mosko SS, Dickel MJ, Ashurst J. Night-to-night variability in sleep apnea and sleep-related periodic leg movements in the elderly. *Sleep* 1988; 11: 340−8.

480. Mukhametov LM. Sleep in marine mammals. In: Borbely AA, Valatx JL. eds. *Sleep mechanisms*. Munich: Springer-Verlag, 1984: 227−38.

481. Mullaney DJ, Kripke DF, Messin S. Wrist actigraphic assessment of sleep time. *Sleep* 1980; 3: 83−92.

482. Murry T, Bone RC. Acoustic characteristics of speech following uvulopalato-pharyngoplasty. *Laryngoscope* 1989; 99: 1217−19.

483. Natori H, Tamaki S, Kira S. Ultrasonographic evaluation of ventilatory effect on inferior vena caval configuration. *Am Rev Respir Dis* 1979; 120: 421−7.

484. Nau SD, Hilliker NA, Schweitzer PK, Stuckey M, Humm T, Moss K, *et al*. Ten years' experience of sleep medicine referrals. *Sleep Res* 1992; 21: 244 (Abstract).

485. Neilly JB, Gaipa EA, Maislin G, Pack AI. Ventilation during early and late rapid-eye-movement sleep in normal humans. *J Appl Physiol* 1991; 71: 1201−15.

486. Newsom Davies J, Goldman M, Loh L, Casson M. Diaphragm function and alveolar hypoventilation. *Q J Med* 1976; 45: 87−100.

487. Newsom Davis JM. Autonomous breathing: report of a case. *Arch Neurol* 1974; 30: 480−3.

488. Nicholson AN, Smith PA, Stone BM, Bradwell AR, Coote JH. Altitude insomnia: studies during an expedition to the Himalayas. *Sleep* 1988; 11: 354—61.

489. Nicholson AN, Stone BM, Wright NA, Belyavin AJ. Daytime sleep latencies: relationships with the electroencephalogram and with performance. *J Psychophysiol* 1989; 3: 387—95.

490. Nickerson BG, Sarkisian C, Tremper K. Bias and precision of pulse oximeters and arterial oximeters. *Chest* 1988; 93: 515—17.

491. Nino-Murcia G, McCann CC, Bliwise DL, Guilleminault C, Dement WC. Compliance and side effects in sleep apnea patients treated with nasal continuous positive airway pressure. *West J Med* 1989; 150: 165—9.

492. Nishino S, Arrigoni J, Shelton J, Dement WC, Mignot E. Further analysis of the effects of serotonergic and noradrenergic uptake inhibitors on canine cataplexy. *Sleep Res* 1992; 21: 66 (Abstract).

493. Nishino S, Arrigoni J, Shelton J, Fruhstorfer B, Guilleminault C, Dement WC, *et al.* Further characterization of the alpha-1 receptor subtype involved in the regulation of cataplexy. *Sleep Res* 1992; 21: 245 (Abstract).

494. Nocturnal oxygen therapy trial group. Continuous or nocturnal oxygen therapy in hypoxemic chronic obstructive lung disease. *Ann Intern Med* 1980; 93: 391—8.

495a. Noonan JA. Reversible cor pulmonale due to hypertrophied tonsils and adenoids. *Circulation* 1965; 32(suppl II): 164 (Abstract).

495b. Norman S, Hesla PA, Nay KN, Kiel M, Mendez A, Coolidge T, Cohn MA. Quantitative changes of sleep parameters and symptoms in obstructive sleep apnea: effect of uvulopalatopharyngoplasty. *Sleep Res* 1985; 14: 194 (Abstract).

496. Norton PG, Dunn EV. Snoring as a risk factor for disease: an epidemiological survey. *Br Med J* 1985; 291: 630—2.

497. O'Ryan FS, Gallagher DM, La Blanc JP, Epker BN. The relationship between nasorespiratory function and dentofacial morphology: a review. *Am J Orthod* 1982; 82: 403—10.

498. Olsen KD. The nose and its impact on snoring and obstructive sleep apnea. In: Fairbanks DNF, Fujita S, Ikematsu T, Simmons FB. eds. *Snoring and obstructive sleep apnea*. New York: Raven Press, 1987: 199—226.

499. Onal E, Burrows DL, Hart RH, Lopata M. Induction of periodic breathing during sleep causes upper airway obstruction in humans. *J Appl Physiol* 1986; 61: 1438—43.

500. Onal E, Leech JA, Lopata M. Relationship between pulmonary function and sleep-induced respiratory abnormalities. *Chest* 1985; 87: 437—41.

501. Onal E, Lopata M, O'Connor T. Pathogenesis of apnea in hypersomnia-sleep apnea syndrome. *Am Rev Respir Dis* 1982; 125: 167—74.

502. Oparil S. The sympathetic nervous system in clinical and experimental hypertension. *Kidney Int* 1986; 30: 437—52.

503. Orem J, Osorio I, Brooks E, Dick T. Activity of the respiratory neurons during NREM sleep. *J Neurophysiol* 1985; 54: 1144—56.

504. Orr WC, Martin RJ, Imes NK, Rogers RM, Stahl ML. Hypersomnolent and nonhypersomnolent patients with upper airway obstruction during sleep. *Chest* 1979; 75: 418—22.

505. Osler W. *The principles and practice of medicine*. 8th edn. New York: Appleton, 1918.

506. Pack AI, Cola MF, Goldszmidt A, Ogilvie MD, Gottschalk A. Correlation between oscillations in ventilation and frequency content of the electroencephalogram. *J Appl Physiol* 1992; 72: 985–92.

507. Pack AI, Millman RP. Changes in control of ventilation, awake and asleep, in the elderly. *J Am Geriatr Soc* 1986; 34: 533–44.

508. Pack AI, Silage DA, Millman RP, Knight H, Shore ET, Chung DC. Spectral analysis of ventilation in elderly subjects awake and asleep. *J Appl Physiol* 1988; 64: 1257–67.

509. Palomaki H, Partinen M, Juvela S, Kaste M. Snoring as a risk factor for sleep-related brain infarction. *Stroke* 1989; 21: 1311–15.

510. Parati G, Casadei R, Groppelli A, Di Rienzo M, Mancia G. Comparison of finger and intra-arterial blood pressure monitoring at rest and during laboratory testing. *Hypertension* 1989; 13: 647–55.

511. Parkes JD. Daytime drowsiness. In: *Sleep and its disorders*. London: W. B. Saunders, 1985: 275–314.

512. Parkes JD. *Sleep and its disorders*. Philadelphia: W. B. Saunders, 1985.

513. Partinen M, Guilleminault C. Daytime sleepiness and vascular morbidity at seven-year follow-up in obstructive sleep apnea patients. *Chest* 1990; 97: 27–32.

514. Partinen M, Guilleminault C. Evolution of obstructive sleep apnea syndrome. In: Guilleminault C, Partinen M. eds. *Obstructive sleep apnea syndrome*. New York: Raven Press, 1990: 15–23.

515. Partinen M, Jamieson A, Guilleminault C. Long-term outcome for obstructive sleep apnea syndrome patients. Mortality. *Chest* 1988; 94: 1200–4.

516. Partinen M, Palomaki H. Snoring and cerebral infarction. *Lancet* 1985; 2: 1325–6.

517. Pasterkamp H. Advances in respiration acoustic monitoring. In: Peter JH, Penzel T, Podszus T, von Wichert P. eds. *Sleep and health risk*. Berlin: Springer-Verlag, 1991: 193–200.

518. Patton TJ, Thawley SE, Waters RC. Expansion hyoidplasty: a potential surgical procedure designed for selected patients with obstructive sleep apnea syndrome. Experimental canine results. *Laryngoscope* 1983; 93: 1387–96.

519. Penzel T, Amend G, Meinzer K, Peter JH, von Wichert P. MESAM: a heart rate and snoring recorder for detection of obstructive sleep apnea. *Sleep* 1990; 13: 175–82.

520. Perks WH, Cooper RA, Bradbury S, Horrocks PM, Baldock N, Allen A, *et al*. Sleep apnoea in Scheie's syndrome. *Thorax* 1980; 35: 85–91.

521. Perks WH, Horrocks PM, Cooper RA. Sleep apnea in acromegaly. *Br Med J* 1980; 280: 894–7.

522. Pezeshkpour GH, Dalakas MC. Long-term changes in the spinal cords of patients with old poliomyelitis—signs of continuous disease activity. *Arch Neurol* 1988; 45: 505–8.

523. Phillips BA, Berry DTR, Schmitt FA, Magan LK, Gerhardstein DC, Cook YR. Sleep-disordered breathing in the healthy elderly. *Chest* 1992; 101: 345–9.

524. Phillips DE, Rogers JH. Down's syndrome with lingual tonsil hypertrophy producing sleep apnoea. *J Laryngol Otol* 1988; 102: 1054–5.
525. Phillipson EA, Bradley TD. *Clinics in chest medicine. Breathing disorders in sleep*. Philadelphia: W.B. Saunders, 1992.
526. Phillipson EA, Kozar LF, Murphy E. Respiratory load compensation in awake and sleeping dogs. *J Appl Physiol* 1976; 40: 895–902.
527. Phillipson EA, Kozar LF, Rebuck AS, Murphy E. Ventilatory and waking responses to CO_2 in sleeping dogs. *Am Rev Respir Dis* 1977; 115: 251–9.
528. Phillipson EA, Remmers JE. Indications and standards for cardiopulmonary sleep studies. American Thoracic Society. Medical Section of the American Lung Association. *Am Rev Respir Dis* 1989; 139: 559–68.
529. Pilcher JJ, Schulz H. The interaction between EEG and transient muscle activity during sleep in humans. *Hum Neurobiol* 1987; 6: 45–9.
530. Pilleri G. The blind Indus dolphin. *Platanista Indi Endeavour* 1979; 3: 48–56.
531. Plum F, Brown HW, Snoep E. Neurological significance of post hyperventilation apnea. *J Am Med Assoc* 1962; 181: 1050–5.
532. Plum F, Swanson AG. Abnormalities in central regulation of respiration in acute convalescent poliomyelitis. *Arch Neurol Psych* 1958; 80: 267–85.
533. Pluto LA, Fahey PJ, Sorenson L, Chandrasekhar AJ. Effect of 8 weeks of intermittent negative pressure ventilation on exercise parameters in patients with severe COLD. *Am Rev Respir Dis* 1985; 131(suppl): A64 (Abstract).
534. Poceta JS, Timms RM, Jeong DU, Ho SL, Erman MK, Mitler MM. Maintenance of wakefulness test in obstructive sleep apnea syndrome. *Chest* 1992; 101: 893–7.
535. Podszus T, Feddersen O, Peter JH, von Wichert P. Cardiovascular risk in sleep-related breathing disorders. In: Gaultier C, Escourrou P, Curzi-Dascalova L. eds. *Sleep and cardiorespiratory control*. Montrouge: INSERM/John Libbey Eurotext, 1991: 177–85.
536. Polo O, Brissaud L, Fraga J, Dejean Y, Billiard M. Partial upper airway obstruction in sleep after uvulopalatopharyngoplasty. *Arch Otolaryngol Head Neck Surg* 1989; 115: 1350–4.
537. Polo O, Brissaud L, Sales B, Besset A, Billiard M. The validity of the static charge sensitive bed in detecting obstructive sleep apnoeas. *Eur Respir J* 1988; 1: 330–6.
538. Polo O, Tafti M, Hamalainen M, Vaahtoranta K, Alihanka J. Respiratory variation of the ballistocardiogram during increased respiratory load and voluntary central apnoea. *Eur Respir J* 1992; 5: 257–62.
539. Pond CD, Mant A, Eyland EA, Saunders NA. Dementia and abnormal breathing during sleep. *Age Ageing* 1990; 19: 247–52.
540. Popkin J, Rutherford R, Lue F, Grossman R, Goldstein R, Hyland R, *et al*. A one year randomized trial of nasal CPAP versus protripyline in the management of obstructive sleep apnea. *Sleep Res* 1988; 17: 237 (Abstract).
541. Potsic WP. Comparison of polysomnography and sonography for assessing regularity of respiration during sleep in adenotonsillar hypertrophy. *Laryngoscope* 1987; 97: 1430–7.
542. Potsic WP. Tonsillectomy and adenoidectomy. *Int Anesthesiol Clin* 1988; 26: 58–60.

543. Potsic WP. Sleep apnea in children. *Otolaryngol Clin North Am* 1989; 22: 537–44.

544. Potsic WP, Pasquariello PS, Baranak CC, Marsh RR, Miller LM. Relief of upper airway obstruction by adenotonsillectomy. *Otolaryngol Head Neck Surg* 1986; 94: 476–80.

545. Powell NB. Speech changes following uvulopalatopharyngoplasty. Complication or acceptable results? *Chest* 1990; 97: 5–6.

546. Powell NB, Riley RW, Guilleminault C. Maxillofacial surgery for obstructive sleep apnea. In: Guilleminault C, Partinen M. eds. *Obstructive sleep apnea syndrome*. New York: Raven Press, 1990: 153–82.

547. Powell NB, Riley RW, Guilleminault C, Murcia GN. Obstructive sleep apnea, continuous positive airway pressure, and surgery. *Otolaryngol Head Neck Surg* 1988; 99: 362–9.

548. Prybylski J, Sabbah HN, Stein PD. Why do patients with essential hypertension experience sleep apnoea syndrome? *Medical Hypothesis* 1980; 20: 173–7.

549. Rauhala E, Polo O, Erkinjuntti M, Sjoholm T, Hasan J. Periodic movements in sleep (PMS) and partial upper airway obstruction. *J Sleep Res* 1992; 1(suppl 1): 191 (Abstract).

550. Rauscher H, Formanek D, Popp W, Zwick H. Nasal CPAP and weight loss in hypertensive patients with obstructive sleep apnoea. *Eur Respir J* 1992; 5(suppl 15): 164s (Abstract).

551. Rauscher H, Popp W, Zwick H. Quantification of sleep-disordered breathing by computerised analysis of oximetry, heart rate and snoring. *Eur Respir J* 1991; 4: 655–9.

552. Rauscher H, Popp W, Zwick H. Systemic hypertension in snorers with and without sleep apnea. *Chest* 1992; 102: 367–71.

553. Rechtschaffen A, Hauri P, Zeitlin M. Auditory awakening thresholds in REM and NREM sleep stages. *Percept Motor Skills* 1966; 22: 927–42.

554. Rechtschaffen A, Kales A. *A manual of standardised terminology, techniques and scoring system for sleep stages of human subjects*. Washington DC: National Institutes of Health, Publication No. 204, 1968.

555. Redmond DP, Hegge FW. Observations on the design and specification of a wrist-worn human activity monitoring system. *Behaviour Research Methods Instrumentation* 1985; 17: 659–69.

556. Reed DJ, Kellog RH. Changes in respiratory response to CO_2 during natural sleep at sea level and at altitude. *J Appl Physiol* 1958; 13: 325–30.

557. Rees PJ, Clark TJH. Paroxysmal nocturnal dyspnoea and periodic respiration. *Lancet* 1979; 2: 1315–17.

558. Reite M, Jackson D, Cahoon RL, Weil JV. Sleep physiology at high altitude. *Electroencephalog Clin Neurophysiol* 1975; 38: 463–71.

559. Remmers JE, Anch AM, deGroot WJ, Baker JP, Sauerland EK. Oropharyngeal muscle tone in obstructive sleep apnea before and after strychnine. *Sleep* 1980; 3: 447–53.

560. Remmers JE, deGroot WJ, Sauerland EK, Anch AM. Pathogenesis of upper airway occlusion during sleep. *J Appl Physiol* 1978; 44: 931–8.

561. Richards JG, Mohler M. Benzodiazepine receptors. *Neuropharmacology* 1984; 23: 233–42.

562. Riemer M, Remmers J. Outcomes of CPAP treatment as perceived by OSA patients and their partners. *Sleep Res* 1991; 20: 316 (Abstract).

563. Rigault JY, Leroy F, Poncey C, Brun J, Mallet JF. [Prolonged mechanical nasal ventilation. Apropos of 27 cases of myopathy]. *Rev Mal Respir* 1991; 8: 479–85.

564. Riley R, Guilleminault C, Herran J, Powell N. Cephalometric analyses and flow–volume loops in obstructive sleep apnea patients. *Sleep* 1983; 6: 303–11.

565. Riley R, Guilleminault C, Powell N, Derman S. Mandibular osteotomy and hyoid bone advancement for obstructive sleep apnea: a case report. *Sleep* 1984; 7: 79–82.

566. Riley R, Guilleminault C, Powell N, Simmons FB. Palatopharyngoplasty failure, cephalometric roentgenograms, and obstructive sleep apnea. *Otolaryngol Head Neck Surg* 1985; 93: 240–4.

567. Riley RW, Powell NB, Guilleminault C. Maxillofacial surgery and nasal CPAP. A comparison of treatment for obstructive sleep apnea syndrome. *Chest* 1990; 98: 1421–5.

568. Riley RW, Powell NB, Guilleminault C. Maxillary, mandibular, and hyoid advancement for treatment of obstructive sleep apnea: a review of 40 patients. *J Oral Maxillofac Surg* 1990; 48: 20–6.

569. Riley RW, Powell NB, Guilleminault C, Nino-Murcia G. Maxillary, mandibular, and hyoid advancement: an alternative to tracheostomy in obstructive sleep apnea syndrome. *Otolaryngol Head Neck Surg* 1986; 94: 584–8.

570. Riley RW, Powell NB, Guilleminault C, Ware W. Obstructive sleep apnea syndrome following surgery for mandibular prognathism. *J Oral Maxillofac Surg* 1987; 45: 450–2.

571. Ringler J, Basner RC, Shannon R, Schwartzstein R, Manning H, Weinberger SE, *et al.* Hypoxemia alone does not explain blood pressure elevations after obstructive apneas. *J Appl Physiol* 1990; 69: 2143–8.

572. Rivlin J, Hoffstein V, Kalbfleisch J, McNicholas W, Zamel N, Bryan AC. Upper airway morphology in patients with idiopathic obstructive sleep apnea. *Am Rev Respir Dis* 1984; 129: 355–60.

573. Robert D, Leger P, Sirodot M, Salord F, Langevin B, Gaussorgues P. [Current modalities of mechanical ventilation for acute respiratory failure in chronic respiratory insufficiency]. *Rev Prat* 1990; 40: 2344–9.

574. Roberts JL, Reed WR, Thach BT. Pharyngeal airway-stabilising function of sternohyoid and sternothyroid muscles in the rabbit. *J Appl Physiol* 1984; 57: 1790–5.

575. Roberts S, Tarassenko L. New method of automated sleep quantification. *Med Biol Eng Comp* 1992; 30: 509–17.

576. Robinson RW, White DP, Zwillich CW. Moderate alcohol ingestion increases upper airway resistance in normal subjects. *Am Rev Respir Dis* 1985; 132: 1238–41.

577. Rodenstein DO, D'Odemont JP, Pieters T, Aubert-Tulkens G. Diurnal and nocturnal diuresis and natriuresis in obstructive sleep apnea. *Am Rev Respir Dis* 1992; 145: 1367–71.

578. Rodenstein DO, Dooms G, Thomas Y, Liistro G, Stanescu DC, Culee C, *et al*. Pharyngeal shape and dimensions in healthy subjects, snorers, and patients with obstructive sleep apnoea. *Thorax* 1990; 45: 722–7.

579. Roehrs T, Zorick F, Wittig R, Conway W, Roth T. Predictors of objective level of daytime sleepiness in patients with sleep-related breathing disorders. *Chest* 1989; 95: 1202–6.

580. Rolfe I, Olson LG, Saunders NA. Long-term acceptance of continuous positive airway pressure in obstructive sleep apnea. *Am Rev Respir Dis* 1991; 144: 1130–3.

581. Rosa RR, Bonnet MH, Bootzin RR, Eastman CI, Monk T, Penn PE, *et al*. Intervention factors for promoting adjustment to nightwork and shiftwork. *Occup Med* 1990; 5: 391–415.

582. Rosenfeld RM, Green RP. Tonsillectomy and adenoidectomy: changing trends. *Ann Otol Rhinol Laryngol* 1990; 99: 187–91.

583. Rosenow EC, Engel AG. Acid maltase deficiency in adults presenting as respiratory failure. *Am J Med* 1978; 64: 485–91.

584. Rowland TW, Nordstrom LG, Bean MS, Burkhardt H. Chronic upper airway obstruction and pulmonary hypertension in Down's syndrome. *Am J Dis Child* 1981; 135: 1050–2.

585. Rubin AE, Eliaschar I, Joachim Z, Alroy G, Lavie P. Effects of nasal surgery and tonsillectomy on sleep apnea. *Bull Eur Physiopathol Respir* 1983; 19: 612–15.

586. Ruckenstein MJ, Macdonald RE, Clarke JT, Forte V. The management of otolaryngological problems in the mucopolysaccharidoses: a retrospective review. *J Otolaryngol* 1991; 20: 177–83.

587. Ruddel H, Curio I. *Non-invasive continuous blood pressure measurement*. Frankfurt: Peter Lang, 1991.

588. Rudman D, Feller AG, Hagraj HS, Gergans GA, Lalitha PY, Goldberg AF, *et al*. Effects of human growth hormone in men over 60 years old. *N Engl J Med* 1990; 323: 1–6.

589. Ryan CF, Dickson RI, Lowe AA, Blokmanis A, Fleetham JA. Upper airway measurements predict response to uvulopalatopharyngoplasty in obstructive sleep apnea. *Laryngoscope* 1990; 100: 248–53.

590. Ryan CF, Lowe AA, Fleetham JA. Nasal continuous positive airway pressure (CPAP) therapy for obstructive sleep apnea in Hallermann–Streiff syndrome. *Clin Pediatr Phila* 1990; 29: 122–4.

591. Ryan CF, Lowe AA, Li D, Fleetham JA. Three-dimensional upper airway computed tomography in obstructive sleep apnea. *Am Rev Respir Dis* 1991; 144: 428–32.

592. Ryan CF, Lowe AA, Li D, Fleetham JA. Magnetic resonance imaging of the upper airway in obstructive sleep apnea before and after chronic nasal continuous positive airway pressure therapy. *Am Rev Respir Dis* 1991; 144: 939–44.

593. Sadeh A, Alster J, Urbach D, Lavie P. Actigraphically based automatic bedtime sleep/wake scoring: validity and clinical applications. *J Amb Mon* 1989; 2: 209–16.

594. Sadeh A, Lavie P, Scher A, Tirosh E, Epstein R. Actigraphic home-monitoring sleep-disturbed and control infants and young children: a new method for pediatric assessment of sleep–wake patterns. *Pediatrics* 1991; 87: 494–9.

595. Sadoul P, Lugaresi E. Hypersomnia with periodic breathing (symposium). *Bull Eur Physiopathol Respir* 1972; 8: 967–1288.

596. Samelson CF. Sequelae and complications of palatopharyngoplasty, impact on vocal trill. *Sleep* 1984; 7: 83–4.

597. Sanders MH. Nasal CPAP effect on patterns of sleep apnea. *Chest* 1984; 86: 839–44.

598. Sangal RB, Thomas L. Obstructive sleep apnea: improvement in somnolence with continuous positive airway pressure. *Sleep Res* 1991; 20: 319 (Abstract).

599. Sangal RB, Thomas L, Mitler MM. Maintenance of wakefulness test and multiple sleep latency test. Measurement of different abilities in patients with sleep disorders. *Chest* 1992; 101: 898–902.

600. Santamaria JD, Prior JC, Fleetham JA. Reversible reproductive dysfunction in men with obstructive sleep apnoea. *Clin Endocrinol Oxf* 1988; 28: 461–70.

601. Sauerland EK, Harper RM. The human tongue during sleep: electromyographic activity of the genioglossus muscle. *Exp Neurol* 1976; 51: 160–70.

602. Saunders KB, Stradling JR. Chemoreceptor drives and short sleep–wake cycles during hypoxia: a simulation study. *Annals of Bio-Medical Engineering* 1993; in press.

603. Saunders NA, Sullivan CE. *Sleep and breathing*. New York: Dekker, 1984.

604. Sawicka EH, Branthwaite MA, Spencer GT. Respiratory failure after thoracoplasty. *Thorax* 1983; 38: 433–5.

605. Scharf SM, Garshick E, Brown R, Tishler PV, Tosteson T, McCarley R. Screening for subclinical sleep-disordered breathing. *Sleep* 1990; 13: 344–53.

606. Schmidt-Nowara WW, Meade TE, Hays MB. Treatment of snoring and obstructive sleep apnea with a dental orthosis. *Chest* 1991; 99: 1378–85.

607. Schmidt-Nowara WW, Coultas DB, Wiggins C, Skipper BE, Samet JM. Snoring in a Hispanic–American population. Risk factors and association with hypertension and other morbidity. *Arch Intern Med* 1990; 150: 597–601.

608. Schoen LS, Anand VK, Weisenberger S. Upper-airway surgery for treating obstructive sleep apnea. *Arch Otolaryngol Head Neck Surg* 1987; 113: 850–3.

609. Scrima L, Broudy M, Nay KN, Cohn MA. Increased severity of obstructive sleep apnea after bedtime alcohol ingestion: diagnostic potential and proposed mechanism of action. *Sleep* 1982; 5: 318–28.

610. Selecky PA, Swancutt MD, Moore RA, Smith HR, Cowen LS. Dental orthotic appliance to treat obstructive sleep apnea. *Am Rev Respir Dis* 1991; 143(No. 4, pt 2): A588 (Abstract).

611. Selinkoff PM. Gastric restrictive surgery and obstructive sleep apnea [letter]. *Tex Med* 1988; 84: 6–7.

612. Semple PD'A, Beastall GH, Watson WS, Hume R. Serum testosterone depression associated with hypoxia in respiratory failure. *Clin Sci* 1980; 58: 105−6.

613. Severinghaus JW, Naifeh KH, Koh SO. Errors in 14 pulse oximeters during profound hypoxia. *J Clin Monit* 1989; 5: 72−81.

614. Sforza E, Krieger J. Daytime sleepiness after long-term CPAP treatment in obstructive sleep apnea patients. *J Sleep Res* 1992; 1(suppl 1): 209 (Abstract).

615. Sforza E, Krieger J, Geisert J, Kurtz D. Sleep and breathing abnormalities in a case of Prader−Willi syndrome. The effects of acute continuous positive airway pressure treatment. *Acta Paediatr Scand* 1991; 80: 80−5.

616. Shapiro CM. Growth hormone−sleep interaction: a review. *Res Commun Psychol Psychiatry* 1981; 6: 115−31.

617. Shapiro GG, Shapiro PA. Nasal airway obstruction and facial development. *Clin Rev Allergy* 1984; 2: 225−35.

618. Sharief MK, Hentges R, Ciardi M. Intrathecal immune response in patients with the post-polio syndrome. *N Engl J Med* 1991; 325: 749−55.

619. Shepard JW. Gas exchange and hemodynamics during sleep. *Med Clin North Am* 1985; 69(No. 6): 1243−64.

620. Shepard JW, Garrison MW, Grither DA, Dolan GF. Relationship of ventricular ectopy to oxyhemoglobin desaturation in patients with obstructive sleep apnea. *Chest* 1985; 88: 335−40.

621. Shepard JW, Olsen KD. Uvulopalatopharyngoplasty for treatment of obstructive sleep apnea. *Mayo Clin Proc* 1990; 65: 1260−7.

622. Sher AE, Shprintzen RJ, Thorpy MJ. Endoscopic observations of obstructive sleep apnea in children with anomalous upper airways: predictive and therapeutic value. *Int J Pediatr Otorhinolaryngol* 1986; 11: 135−46.

623. Sher HE, Thorpy MJ, Shprintzen RJ, Speilman AJ, Burack B, McGregor PA. Predictive value of Mueller manoeuvre in selection of patients for uvulopalatopharyngoplasty. *Laryngoscope* 1985; 95: 1483−7.

624. Shimizu T, Kogawa S, Tashiro T, Sato Y, Shibayama H, Sugawara J, *et al.* Mechanisms of transient marked elevations of arterial pressure in patients with sleep apnea syndrome. In: Horne J. ed. *Sleep '90*. Bochum: Pontenagel Press, 1990: 182−4.

625. Shneerson J. *Disorders of ventilation*. Oxford: Blackwell Scientific, 1988.

626. Shore ET, Millman RP, Silage DA, Chung DC, Pack AI. Ventilatory and arousal patterns during sleep in normal young and elderly subjects. *J Appl Physiol* 1985; 59: 1607−15.

627. Silverman M. Airway obstruction and sleep disruption in Down's syndrome. *Br Med J* 1988; 296: 1618−19.

628. Simmons FB. Tracheostomy in obstructive sleep apnea patients. *Laryngoscope* 1979; 89: 1702−3.

629. Simmons FB, Guilleminault C, Silvestri R. Snoring, and some obstructive sleep apnea can be cured by oropharyngeal surgery. *Arch Otolaryngol* 1983; 109: 503−7.

630. Simonds A. *The role of negative pressure ventilation in restrictive chest wall disease* (MD thesis, section 4). University of London, 1988.

631. Simonds AK, Branthwaite MA. Efficiency of negative pressure ventilatory equipment. *Thorax* 1985; 40: 213 (Abstract).

632. Simonds AK, Parker RA, Branthwaite MA. Effects of protriptyline on sleep related disturbances of breathing in restrictive chest wall disease. *Thorax* 1986; 41: 586–90.

633. Skatrud J, Iber C, McHugh W, Rasmussen H, Nichols D. Determinants of hypoventilation during wakefulness and sleep in diaphragmatic paralysis. *Am Rev Respir Dis* 1980; 121: 587–93.

634. Skatrud JB, Dempsey JA. Interaction of sleep state and chemical stimuli in sustaining rhythmic ventilation. *J Appl Physiol* 1983; 55: 813–22.

635. Skatrud JB, Dempsey JA. Airway resistance and respiratory muscle function in snorers during NREM sleep. *J Appl Physiol* 1985; 59: 328–35.

636. Smith PE, Calverley PM, Edwards RH. Hypoxemia during sleep in Duchenne muscular dystrophy. *Am Rev Respir Dis* 1988; 137: 884–8.

637. Smith PE, Edwards RH, Calverley PM. Ventilation and breathing pattern during sleep in Duchenne muscular dystrophy. *Chest* 1989; 96: 1346–51.

638. Smith PL, Haponik EF, Bleeker ER. The effects of oxygen in patients with sleep apnea. *Am Rev Respir Dis* 1984; 130: 958–63.

639. Smith PL, Wise RA, Gold AR, Schwartz AR, Permutt S. Upper airway pressure–flow relationships in obstructive sleep apnea. *J Appl Physiol* 1988; 64: 789–95.

640. Somers VK, Mark AL, Abboud FM. Sympathetic activation by hypoxia and hypercapnia—implications for sleep apnea. *Clin Exp Hypertens A* 1988; 10(suppl 1): 413–22.

641. Southall DP. Role of apnea in the sudden infant death syndrome: a personal view. *Pediatrics* 1988; 81: 73–84.

642. Southall DP, Stebbens VA, Mirza R, Lang MH, Croft CB, Shinebourne EA. Upper airway obstruction with hypoxaemia and sleep disruption in Down syndrome. *Dev Med Child Neurol* 1987; 29: 734–42.

643. Spitzer SA, Korczyn AD, Kalaci J. Transient bilateral diaphragmatic paralysis. *Chest* 1973; 64: 355–7.

644. Spriggs DA, French JM, Murdy JM, Bates D, James OFW. Historical risk factors for stroke: a case control study. *Age Ageing* 1990; 19: 280–7.

645. Staats BA, Bonekat HW, Harris CD, Offord KP. Chest wall motion in sleep apnea. *Am Rev Respir Dis* 1984; 130: 59–63.

646. Stebbens VA, Dennis J, Samuels MP, Croft CB, Southall DP. Sleep related upper airway obstruction in a cohort with Down's syndrome. *Arch Dis Child* 1991; 66: 1333–8.

647. Stolz SE, Aldrich MS. Serious injuries from motor vehicle accidents as a presentation of sleep apnea syndrome. *Sleep Res* 1991; 20: 342 (Abstract).

648. Stoohs R, Guilleminault C. Obstructive sleep apnea syndrome or abnormal upper airway resistance during sleep? *J Clin Neurophysiol* 1990; 7: 83–92.

649. Stoohs R, Guilleminault C. Snoring during NREM sleep: respiratory timing, esophageal pressure and EEG arousal. *Respir Physiol* 1991; 85: 151–67.

650. Stoohs R, Guilleminault C. Mesam 4: an ambulatory device for the detection of patients at risk for obstructive sleep apnea syndrome (OSAS). *Chest* 1992; 101: 1221–7.

651. Stradling J, Davies R, Pitson D, Crosby J. Verification of snoring at home in snorers, control subjects and patients with obstructive sleep apnoea. *J Sleep Res* 1992; 1(suppl): 222 (Abstract).

652. Stradling JR. Avoidance of tracheostomy in sleep apnoea syndrome. *Br Med J* 1982; 285: 407–8.

653. Stradling JR. The accuracy of the Hewlett-Packard oximeter below 50 per cent S_{ao_2}. *Clin Respir Physiol* 1982; 18: 791–4.

654. Stradling JR. Obstructive sleep apnoea and driving. *Br Med J* 1989; 298: 904–5.

655. Stradling JR. Sleep apnoea and systemic hypertension. *Thorax* 1989; 44: 984–9.

656. Stradling JR. Sleep studies for sleep-related breathing disorders. A consensus report. *J Sleep Res* 1992; 1: 223–30.

657. Stradling JR, Chadwick G, Quirk C, Phillips T. Respiratory inductive plethysmography: calibration techniques, their validation and the effects of posture. *Bull Eur Physiopathol Respir* 1985; 21: 317–24.

658. Stradling JR, Chadwick GA, Frew AJ. Changes in ventilation and its components in normal subjects during sleep. *Thorax* 1985; 40: 364–70.

659. Stradling JR, Crosby J. Prevalence of sleep apnea in 1001 men aged years 35–65. In: Horne J. ed. *Sleep '90*. Bochum: Pontenagel Press, 1990: 170–3.

660. Stradling JR, Crosby JH. Relation between systemic hypertension and sleep hypoxaemia or snoring: analysis in 748 men drawn from general practice. *Br Med J* 1990; 300: 75–8.

661. Stradling JR, Crosby JH. Predictors and prevalence of obstructive sleep apnoea and snoring in 1001 middle aged men. *Thorax* 1991; 46: 85–90.

662. Stradling JR, Crosby JH, Payne CD. Self-reported snoring and daytime sleepiness in men aged 35-65 years. *Thorax* 1991; 46: 807–10.

663. Stradling JR, England SJ, Harding R, Kozar LF, Andrey S, Phillipson EA. Role of upper airway in ventilatory control in awake and sleeping dogs. *J Appl Physiol* 1987; 62: 1167–73.

664. Stradling JR, Huddart S, Arnold AG. Sleep apnoea syndrome caused by neurofibromatosis and superior vena caval obstruction. *Thorax* 1981; 36: 634–5.

665. Stradling JR, Kozar L, Andrey S, Phillipson EA. Steady state responses to hypercapnia and added deadspace in awake and sleeping dogs. *Thorax* 1986; 41: 724 (Abstract).

666. Stradling JR, Kozar LF, Dark J, Kirby T, Andrey SM, Phillipson EA. Effect of acute diaphragm paralysis on ventilation in awake and sleeping dogs. *Am Rev Respir Dis* 1987; 136: 633–7.

667. Stradling JR, Lane DJ. Nocturnal hypoxaemia in chronic obstructive pulmonary disease. *Clin Sci* 1983; 64: 213–22.

668. Stradling JR, Mitchell J. Reproducibility of home oximetry tracings. *J Amb Mon* 1989; 2: 203–8.

669. Stradling JR, Thomas G, Belcher R. Analysis of overnight sleep patterns by automatic detection of movement on video recordings. *J Amb Mon* 1988; 1: 217–22.

670. Stradling JR, Thomas G, Warley ARH, Williams P, Freeland A. Effect of adenotonsillectomy on nocturnal hypoxaemia, sleep disturbance, and symptoms in snoring children. *Lancet* 1990; 335: 249–53.

671. Stradling JR, Warley A, Sharpley A. Wrist actigraphic assessment of sleep. *Sleep Res* 1987; 16: 586 (Abstract).

672. Stradling JR, Warley AR. Bilateral diaphragm paralysis and sleep apnoea without diurnal respiratory failure. *Thorax* 1988; 43: 75–7.

673. Stradling JR, Warley ARH, Sharpley A, Apps M, Calverley PMA, Chadwick G, *et al.* Oximetry versus polysomnography in the diagnosis of sleep disorders. *J Amb Mon* 1989; 2: 197–201.

674. Strelzow VV, Blanks RH, Basile A, Strelzow AE. Cephalometric airway analysis in obstructive sleep apnea syndrome. *Laryngoscope* 1988; 98: 1149–58.

675. Strohl KP, Hensley MJ, Hallett M, Saunders NA, Ingram RH. Activation of upper airway muscles before onset of inspiration in normal humans. *J Appl Physiol* 1980; 49: 638–42.

676. Strohl KP, Redline S. Nasal CPAP therapy, upper airway muscle activation, and obstructive sleep apnea. *Am Rev Respir Dis* 1986; 134: 555–8.

677. Stuart-Harris C, Flenley DC, Bishop JM, Howard P, Oldham PD. Long term domiciliary oxygen therapy in chronic hypoxic cor pulmonale complicating chronic bronchitis and emphysema. *Lancet* 1981; 1: 681–6.

678. Sullivan CE, Grunstein RR. Continuous positive airways pressure in sleep-disordered breathing. In: Kryger MH, Roth T, Dement WC. eds. *Principles and practice of sleep medicine*. Philadelphia: W.B. Saunders, 1989: 559–70.

679. Sullivan CE, Grunstein RR, Marrone O, Berthon-Jones M. Sleep apnea-pathophysiology: upper airway and control of breathing. In: Guilleminault C, Partinen M. eds. *Obstructive sleep apnea syndrome*. New York: Raven Press, 1990: 49–69.

680. Sullivan CE, Issa FG, Berthon-Jones M, Eves L. Reversal of obstructive sleep apnoea by continuous positive airway pressure applied through the nares. *Lancet* 1981; 1: 862–5.

681. Sullivan CE, Kozar LF, Murphy E, Phillipson EA. Primary role of respiratory afferents in sustaining breathing rhythm. *J Appl Physiol* 1978; 45: 11–17.

682. Sullivan CE, Kozar LF, Murphy E, Phillipson EA. Arousal, ventilatory and airway responses to bronchopulmonary stimulation in sleeping dogs. *J Appl Physiol* 1979; 47: 17–25.

683. Sullivan CE, Murphy E, Kozar LF, Phillipson EA. Waking and ventilatory responses to laryngeal stimulation in sleeping dogs. *J Appl Physiol* 1978; 45: 681–9.

684. Sullivan CE, Murphy E, Kozar LF, Phillipson EA. Ventilatory responses to CO_2 and lung inflation in tonic versus phasic REM sleep. *J Appl Physiol* 1979; 47: 1304–10.

685. Summers CL, Stradling JR, Baddeley RM. Treatment of sleep apnoea by vertical gastroplasty. *Br J Surg* 1990; 77: 1271–2.

686. Suratt PM, McTier RF, Wilhoit SC. Upper airway muscle activation is augmented in patients with obstructive sleep apnea compared with that in normal subjects. *Am Rev Respir Dis* 1988; 137: 889–94.

687. Sutton FD, Zwillich CW, Creagh CE, Pierson DJ, Weil JV. Progesterone for outpatient treatment of Pickwickian syndrome. *Ann Intern Med* 1975; 83: 476–9.

688. Svanborg E, Larsson H, Carlsson-Nordlander B, Pirskanen R. A limited diagnostic investigation for obstructive sleep apnea syndrome. Oximetry and static charge sensitive bed. *Chest* 1990; 98: 1341–5.

689. Swift AC. Upper airway obstruction, sleep disturbance and adenotonsillectomy in children. *J Laryngol Otol* 1988; 102: 419–22.

690. Taasan VC, Block AJ, Boysen PG, Wynne JW. Alcohol increases sleep apnea and oxygen desaturation in asymptomatic men. *Am J Med* 1981; 71: 240–5.

691. Taasan VC, Wynne JW, Cassisi N, Block AJ. The effect of nasal packing on sleep-disordered breathing and nocturnal oxygen desaturation. *Laryngoscope* 1981; 91: 1163–72.

692. Tabachnik E, Muller NL, Bryan AC, Levison H. Changes in ventilation and chest wall mechanics during sleep in normal adolescents. *J Appl Physiol* 1981; 51: 557–64.

693. Takasaki Y, Orr D, Popkin J, Rutherford R, Liu P, Bradley TD. Effect of nasal continuous positive airway pressure on sleep apnea in congestive heart failure. *Am Rev Respir Dis* 1989; 140: 1578–84.

694. Tan ETH, Lambie DG, Johnson RH, Robinson BJ, Whiteside EA. Sleep apnoea in alcoholic patients after withdrawal. *Clin Sci* 1985; 69: 655–61.

695. Tangel DJ, Mezzanotte WS, White DP. The effect of sleep on inspiratory phasic vs. tonic postural muscles in normal subjects. *Am Rev Respir Dis* 1991; 143(No. 4, pt 2): A793 (Abstract).

696. Tangel DJ, Mezzanotte WS, White DP. Influence of sleep on tensor palatini EMG and upper airway resistance in normal men. *J Appl Physiol* 1991; 70: 2574–81.

697. Tashiro T, Shimizu T, Iijima S, Kogawa S, Hishikawa Y. Increased urinary noradrenaline excretion during sleep in patients with sleep apnea syndrome. *Sleep Res* 1989; 18: 312 (Abstract).

698. Taylor L, Santiago S, Williams A. Correlation of the level of nasal CPAP with body weight. *Am Rev Respir Dis* 1991; 143(No. 4, pt 2): A591 (Abstract).

699. Telakivi T, Partinen M, Koskenvuo M, Kaprio J. Snoring and cardiovascular disease. *Compr Ther* 1987; 13: 53–7.

700. Telakivi T, Partinen M, Koskenvuo M, Salmi T, Kaprio J. Periodic breathing and hypoxia in snorers and controls: validation of snoring history and association with blood pressure and obesity. *Acta Neurol Scand* 1987; 76: 69–75.

701. Telakivi T, Partinen M, Salmi T, Leinonen L, Harkonen T. Nocturnal periodic breathing in adults with Down's syndrome. *J Ment Defic Res* 1987; 31: 31–9.

702. Thawley SE, Shepard JW. Understanding the sleep apnea syndrome: causes and treatment. *VA Practitioner* 1985; Jan: 60–83.

703. Thorpy MJ, Ledereich PS. Follow-up of patients with obstructive sleep apnea. In: Horne J. ed. *Sleep '88.* Stuttgart: G.F.Verlag, 1989: 279–81.

704. Thorpy MJ (Chairman). *The international classification of sleep disorders. Diagnostic and coding manual.* Rochester, Minnesota: American Sleep Disorders Association, 1990.

705. Tishler PV, Browner I, Ferrette V. Risk factors for sleep apnea (SA) in a genetic—epidemiologic study: variation by age. *Am Rev Respir Dis* 1992; 145: A866 (Abstract).

706. Tolle FA, Judy WV, Yu PL, Markand ON. Reduced stroke volume related to pleural pressure in obstructive sleep apnea. *J Appl Physiol* 1983; 55: 1718—24.

707. Trask CH, Cree EM. Oximeter studies on patients with chronic obstructive emphysema awake and during sleep. *N Engl J Med* 1962; 266: 639—42.

708. van der Schaar A, Roberts SJ, Davies WL. Repeatability studies on the Oxford Medilog SS90 sleep stager. *J Amb Mon* 1989; 2: 217—25.

709. van-Someren VH, Hibbert J, Stothers JK, Kyme MC, Morrison GA. Identifying hypoxaemia in children admitted for adenotonsillectomy. *Br Med J* 1989; 298: 1076.

710. Vela-Bueno A, Kales A, Soldatos CR, Dobladez-Blanco B, Campos-Castell J, Espino-Hurtado P, *et al.* Sleep in the Prader—Willi syndrome. *Arch Neurol* 1984; 41: 294—6.

711. Verdecchia P, Schillaci G, Guerrieri M, Gatteschi C, Benemio G, Boldrini F, *et al.* Circadian blood pressure changes and left ventricular hypertrophy in essential hypertension. *Circulation* 1990; 81: 528—36.

712. Viner S, Szalai JP, Hoffstein V. Are history and physical examination a good screening test for sleep apnea? *Ann Intern Med* 1991; 115: 356—9.

713. Vitiello MV, Prinz PN, Personius JP, Vitaliano PP, Nuccio MA, Koerker R. Relationship of alcohol abuse history to nighttime hypoxaemia in abstaining chronic alcoholic men. *J Stud Alcohol* 1990; 51: 29—33.

714. Vlachogianni ED, Sandhagen B, Gislason T, Stalenheim G. High ventilatory response to hypoxia in hypertensive patients with sleep apnea. *Ups J Med Sci* 1989; 94: 89—94.

715. Vos PJE, Stradling JR. Assessment of sleep times and movement arousals from video recordings. *J Amb Mon* 1991; 4: 35—42.

716. Waggener TB, Brusil PJ, Kronauer RE, Gabel RA, Inbar GF. Strength and cycle time of high-altitude ventilatory patterns in unacclimatized humans. *J Appl Physiol* 1984; 56: 576—81.

717. Wagner PD, Dantzker DR, Dueck R, Clausen JL, West JB. Ventilation—perfusion inequality in chronic obstructive pulmonary disease. *J Clin Invest* 1977; 59: 203—16.

718. Waite PD, Wooten V, Lachner J, Guyette RF. Maxillomandibular advancement surgery in 23 patients with obstructive sleep apnea syndrome. *J Oral Maxillofac Surg* 1989; 47: 1256—61.

719. Wakai Y, Welsh MM, Leevers AM, Road JD. Expiratory muscle activity in the awake and sleeping human during lung inflation and hypercapnia. *J Appl Physiol* 1992; 72: 881—7.

720. Waldhorn RE. Nocturnal nasal intermittent positive pressure ventilation with bi-level positive airway pressure (BiPAP) in respiratory failure. *Chest* 1992; 101: 516—21.

721. Waldhorn RE, Herrick TW, Nguyen MC, O'Donnell AE, Sodero J, Potolicchio SJ. Long-term compliance with nasal continuous positive airway pressure therapy of obstructive sleep apnea. *Chest* 1990; 97: 33—8.

722. Walker EB, Frith RW, Harding DA, Cant BR. Uvulopalatopharyngoplasty in severe idiopathic obstructive sleep apnoea syndrome. *Thorax* 1989; 44: 205–8.

723. Warley AR, Mitchell JH, Stradling JR. Evaluation of the Ohmeda 3700 pulse oximeter. *Thorax* 1987; 42: 892–6.

724. Warley AR, Mitchell JH, Stradling JR. Prevalence of nocturnal hypoxaemia amongst men with mild to moderate hypertension. *Q J Med* 1988; 68: 637–44.

725. Warley AR, Stradling JR. Abnormal diurnal variation in salt and water excretion in patients with obstructive sleep apnoea. *Clin Sci* 1988; 74: 183–5.

726. Warley ARH, Clarke M, Phillips T, Stradling JR. Ventilatory response to a steady state CO_2 load and added deadspace in man, awake and asleep. *Respir Physiol* 1989; 75: 183–92.

727. Warley ARH, Morice A, Stradling JR. Plasma levels of atrial natriuretic peptide (ANP) in obstructive sleep apnoea (OSA). *Thorax* 1988; 18: 195 (Abstract).

728. Weil JV, Cherniack NS, Dempsey JA, Edelman NH, Phillipson EA, Remmers JE, *et al.* NHLBI workshop summary. Respiratory disorders of sleep. Pathophysiology, clinical implications, and therapeutic approaches. *Am Rev Respir Dis* 1987; 136: 755–61.

729. Weiner D, Mitra J, Salamone J, Cherniack NS. Effect of chemical stimuli on nerves supplying upper airway muscles. *J Appl Physiol* 1982; 52: 530–6.

730. Weinsier RL, Norris DJ, Birch R, Bernstein RS, Wang J, Yang M, *et al.* The relative contribution of body fat and fat pattern to blood pressure level. *Hypertension* 1984; 7: 578–85.

731. Weitzenblum E, Krieger J, Apprill M, Vallee E, Ehrhart M, Ratomaharo J, *et al.* Daytime pulmonary hypertension in patients with obstructive sleep apnea syndrome. *Am Rev Respir Dis* 1988; 138: 345–9.

732. Weitzman ED, Kahn E, Pollack CP. Quantitative analysis of sleep and sleep apnea before and after tracheostomy in patients with the hypersomnia sleep apnea syndrome. *Sleep* 1980; 3: 407–23.

733. Weitzman ED, Pollak CP, Borowiecki B, Burack B, Shprintzen R, Rakoff S. The hypersomnia-sleep apnea syndrome: site and mechanism of upper airway obstruction. In: Guilleminault C, Dement WC. eds. *Sleep apnea syndromes*. New York: Alan R. Liss, 1978: 243.

734. Welin L, Svardsudd K, Wilhelmsen L, Larsson B, Tibblin G. Analysis of risk factors for stroke in a cohort of men born in 1913. *N Engl J Med* 1987; 317: 521–6.

735. Wesseling KH, Settels JJ, van-der-Hoeven GM, Nijboer JA, Butijn MW, Dorlas JC. Effects of peripheral vasoconstriction on the measurement of blood pressure in a finger. *Cardiovasc Res* 1985; 19: 139–45.

736. West JB, Peters RMJ, Aksnes G, Maret KH, Milledge JS, Schoene RB. Nocturnal periodic breathing at altitudes of 6,300 and 8,050 m. *J Appl Physiol* 1986; 61: 280–7.

737. Wetmore SJ, Scrima L, Hiller C. Sleep apnea in epistaxis patients treated with nasal packing. *Otolaryngol Head Neck Surg* 1988; 98: 596–9.

738. White D, Miller F, Erikson R. Sleep apnea and nocturnal hypoventilation following western equine encephalitis. *Am Rev Respir Dis* 1983; 127: 132–3.

739. White DP, Ballard RD. Pharyngeal muscle activity and upper airway resistance in obstructive sleep apnea patients versus controls. In: Issa FG, Suratt PM, Remmers JE. eds. *Sleep and respiration.* New York: Wiley-Liss, 1990: 243–251.

740. White DP, Douglas NJ, Pickett CK, Weil JV, Zwillich CW. Sleep deprivation and the control of breathing. *Am Rev Respir Dis* 1983; 128: 984–6.

741. White DP, Zwillich CW, Pickett CK, Douglas NJ, Findley LJ, Weil JV. Central sleep apnea: improvement with acetazolamide therapy. *Arch Intern Med* 1982; 142: 1816–19.

742. Whyte KF, Allen MB, Jeffrey AA, Gould GA, Douglas NJ. Clinical features of the sleep apnoea/hypopnoea syndrome. *Q J Med* 1989; 72: 659–66.

743. Whyte KF, Gould GA, Airlie MA, Shapiro CM, Douglas NJ. Role of protriptyline and acetazolamide in the sleep apnea/hypopnea syndrome. *Sleep* 1988; 11: 463–72.

744. Wickwire NA, White RP, Proffit WR. The effect of mandibular osteotomy on tongue position. *J Oral Surg* 1972; 30: 184–90.

745. Wiegand L, Zwillich CW, White DP. Collapsibility of the human upper airway during normal sleep. *J Appl Physiol* 1989; 66: 1800–8.

746. Wiegand L, Zwillich CW, White DP. Sleep and the ventilatory response to resistive loading in normal men. *J Appl Physiol* 1988; 64: 1186–95.

747. Wiers PWJ, Le Coultre R, Dallinga OT, Van Dijl W, Meinesz AF, Sluiter HJ. Cuirass respirator treatment of chronic respiratory failure in scoliotic patients. *Thorax* 1977; 32: 221–8.

748. Wilcox PG, Pare PD, Fleetham JA. Conditioning of the diaphragm by phrenic nerve pacing in primary alveolar hypoventilation. *Thorax* 1988; 43: 1017–18.

749. Wilde-Frenz J, Schulz H. Rate and distribution of body movements during sleep in humans. *Percept Motor Skills* 1983; 56: 275–83.

750. Wilkinson AR, McCormick MS, Freeland AP, Pickering D. Electrocardiographic signs of pulmonary hypertension in children who snore. *Br Med J* 1981; 282: 1579–82.

751. Wilkinson RT. Sleep deprivation: performance tests for partial and selective sleep deprivation. In: Abt L, Riess B. eds. *Progress in clinical psychology.* Vol 8. New York: Grune & Stratton, 1968: 28–43.

752. Wilkinson RT, Houghton D. Field test of arousal: a portable reaction timer with data storage. *Human Factors* 1982; 24: 487–93.

753. Williams A, Santiago S, Stein M. Screening for sleep apnea. *Chest* 1989; 96: 451–3.

754. Williams AJ, Houston D, Finberg S, Lamb C, Kinney JL, Santiago S. Sleep apnoea syndromes and essential hypertension. *Am J Cardiol* 1985; 55: 1019–22.

755. Williams AJ, Yu G, Santiago S, Stein M. Screening for sleep apnea using pulse oximetry and a clinical score. *Chest* 1991; 100: 631–5.

756. Williams BE, Ali NJ, Stradling JR. Autonomic function in patients with obstructive sleep apnoea. *Thorax* 1993; 48: 447 (Abstract).

757. Williams DL, MacLean AW, Cairns J. Dose–response effects of ethanol on the sleep of young women. *J Stud Alcohol* 1983; 44: 515–23.

758. Williams EF, Woo P, Miller R, Kellman RM. The effects of adenotonsillectomy on growth in young children. *Otolaryngol Head Neck Surg* 1991; 104: 509–16.

759. Wilson P, Skatrud JB, Dempsey JA. Effects of slow-wave sleep on ventilatory compensation to inspiratory elastic loading in humans. *Respir Physiol* 1984; 55: 103–20.

760. Winter JH, Neilly JB, Henderson AF, Stevenson RD, Doyle D, Wiles CM, *et al*. Life-threatening respiratory failure due to a previously undescribed myopathy. *Q J Med* 1986; 61: 1171–8.

761. Wynne JW, Block AJ, Hemenway J, Hunt LA, Flick MR. Disordered breathing and oxygen desaturation during sleep in patients with chronic obstructive lung disease (COLD). *Am J Med* 1979; 66: 573–9.

762. Wynter J, Milner B, Brennan S, Kapen S. Occupational hazards for obstructive sleep apnea. *Sleep Res* 1991; 20: 353 (Abstract).

763. Yasuma F, Kozar LF, Kimoff J, Bradley TD, Phillipson EA. Interaction of chemical and mechanical respiratory stimuli in the arousal response to hypoxia in sleeping dogs. *Am Rev Respir Dis* 1991; 143: 1274–7.

764. Young DK, Atkinson AM, Hulce VD, Fish S, Jaglowski D. Sleep disorders in a community hospital: 18 months experience. *Sleep Res* 1992; 21: 283 (Abstract).

765. Young T, Palta M, Badr S, Weber S, Zaccaro D. Sleep disordered breathing occurrence among employed adults: interim report from the University of Wisconsin sleep cohort study. *Sleep Res* 1992; 21: 284 (Abstract).

766a. Zorick F, Roehrs T, Wittig R, Lamphere J, Sicklesteel J, Roth T. Sleep–wake abnormalities in narcolepsy. *Sleep* 1986; 9: 189–93.

766b. Zorick F, Roehrs T, Conway W, Fujita S, Wittig R, Roth T. Effects of uvulopalatopharyngoplasty on the daytime sleepiness associated with the sleep apnea syndrome. *Bull Eur Physiopathol Respir* 1983; 19: 600–3.

767. Zorick R, Roth T, Kramer M, Flessa H. Intensification of excessive daytime sleepiness by lymphoma. *Sleep Res* 1977; 6: 199 (Abstract).

768. Zwillich C, Devlin T, White D, Douglas N, Weil J, Martin R. Bradycardia during sleep apnea: characteristics and mechanism. *J Clin Invest* 1982; 69: 1286–92.

769. Zwillich CW, Pickett C, Hanson FN, Weil JV. Disturbed sleep and prolonged apnea during nasal obstruction in normal men. *Am Rev Respir Dis* 1981; 124: 158–60.

Index

DATE DUE

SEP 0 7 1994			
JAN. 0 5 1995			
FEB 1 6 1995			
FEB 1 6 1995 MAR 2 0 1995			
APR 13 1995			
MAY 1 1995 JUN 0 3 1997			
MAY 1 9 1997 NOV 1 9 1997			
MAR 1 5 2007			

DEMCO 38-297

DE PAUL UNIVERSITY LIBRARY

30511000141484

616.2S895H1993 C001
LPX HANDBOOK OF SLEEP-RELATED BREATHING